T0077264

Pathology of Challenging Melanocytic Neoplasms

Christopher R. Shea • Jon A. Reed
Victor G. Prieto
Editors

Pathology of Challenging Melanocytic Neoplasms

Diagnosis and Management

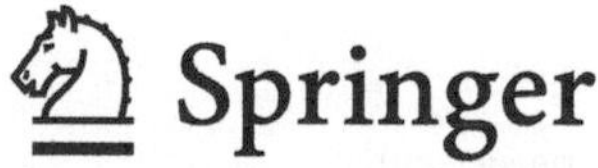

Editors
Christopher R. Shea
Section of Dermatology
University of Chicago Medicine
Chicago, IL, USA

Victor G. Prieto
Department of Pathology
University of Texas
MD Anderson Cancer
Houston, TX, USA

Jon A. Reed, M.D.
Department of Pathology
Baylor College of Medicine
Houston, TX, USA

CellNetix Pathology
Seattle, WA, USA

ISBN 978-1-4939-1443-2 ISBN 978-1-4939-1444-9 (eBook)
DOI 10.1007/978-1-4939-1444-9
Springer New York Heidelberg Dordrecht London

Library of Congress Control Number: 2014948771

Printed on acid-free paper

Springer is part of Springer Science+Business Media (www.springer.com)

The editors wish to thank our master teacher, Prof. N. Scott McNutt, M.D., who imparted to us his ideals in pathology: a scientific approach to diagnostic problems, clear communication, dedication, and professionalism.

We also wish to express to our wives Kuri (Shea), Nobuko (Reed), and Eugenia (Prieto) our deepest gratitude, love, and appreciation for their endless patience and support.

Christopher R. Shea, M.D.
Jon A. Reed, M.D.
Victor G. Prieto, M.D., Ph.D.

Contents

Contributors

Juliana L. Basko-Plluska, M.D. University of Chicago Medicine, Chicago, IL, USA

Alexander D. Means University of Chicago Medicine, Chicago, IL, USA

Eduardo K. Moioli University of Chicago Medicine, Chicago, IL, USA

Adaobi I. Nwaneshiudu University of Chicago Medicine, Chicago, IL, USA

Kristen M. Paral University of Chicago Medicine, Chicago, IL, USA

Penvadee Pattanaprichakul Faculty of Medicine Siriraj Hospital, Mahidol University, Bangkok, Thailand

Victor G. Prieto, M.D., Ph.D. MD Anderson Cancer Center, University of Houston, Houston, TX, USA

Jon A. Reed, M.S., M.D. CellNEtix Pathology & Laboratories, Seattle, WA, USA

Christopher R. Shea, M.D. University of Chicago Medicine, Chicago, IL, USA

Jamie L. Steinmetz University of Chicago Medicine, Chicago, IL, USA

Part I

Introductory Chapters

Gross Prosection of Melanocytic Lesions

1

Jon A. Reed, Victor G. Prieto, and Christopher R. Shea

Introduction

Accurate diagnosis of a challenging melanocytic neoplasm requires adequate (i.e., representative) clinical sampling of the lesion and careful microscopic examination of histological sections. Adequate microscopic examination of a lesion in turn depends on the proper transport, gross prosection, and tissue processing of the clinical specimen to assure optimum histology. These technical considerations also are important to preserve tissues for additional immunohistochemical or molecular diagnostic studies if required. As such, tissue handling is becoming an increasingly important variable as newer, more sophisticated molecular tests are developed to provide better diagnostic and prognostic information and to identify specific aberrations with actionable treatment options for individual patients. Many of the newer molecular diagnostic tests have been developed for use on formalin-fixed, paraffin-embedded tissues [1–4]. The objective of this chapter is to summarize current best practice techniques for the gross examination and prosection of formalin-fixed, paraffin-embedded cutaneous specimens containing melanocytic lesions.

J.A. Reed, M.S., M.D. (✉)
Baylor College of Medicine, 1 Baylor Plaza, Houston, TX 77030, USA

CellNetix Pathology & Laboratories, 1124 Columbia St., Suite 200, Seattle, WA 98117, USA
e-mail: jreed@bcm.edu; jreed@cellnetix.com

V.G. Prieto, M.D., Ph.D.
MD Anderson Cancer Center, University of Houston, 1515 Holcombe Blvd., Unit 85, Houston, TX 77030, USA

C.R. Shea, M.D.
University of Chicago Medicine, 5841 S. Maryland Ave., MC 5067, L502, Chicago, IL 60637, USA

Biopsy/Surgical Techniques

Proper handling of tissues containing melanocytic neoplasms requires an understanding of the types of specimens commonly submitted to the laboratory for pathologic examination. Most cutaneous specimens can be divided into two broad categories: diagnostic biopsies and therapeutic excisions. Cutaneous melanocytic lesions often are sampled first by shave biopsy or punch biopsy to establish a diagnosis. Subsequent (or primary) therapeutic procedures may include deeper shaves (tangential excisions/saucerizations), larger punches, and deeper elliptical or cylindrical surgical excisions. Melanocytic lesions are seldom intentionally sampled by curettage because of diagnostic limitations related to tissue orientation in histological sections.

A considerable body of literature already exists concerning the benefits and limitations of frozen section diagnosis of melanocytic lesions

C.R. Shea et al. (eds.), *Pathology of Challenging Melanocytic Neoplasms: Diagnosis and Management*,
DOI 10.1007/978-1-4939-1444-9_1, © Springer Science+Business Media New York 2015

treated by Mohs micrographic surgery in a clinical office setting and will not be further discussed in this introductory chapter. Similarly, diagnostic and therapeutic procedures (such as needle core biopsies, fine needle aspiration cytology, surgical de-bulking procedures, and regional lymphadenectomies) commonly used to evaluate extracutaneous deposits of metastatic melanomas are not included. The handling of sentinel lymph node biopsies related to the challenging differential diagnosis of metastatic melanoma versus capsular nevus is addressed in Chap. 17.

Punch Biopsies/Punch Excisions

Punch biopsies of skin produce a cylindrical portion of tissue that is oriented perpendicular to the epidermal surface. Punch biopsies often are performed to diagnose inflammatory dermatoses because they allow histological examination of epidermis, superficial and deep dermis, and possibly superficial subcutaneous adipose tissue. Similarly, a punch biopsy may be used for a melanocytic lesion that is suspected of having a deeper dermal or subcutaneous component. Larger punches also may used to completely remove a lesion that was previously biopsied by a smaller diameter punch biopsy or by a superficial shave biopsy (see below).

Small punch biopsies should be used with caution when sampling a melanocytic neoplasm [5]. A single small punch biopsy may yield a nonrepresentative sample form a large atypical melanocytic neoplasm. Multiple smaller punches may be used; however, to "map" peripheral spread of a large lesion such as lentigo maligna that has previously been diagnosed by another biopsy.

Handling of a punch biopsy is straightforward. Punches intended to completely remove a lesion should be marked with indelible ink along the entire dermal surface including periphery and base, sparing only the epidermal surface. Specimens larger than 3 mm in diameter are bisected, and very large specimens, serially sectioned along the long axis (i.e., perpendicular to the epidermal surface). After routine tissue processing, histological sections cut perpendicular to the epidermis will thus have a perimeter marked by ink that defines the surgical margin (Fig. 1.1).

Shave Biopsies/Shave Excisions (Saucerizations, Tangential Excisions)

Shave biopsies represent a sampling of epidermis and superficial dermis taken in a plane parallel to the epidermal surface. Deeper shaves may include superficial reticular dermis, but subcutis is almost never sampled by this technique. Deeper shave biopsies (tangential excisions/saucerizations) intended to completely remove a lesion are

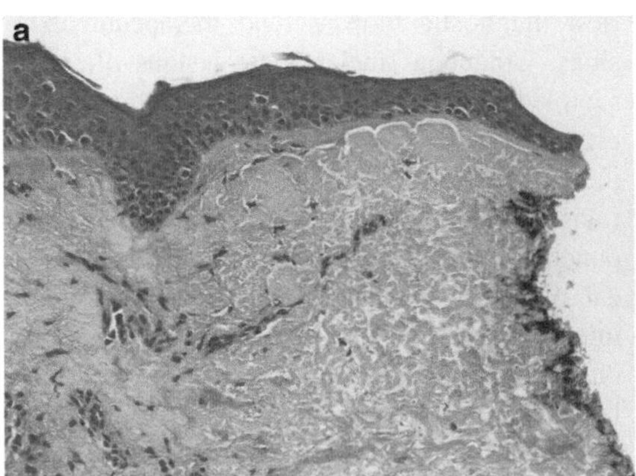

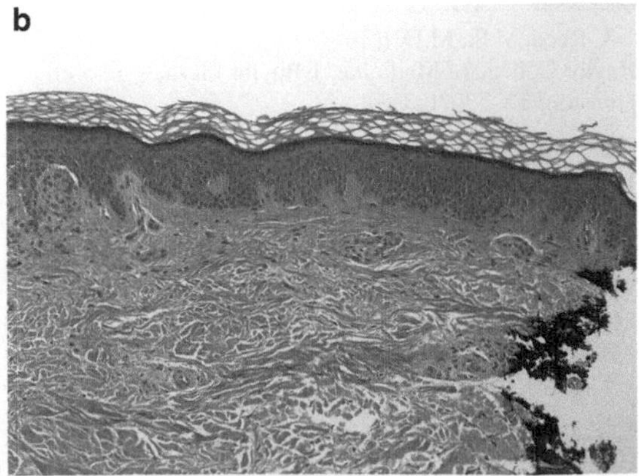

Fig. 1.1 Microscopic evaluation of peripheral margins. (**a**) Melanoma in situ involving the inked peripheral margin of a specimen (×20). (**b**) Atypical nevus excised with a margin of un-involved skin (×10)

marked with indelible ink along the entire margin sparing only the epidermal surface. Depending on the size, shave biopsies may be bisected along the long axis or serially sectioned. The tissue is then embedded on edge so that the inked peripheral and deep margin is entirely represented in the histological section. Larger shaves may be divided between cassettes so that the tip (third dimension) margins can be evaluated independent of sections from the middle of the lesion.

Elliptical (and Cylindrical) Excisions

Excisions are, by definition, specimens intended to excise a lesion. As such, assessment and reporting of margins is usually required. Most excisions are elliptical; however, cylindrical specimens may be taken from certain anatomic sites where optimum lines of surgical closure are not clinically evident prior to the procedure. In this case, additional detached tips ("dog ears") may be submitted separately, and should be treated as true "tip" margins. Larger excisional specimens often are oriented to identify a specific anatomic site on the patient such that a positive margin may be treated locally and less aggressively. Any surface lesion should be described noting its size, circumscription, color(s), and proximity to the peripheral margins.

Un-oriented specimens are marked with indelible ink along the entire peripheral and deep surgical margin similar to a shave biopsy. The ellipse (or cylinder) is then serially sectioned along the entire specimen (bread-loafed) to produce parallel sections perpendicular to the epidermal surface. Each section should be no greater than 2–3 mm in thickness to facilitate optimum tissue fixation and to allow examination of a larger area of surgical margin. Any lesion present on the cut surface should be noted, especially satellite lesions outside of the prior biopsy site in larger excisions.

Larger oriented specimens are treated somewhat differently than un-oriented excisions.

A suture often is used to orient an excisional specimen. The suture may be placed at one end (on a tip) and/or along one long axis (edge). Occasionally, two sutures may be used (different colors or lengths to differentiate). Some surgeons use a standard designation of "**S**hort suture—**S**uperior, **L**ong suture—**L**ateral" to simplify communication with the laboratory. Others may place a nick/slice along one border to designate orientation, but this practice is not advised as formalin fixation may result in tissue shrinkage that obscures the mark [6].

Regardless of the method used to identify a specific margin, specimens are differentially inked to reflect the orientation. The easiest way to orient an excisional specimen is by quadrant using a clock face for landmarks. Assuming that a marking suture at one tip of an ellipse is designated 12 o'clock, the specimen can be divided into 12–3, 3–6, 6–9, and 9–12 o'clock quadrants. Each quadrant could then be marked with a different color of indelible ink along the peripheral and deep surgical margin.

Another approach using only three colors of ink produces similar results. The 12–3 and 3–6 o'clock quadrants are differentially inked, whereas the 6–9–12 o'clock half is marked with one color. As such, the 12 o'clock half can be distinguished from the 6 o'clock half based on the unique pairing of the ink colors.

Very Large Re-excision Specimens

Very large excisional specimens, often taken for treatment of broad malignant melanomas, pose a unique challenge. These specimens may be marked with ink to reflect orientation similar to a small excision, but serial sectioning may result in pieces of tissue still too large to fit into a cassette for tissue processing. In this scenario, the prior biopsy site and residual primary tumor should be removed en bloc, serially sectioned, and entirely submitted as if it was an elliptical excision. Peripheral margins closet to the en bloc excision are then serially sectioned to document the peripheral margins. *En face* peripheral margins may be employed for extremely large specimens in which serial sections perpendicular to the primary lesion are still too large. *En face* sections, however, are not optimum for evaluating margins of lentigo maligna as distinction from melanocyte hyperplasia reflective of the background actinic changes may be difficult without use of additional special studies such as immunohistochemistry [7, 8].

Interpretation of Surgical Margins

Each of the procedures described above produces a specimen that can be assessed for adequacy of local therapy. Chapter 2 will address the reporting of melanocytic lesions including recommendations for adequacy of surgical margins. Surgical margins can be evaluated for most specimens regardless of biopsy/surgical technique. A microscope fitted with a calibrated ocular micrometer facilitates measurement of distance between the lesion and the surgical margin. Larger excisions may be measured with a ruler after marking the coverslip above the peripheral extension of the lesion under low magnification. These measurements may be reported directly or incorporated with a recommendation for further therapy based upon current consensus [9–19].

Conclusions

Proper handling of melanocytic lesions is necessary to assure accurate diagnosis and to allow additional special studies if necessary. Punch biopsies and shave biopsies are appropriate for sampling melanocytic neoplasms, whereas larger punches and elliptical excisions are best performed to ensure complete removal of a lesion. Surgical margin status should be reported for specimens intended as complete removal of a lesion.

References

1. Busam KJ. Molecular pathology of melanocytic tumors. Semin Diagn Pathol. 2013;30:362–74.
2. Gerami P, Li G, Pouryazdanparast P, et al. A highly specific and discriminatory FISH assay for distinguishing between benign and malignant melanocytic neoplasms. Am J Surg Pathol. 2012;36:808–17.
3. Jeck WR, Parker J, Carson CC, et al. Targeted next generation sequencing identifies clinically actionable mutations in patients with melanoma. Pigment Cell Melanoma Res. 2014;27(4):653–63.
4. North JP, Garrido MC, Kolaitis NA, Leboit PE, McCalmont TH, Bastian BC. Fluorescence in situ hybridization as an ancillary tool in the diagnosis of ambiguous melanocytic neoplasms: a review of 804 cases. Am J Surg Pathol. 2014;38(6):824–31.
5. Stevens G, Cockerell CJ. Avoiding sampling error in the biopsy of pigmented lesions. Arch Dermatol. 1996;132:1380–2.
6. Kerns MJ, Darst MA, Olsen TG, Fenster M, Hall P, Grevey S. Shrinkage of cutaneous specimens: formalin or other factors involved? J Cutan Pathol. 2008;35:1093–6.
7. Prieto VG, Argenyi ZB, Barnhill RL, et al. Are en face frozen sections accurate for diagnosing margin status in melanocytic lesions? Am J Clin Pathol. 2003;120:203–8.
8. Trotter MJ. Melanoma margin assessment. Clin Lab Med. 2011;31:289–300.
9. NIH Consensus conference. Diagnosis and treatment of early melanoma. JAMA. 1992;268:1314–9.
10. Ivan D, Prieto VG. An update on reporting histopathologic prognostic factors in melanoma. Arch Pathol Lab Med. 2011;135:825–9.
11. Kmetz EC, Sanders H, Fisher G, Lang PG, Maize JCS. The role of observation in the management of atypical nevi. South Med J. 2009;102:45–8.
12. Kolman O, Hoang MP, Piris A, Mihm MCJ, Duncan LM. Histologic processing and reporting of cutaneous pigmented lesions: recommendations based on a survey of 94 dermatopathologists. J Am Acad Dermatol. 2010;63:661–7.
13. Kunishige JH, Brodland DG, Zitelli JA. Surgical margins for melanoma in situ. J Am Acad Dermatol. 2012;66:438–44.
14. Scolyer RA, Judge MJ, Evans A, et al. Data set for pathology reporting of cutaneous invasive melanoma: recommendations from the international collaboration on cancer reporting (ICCR). Am J Surg Pathol. 2013;37:1797–814.
15. Sellheyer K, Bergfeld WF, Stewart E, Roberson G, Hammel J. Evaluation of surgical margins in melanocytic lesions: a survey among 152 dermatopathologists. J Cutan Pathol. 2005;32:293–9.
16. Shors AR, Kim S, White E, et al. Dysplastic naevi with moderate to severe histological dysplasia: a risk factor for melanoma. Br J Dermatol. 2006;155:988–93.
17. Tallon B, Snow J. Low clinically significant rate of recurrence in benign nevi. Am J Dermatopathol. 2012;34:706–9.
18. Weinstein MC, Brodell RT, Bordeaux J, Honda K. The art and science of surgical margins for the dermatopathologist. Am J Dermatopathol. 2012;34:737–45.
19. Reddy KK, Farber MJ, Bhawan J, Geronemus RG, Rogers GS. Atypical (dysplastic) nevi: outcomes of surgical excision and association with melanoma. JAMA Dermatol. 2013;149:928–34.

Histopathologic Staging and Reporting of Melanocytic Lesions

2

Eduardo K. Moioli, Jon A. Reed, Victor G. Prieto, and Christopher R. Shea

Introduction

The accurate pathologic staging and reporting of melanocytic lesions is crucial for guiding effective therapy, providing useful prognostic information, and facilitating sound clinicopathologic correlation. Moreover, in our fragmented American healthcare system and mobile workplace, in which many patients change healthcare providers from year to year, a clear and intelligible pathology report may be the best means of ensuring appropriate care through years of follow-up. Also, because some laboratories and hospitals destroy slides and blocks after a number of years (a deplorable practice), the pathology report may survive as the sole reliable documentation of a dangerous melanoma having a risk of recurrence over time. Finally, because melanoma is a leading cause of medicolegal liability, a clearly stated report, carefully documenting pertinent positive and negative findings, is often the pathologist's best defense, even in cases eventuating in a poor outcome.

There is no single standard for what constitutes an acceptable pathology report, and many pathologists undoubtedly simply follow whatever format they learned during their training. Thus, many pathologists state the diagnosis near the top of their reports, presumably on the principle that busy clinicians may prefer to get to the diagnosis quickly and skip the subsequent details of gross description, prosection, microscopic description, results of special studies, etc. We, on the contrary, prefer a reporting style that more logically replicates the actual flow of information during the course of processing a specimen and reaching a diagnosis. Thus, our reports first state the information received on the requisition sheet regarding patient name and demographics, requests if any from the provider (e.g., reporting on margins, requests for special studies or expedited service), clinical history, and clinical diagnosis. We next provide the gross description, giving details of any gross lesions and their distance from the deep and peripheral margins; describe the scheme, if any, used for inking the margins; and summarize the prosection method, covering the thoroughness of sampling, numbering of blocks, etc.

Next, it is our practice to provide a microscopic description for every specimen, generally proceeding from the epidermal surface down to the deepest tissue represented, and going from

E.K. Moioli • C.R. Shea, M.D. (✉)
University of Chicago Medicine,
5841 S. Maryland Ave., Chicago, IL 60637, USA
e-mail: cshea@medicine.bsd.uchicago.edu

J.A. Reed
CellNEtix Pathology & Laboratories,
1124 Columbia St., Suite 200, Seattle,
WA 98117, USA

V.G. Prieto
MD Anderson Cancer Center, University of Houston,
1515 Holcombe Blvd., Unit 85, Houston,
TX 77030, USA

C.R. Shea et al. (eds.), *Pathology of Challenging Melanocytic Neoplasms: Diagnosis and Management*,
DOI 10.1007/978-1-4939-1444-9_2, © Springer Science+Business Media New York 2015

low-power (architecture, silhouette) to high-power (cytologic) findings. Admittedly, many very distinguished pathologists do not routinely provide microscopic descriptions, instead inserting a comment on selected cases to make pertinent microscopic observations; such reports often include the simple statement, "Microscopic examination was performed," which clearly is included merely to meet the minimal reporting standards to justify a gross/microscopic CPT billing code. It is probably true that if one had to sacrifice one component of the report, a good gross description would win out over the microscopic description, at least for larger or more complex specimens. Nonetheless, pathologists whose clientele is mainly composed of surgeons should be aware that most dermatologists have different expectations, and may prefer to receive a microscopic description. All dermatologists receive extensive training in cutaneous histopathology, many actively practice diagnostic dermatopathology, and most find it very useful if not essential to read the microscopic findings so that they may correlate them with what they saw in the clinic—their in vivo gross examination.

Going through the exercise of providing a brief, pointed microscopic description also serves as a very important check for pathologists, forcing them to provide criteria and rationales for their diagnosis rather than relying excessively on intuition or *Gestalt* psychology (as useful as these also may be). In this regard, the use of macros or "canned" descriptive phrases bears some discussion. We routinely use them, as do most of our colleagues; but there is no doubt that they can be dangerous unless used with care. They can have the undesirable effect of short-circuiting the intellectual process by letting one evade the crucial, explicit step of describing findings. Indeed, one of the more common problems seen in training residents and fellows is their tendency to jump at a diagnosis (often reaching the correct conclusion), and then simply to reach for whichever canned microscopic description corresponds with that diagnosis, thus avoiding a more explicit, lengthy, but ultimately rewarding method of searching for pertinent diagnostic findings, assigning them due weight, and finally arriving at a balanced and deliberate conclusion. Also, in cases of error leading to misdiagnosis, it is very difficult to defend a statement (such as "mitotic figures are not identified") that can be readily contradicted upon subsequent review with the benefit of hindsight; it is perhaps out of concern for saying too much, as well as a desire for speed and concision, that many pathologists eschew microscopic descriptions altogether. To the contrary, we use our macros as a checklist of essential findings, and we rapidly run through each description in our minds, before deciding whether to apply it. For example, a standard microscopic description of a compound (non-dysplastic/non-atypical) nevus may state, "Nests of melanocytes without significant atypia or mitotic figures are present both at the dermo-epidermal junction and in the dermis. There is no significant architectural disorder or inflammatory response." That simple description contains a wealth of positive and negative criteria, and a rapid consideration of its elements can usefully prompt the careful pathologist to rethink the diagnosis, in cases where discordant features are present. The best advice is: If you choose to use canned microscopic descriptions, be sure that you know exactly what they say, and that they accurately describe the case at hand; if not, modify them, omit them, or write individual descriptions as needed.

The heart of the report is, of course, the diagnosis. Similar to a clinical progress note, where the subjective evaluation and objective data precedes the final assessment and plan, we prefer to present the final pathologic diagnosis at the end of the report, to complete a logical progression of information that the clinician can easily follow. The diagnosis line should be clear, readily found within the report, and indicate associated data when appropriate. For instance, following the diagnosis line that reads "Melanoma, Invasive", the histogenetic type, Breslow thickness, mitotic figure count, staging information and other pertinent data are presented.

Other useful information, when appropriate, may be added in comments and notes that follow the diagnosis line. Under comments, one may add details about margin involvement of relevance and suggestions for the clinician, such as management recommendations when appropriate. Areas of uncertainty should be described, and evidence in favor and against the diagnosis presented. Lastly, consultations for collaborative diagnosis with multidisciplinary teams, and pertinent references from the published literature, may also be noted in this section.

More standardized pathology reports may lead to better efficiency, more accurate reporting, and reliability. Regardless of the layout chosen for the report, one of the pathologist's principal tasks is to include information that will help the clinician and patient decide on appropriate treatment. Reporting out a diagnosis of melanoma can be especially challenging. Some of the features currently understood to influence estimated prognosis may not remain the same in the decades to come. Accordingly, the pathologist may consider including some criteria (i.e., histogenetic type) not currently used for staging or treatment planning, with the expectation that they may become of value for future applications. In addition, the advancement of our understanding of melanocytic lesion behavior depends on research, which often relies on the retrospective evaluation of data obtained from pathology reports. In an attempt to help shed light on some of these important microscopic features of melanocytic lesions, the current chapter highlights data that support the inclusion of selected histopathologic characteristics in the reporting of melanoma.

Table 2.1 Pathologic staging of melanomas for primary tumors

Stage	Description
pTX	Primary tumor cannot be assessed
pT0	No evidence of primary tumor
pTis	Melanoma in situ
pT1a	Melanoma 1.0 mm or less in thickness, no ulceration, <1 mitoses/mm^2
pT1b	Melanoma 1.0 mm or less in thickness with ulceration and/or 1 or more mitoses/mm^2
pT2a	Melanoma 1.01–2.0 mm in thickness, no ulceration
pT2b	Melanoma 1.01–2.0 mm in thickness, with ulceration
pT3a	Melanoma 2.01–4.0 mm in thickness, no ulceration
pT3b	Melanoma 2.01–4.0 mm in thickness, with ulceration
pT4a	Melanoma >4.0 mm in thickness, no ulceration
pT4b	Melanoma >4.0 mm in thickness, with ulceration

Table content adapted from the American Joint Committee on Cancer

Staging and Reporting of Melanoma

The multidisciplinary clinical management, staging, and assessment of prognosis of melanoma are largely based on the histopathologic assessment of tissue biopsy specimens. Parameters of the skin lesion predict outcome and affect management. Hence, many international groups, including The College of American Pathologists (CAP), The Royal College of Pathologists of Australasia, and The Royal College of Pathologists, have proposed reporting guidelines for pathology reports. These guidelines were selected based on their correlation to tumor behavior, interobserver reproducibility of results, and impact on clinical management, among other issues [1]. Some of the clinical and histopathologic parameters recommended include: tumor site, specimen laterality, specimen type, Breslow thickness, margins, ulceration, mitotic rate, lymphovascular invasion, neurotropism, satellites, and desmoplastic component. These pathology data elements are either fully or mostly concordant among the three colleges [2], and some of these are included in current melanoma staging [3].

Histogenetic Type

Multiple histologic subtypes of malignant melanocytic neoplasms have been described. According to the CAP, the World Health Organization classification of tumor variants include a non-exhaustive list of subtypes consisting of: superficial spreading melanoma, nodular melanoma, lentigo maligna melanoma, mucosal-lentiginous melanoma, desmoplastic melanoma, melanoma arising from blue nevus, melanoma arising from giant congenital nevus, melanoma in childhood, nevoid melanoma, persistent melanoma, and melanoma not otherwise classified (Fig. 2.1). Each of these variants has specific

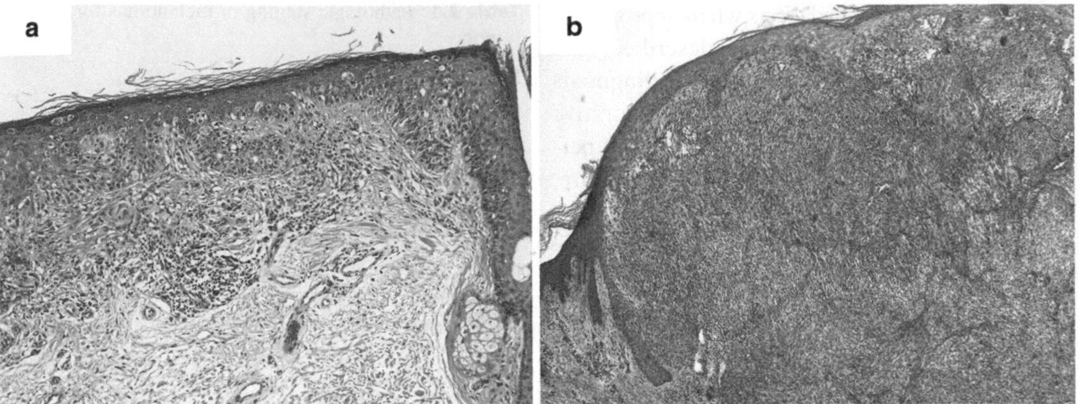

Fig. 2.1 Histogenetic types of melanoma. (**a**) Superficial spreading melanoma. (**b**) Nodular melanoma

histopathologic characteristics. For instance, desmoplastic melanoma classically demonstrates a dense desmoplastic stroma with nodular lymphoid aggregates, atypical spindle cells, and perineural extension, while a nodular melanoma shows no radial growth phase, appears relatively symmetrical, may have areas of necrosis, and is often rich in plasma cells. These features however, are not specific, are overlapping, and do not carry reliable prognostic value.

The use of histogenetic type for prognosticating melanomas is not commonplace given the overlap of defining characteristics, minimal relevance in treatment planning, reliance on tumor site for certain types, among other issues [4]. However, subclassification provides clinicians with a clinicopathologic correlation that may aid in the early recognition of clinical lesions.

The genetic basis for melanoma is becoming increasingly well described, and some of these subtypes have been associated with specific genetic mutations [5]. For instance, acral-lentiginous melanoma and mucosal melanoma are often found to have mutations in KIT. Alternatively, the chronically sun-exposed region-associated lentigo maligna melanoma more commonly has NRAS mutations than KIT mutations. The most commonly observed mutation overall, in BRAF, is particularly associated with superficial spreading melanomas found in skin of intermittently sun-exposed areas. In addition, GNAQ/GNA11 mutations are found in approximately 50 % of uveal melanomas. It is prudent however, to note that histopathologic subtype only loosely predicts a gene mutation, and does not replace genetic testing. As new data on the genetic and molecular fingerprint of specific melanoma subtypes are elucidated, consideration of their inclusion in pathology reports should take place.

Breslow Thickness

Breslow thickness is currently the most important prognostic factor for localized primary melanoma [6]. Tumor invasion as assessed by this method correlates to the risk of regional and distant metastases, and to mortality [7, 8]. Tumor thickness is currently the major consideration when physician and patient discuss sentinel lymph node biopsy; therefore, the Breslow thickness has a significant impact not only on clinical management, but also on potential morbidity and healthcare costs [9]. Thus, standardization and accuracy regarding thickness are of critical importance in the pathologist's report.

Tumor thickness is to be measured with an ocular micrometer at a right angle to the epidermal surface, from the top of the granular layer to the deepest point of tumor invasion. If the lesion is ulcerated, the upper point of reference is the base of the ulcer, and special consideration should be taken given that it will likely underestimate "true" depth (Figs. 2.2 and 2.3). The lower point of reference should be the leading edge of a single mass or an isolated cell or group of melanoma cells deep to the main mass [8].

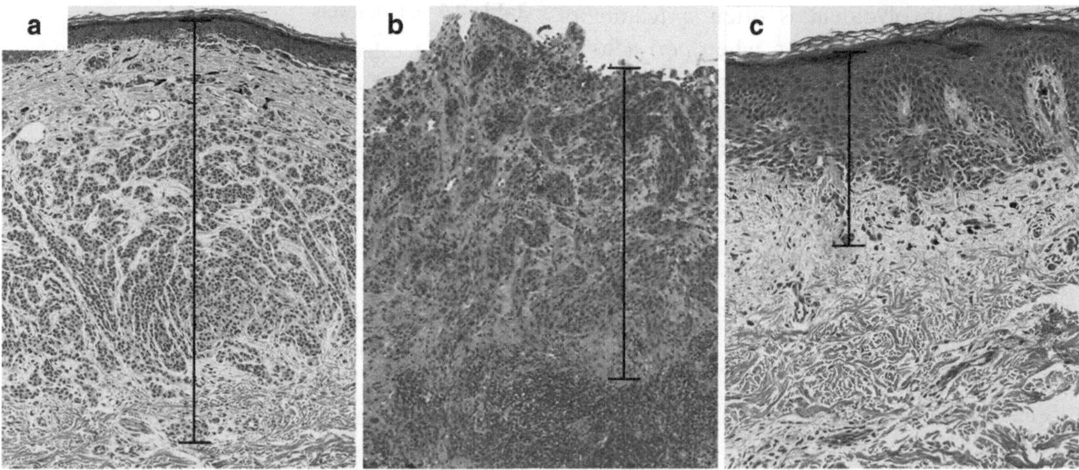

Fig. 2.2 Breslow thickness measurement in various histopathologic settings. (**a**) Melanoma displaying intact epidermis and no ulceration. The granular layer serves as the upper margin of the measurement. (**b**) Ulcerated melanoma with lack of granular layer. The base of the ulcer serves as the upper margin of the measurement. (**c**) Melanoma with hyperplastic epidermis. Note that a significant portion of the Breslow thickness corresponds to the epidermal component

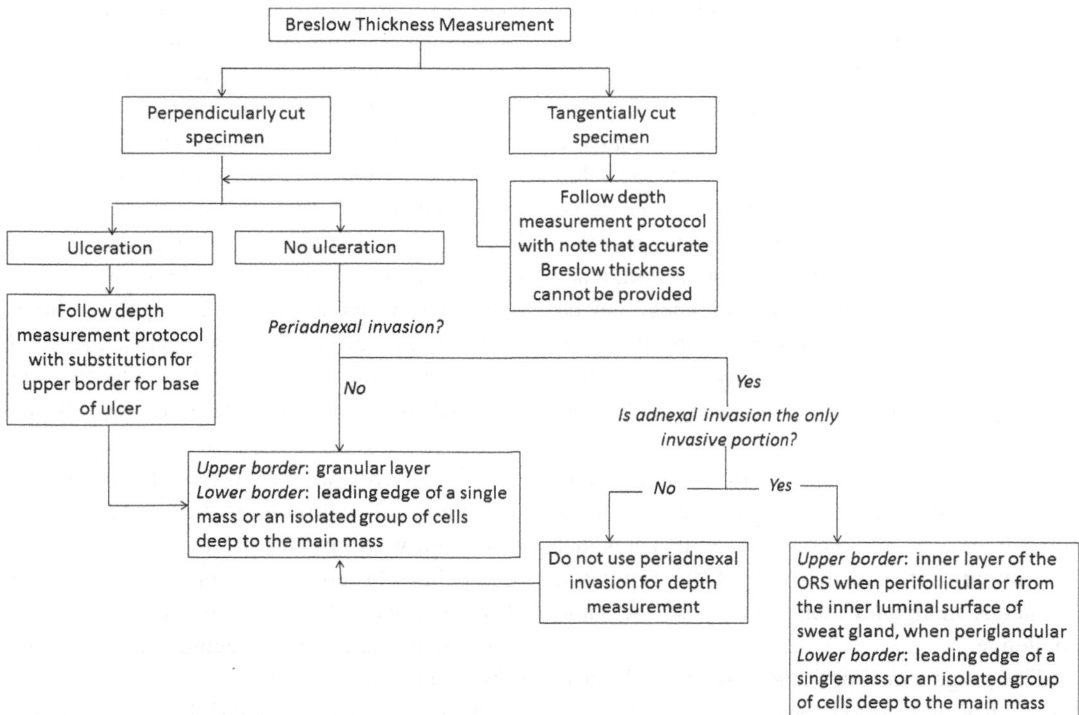

Fig. 2.3 Flowchart for the measurement of the Breslow thickness

Tangentially cut sections should be reported with a comment noting that an accurate Breslow thickness cannot be provided. If the epidermis cannot be visualized, no accurate tumor thickness can be provided, and other prognostic information such as mitotic rate and Clark level may be required to infer stage, prognosis, and clinical management.

Adnexal involvement is often a feature of melanoma in situ. However, when *peri*-adnexal invasion is the only focus of invasion, Breslow thickness can be measured from the inner layer of the outer root sheath when perifollicular, or from the inner luminal surface of sweat glands, when periglandular, to the farthest peripheral infiltration into the dermis (Fig. 2.2). If the peri-adnexal invasion is not the only focus of invasion, it should not be utilized for Breslow thickness reporting (Fig. 2.3) [2].

In cases where the deepest portion of the biopsy specimen is transected, the report should so indicate, with a note that the Breslow thickness is "at least" a certain value. Other factors that may influence accurate reporting of tumor thickness include when melanomas arise in association with a nevus. Architectural and cytologic feature assessment is difficult and prone to observer bias.

Since the Breslow thickness is measured from the granular layer, samples with epidermal hyperplasia may seemingly overestimate the depth of invasion (Fig. 2.2). The Breslow thickness includes viable epidermis and dermis, and the contribution of each layer to the prognostic value of the thickness is not entirely clear. The viable epidermis of normal, non-acral skin may measure approximately 0.1 mm. In melanomas with reactive epidermal hyperplasia, this thickness may be increased significantly, thus increasing the measured total depth of melanoma invasion. Breslow considered the difficulty of assessing melanoma thickness in this scenario and noted that, especially in thin tumors, hyperplastic epidermis may represent a significant portion of the total measured thickness, and recommended that this fact be communicated in the report [10]. Similarly, verrucous malignant melanomas pose the same challenge.

The prognostic implication of hyperplasia is not clearly understood. Some studies have suggested that epidermal hyperplasia results in a change in the local cytokine milieu including a decrease in interferon-beta (IFN-β), which is an anti-angiogenic factor produced by keratinocytes [11]; it was postulated that this decrease in anti-angiogenic factors may promote tumor growth.

Table 2.2 Clark levels

Clark level I	Intraepidermal tumor only
Clark level II	Tumor present in but does not fill and expand papillary dermis
Clark level III	Tumor fills and expands papillary dermis
Clark level IV	Tumor invades reticular dermis
Clark level V	Tumor invades subcutis

One can speculate that there is cross-talk between normal cells of the epidermis and melanoma cells. There is likely a temporal response from keratinocytes to the alteration of the microenvironment during melanoma tumor formation; whether keratinocyte hyperproliferation is pro- or anti-tumorigenic in different growth stages remains uncertain.

Clark Level

Recent trends have led to the exclusion of the Clark level as a primary method of categorizing melanomas and guiding their treatment. Specifically, under current AJCC guidelines, the Clark level is no longer the primary histopathologic feature utilized to define T1b tumors, which are now determined by the presence of ulceration or dermal mitotic rate of 1 or more per mm^2. Evidence-based studies have suggested that the Breslow thickness predicts prognosis more accurately than Clark level [6, 12, 13]. In addition, some of the current disfavor against the Clark level stems from interobserver variability, especially when distinguishing between level III and level IV (Table 2.2). Here, the papillary dermis must be differentiated from the reticular dermis, which may prove difficult in the setting of scar or regression with fibrosis, presence of a precursor nevus that obscures the interface, and lack of clear interface between the two dermal components in palmar, plantar, genital, mucosal, and subungual sites [14, 15].

Instances where the Clark level may be useful include when an accurate Breslow thickness cannot be determined, as well as in T1 melanomas where ulceration and mitotic rate cannot be determined. When ulceration is not present and mitotic rate is not obtainable, a Clark level IV or V invasion should be used as a tertiary criterion for upgrading a T1a lesion to T1b. This is of clinical significance given that the AJCC recommends sentinel lymph node exploration for melanomas stage T1b and above.

Mitotic Index

The mitotic index observed in melanoma sections has been extensively studied as a prognostic factor and, more recently, adopted as one of the major histopathologic features influencing surgical management. In the seventh edition staging system for melanomas from the AJCC, mitotic rate replaced the Clark level of invasion for T1 melanomas. A mitotic rate of 1 or more per mm^2 indicates an upstage for pT1 lesions from pT1a to pT1b. This recommendation stems from data in multiple studies that indicate that the presence of mitotic figures seems to have a direct correlation to the rate of positive sentinel lymph node biopsies [16–18]. It is currently advocated by some that patients with thin melanomas of <1 mm depth with a mitotic rate of >1 per mm^2 should be offered a lymph node biopsy [19]. Interestingly, it has been shown that there were no significant patient survival differences between melanomas with increasing number of mitotic figures beyond 1 per mm^2 [6].

In years past the mitotic index was reported as the number of mitotic figures per high-power field. This reporting was later standardized to the current accepted format of mitotic number per square millimeter (mm^2). Given the variability between objectives in different microscopes, the field diameter of each microscope must be calibrated with a stage micrometer in order to accurately and reproducibly determine the number of high-power fields that equates to 1 mm^2.

Mitotic figures are best enumerated by first determining the "hot spot" of the lesion; i.e., the focus in vertical growth phase containing the greatest number of mitotic figures. The number of mitoses in the hot-spot field is counted, and the observer then repeats the count on immediately adjacent, non-overlapping areas until an area of 1 mm^2 is covered (approximately 5–6 high-power fields using ×400 magnification, depending on the microscope employed). In cases where the invasive component is <1 mm^2, an average for a 1 mm^2 area is then inferred based on the available area of invasion. In cases where there is no prominent invasive focus that can serve as the "hot spot," the average of mitotic cells from several independent random areas that add up to 1 mm^2 of the tissue section is used. The final report should indicate a whole number of mitoses per mm^2; if no mitotic figures are found, 0 per mm^2 may be reported. If a single dermal mitotic figure is observed, 1 per mm^2 is reported. Similar standardized methodologies have been shown to result in an interobserver correlation coefficient of 0.76 among trained pathologists [20].

The counting of mitotic figures and finding the mitotic hot spot may be challenging in hematoxylin and eosin (H&E)-stained slides as the pathologist relies on the observation of condensed chromosomes to identify a mitotic figure. Common problems with this technique include staining artifacts, suboptimal histology preparation, and occasionally, apoptotic figures can be confused with mitosis. Some studies comparing the use of H&E slides and immunohistochemical labels used as markers of proliferation for determining the mitotic index did not offer significant advantage over conventional H&E [18]. However, other immunohistochemical labels have been suggested to improve the detection of mitotic figures, such as the use of phosphohistone H3 (pHH3) labeling [21–23]. pHH3 plays an important role in cell cycling and highlights cells more selectively in the M phase. Visualization of mitotic figures can be highly improved using this technique and aid in finding the hot spot in difficult cases where condensed chromatin within nuclei of melanocytes is not readily observed. The search for the mitotic hot spot is often performed by scanning the entire slide at relatively low magnification. At low magnification, mitotic figures may not be readily observed, but on pHH3 stained slides, the mitotic figures stand out even at low magnifications improving the yield of finding the true hot spot (Fig. 2.4).

It is important to highlight that the prognostic significance of the mitotic index stems from studies of mitotic counts using H&E-stained slides.

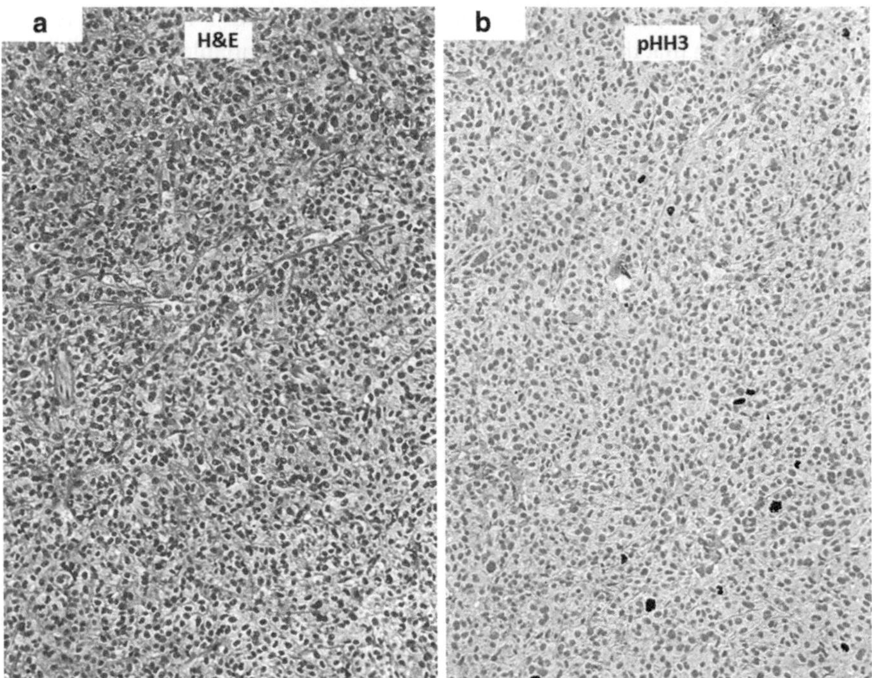

Fig. 2.4 Aid in finding the mitotic hot spot using immunostaining. (**a**) Hematoxylin and eosin (H&E)-stained slide at low magnification (×10) with difficult-to-see mitotic figures. (**b**) Phosphohistone H3 (pHH3)-immunostained slide (*dark brown*) with readily observed cells in the M phase

Hence, at this time, H&E slides should be used to determine the index in order to maintain standardization. However, immunostains may be helpful in identifying the mitotic hot spot and improve interobserver correlation in challenging cases.

Tumor growth and expansion are obviously dependent on mitosis of cells forming the tumor. Hence, one can expect that if a thorough search for mitotic figures is performed in multiple sections with the aid of immunohistochemical staining, mitotic figures will likely be found. Accordingly, as the protocol for mitotic rate determination is modified to optimize capture of mitotic figures (i.e., addition of immunostaining, deviating from the studies that led to the inclusion of mitotic index in melanoma staging), the translation of mitotic index to melanoma staging should be adjusted.

Ulceration

Together with tumor thickness, the presence of ulceration is one of the two most powerful independent variables of primary melanoma lesions when compared to other histopathologic prognostic variables [13]. There are likely multiple reasons why ulceration is a poor prognostic factor. Ulceration may impact measurement of the Breslow thickness as discussed previously and underestimate this important prognostic value. Moreover, ulceration often results from increased growth and expansion of the tumor, likely representing more malignant intrinsic properties. For patients with ulcerated melanoma, there was a twofold increased hazard ratio when compared to those with non-ulcerated tumors. In patients with thin melanomas that demonstrated ulceration, survival rates decreased to levels near those of thicker melanomas. In patients with melanomas of <1 mm depth with ulceration, survival (near 85 % at 10-years) was similar to those with depth of 1.1–2.0 mm without ulceration. Similarly, tumors with depth of 2.1–4.0 mm with ulceration, had similar survival rates (near 55 % at 10-years) to thicker tumors of >4 mm depth without ulceration [13]. Based on these data, similar to the mitotic index, presence of ulceration affects tumor staging.

Ulceration, when visualized on histopathologic sections of melanomas, upgrades a pT1 lesion from pT1a to pT1b, regardless of the mitotic index. Similarly, for T2, T3, and T4 tumors, the presence of ulceration determines whether the lesion is a T2a or T2b, and so forth. In fact, for thicker melanomas, the presence of ulceration has been shown to have more prognostic import than tumor depth [13]. Moreover, the thicker the tumor, the more likely it is to show presence of ulceration. For instance, tumors of less than 1 mm depth showed 6 % ulceration rate whereas tumors with depth of 1.1–2.0 mm, 2.1–4.0, or >4 mm showed 23 %, 47 %, or 63 % ulceration rates, respectively [13]. On the other hand, studies in patients with thin melanomas of <1 mm in depth demonstrate that thickness is more predictive for survival than ulceration.

Assessing ulceration may prove to be a difficult task and the pathologist, aware of the importance of this prognostic histologic factor, may spend considerable time determining its presence or absence in certain sections. For instance, cases with only a focal loss of epidermis pose a dilemma where the defect could be considered artifactual versus a true ulceration. Certain features may clue in the astute pathologist as to the true state of the lesion. For example, the presence of fibrin or granulation tissue may indicate a true ulcer. Moreover, distinguishing traumatic (exogenous) from non-traumatic (endogenous) ulceration is indeed also important, as the former would have less prognostic significance [24]. Clinical history is of key importance but the pathologist often relies on the description provided by the clinical dermatologist who performed the biopsy. Lesion site is also another consideration when determining whether the ulceration is traumatic, as areas prone to trauma have higher risk of traumatic ulceration, albeit limited by speculation. Characteristics of the ulceration should be considered, such as sharp border demarcation and wedge-shaped granulation tissue pointing towards a traumatic ulceration. In addition, the presence of scar in the dermis may help make this distinction, as scars would be more characteristic of trauma [20]. True intrinsic ulcerations have been described in two principal settings. First is an ulcer formed from invasion of melanoma cells through the epidermis disturbing the desmosomal junctions of keratinocytes. Second is the ulcer formed by larger nodular melanomas, where nodular expansion may force the epidermis into an effaced state resulting in thinning and ulceration [20].

Currently, pathology reports include merely the presence or absence of ulceration. However, the extent of ulceration may also have prognostic relevance. Multiple studies have evaluated quantitative outcome measures of ulceration and suggested their inclusion in the pathology report [25, 26]. Extent of ulceration may be measured as total absolute diameter or as a percentage of tumor width. Melanomas with ulceration of either less than 70 % of total width or less than 5 mm diameter showed a 5-year melanoma-specific survival (MSS) of 80.4 % and 82.7 %, respectively. Remarkably, the 5-year MSS of melanomas with ulceration of >70 % of total width or>5 mm were 66.4 % and 59.3 %, respectively. These data along with further studies may influence pathologists to consider the addition of qualifiers and quantifiers of ulceration given possible prognostic impact.

Tumor-Infiltrating Lymphocytes and Tumor Regression

Melanoma regression is a histopathologic characteristic that spans a spectrum of microscopic findings. Early regression represents the presence of tumor-infiltrating lymphocytes. Intermediate and late regression is the replacement of melanoma tumor tissue by fibrosis in the dermis, either immature when intermediate or mature when late. Along with haphazard dermal fibroplasia, the pathologist can often observe melanophages, variable edema, telangiectasia, and epidermal effacement in intermediate and late regression. Blood vessels may also assume a perpendicular orientation [27].

Importantly, the prognostic value of early versus intermediate/late regression varies. For early regression, which is characterized by tumor-infiltrating lymphocytes that disrupt tumor nests or oppose melanoma cells, the prognosis may be more favorable [28–30]. However, it is important

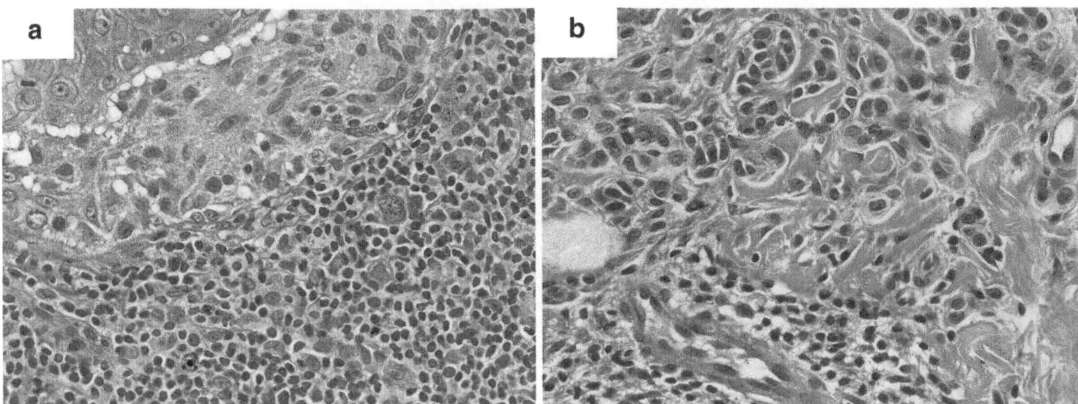

Fig. 2.5 Tumor-infiltrating lymphocytes. (**a**) Brisk infiltrate with tumor-infiltrating lymphocytes surrounding the base of the tumor. (**b**) Non-brisk infiltrate with relatively few, scattered tumor-infiltrating lymphocytes

to note that the level of lymphocyte infiltration must be graded and, if accurately described, may predict survival rates. A "brisk" lymphocytic infiltrate is characterized by diffuse infiltration of the entire base of the vertical growth phase or throughout the entire invasive component of the melanoma (Fig. 2.5). On the contrary, a non-brisk infiltrate is found only focally. When the infiltrate of melanoma with vertical growth phase is brisk, the 5-year survival rate was 77 % and the 10-year rate 55 %. When compared to a non-brisk infiltrate, these rates declined to 53 % and 45 %, respectively. If no tumor-infiltrating lymphocytes were sighted, these rates declined further to 37 % and 27 %, respectively [29]. Hence, a brisk infiltrate may be considered as a positive prognostic factor. Of note, one should bear in mind that the type of lymphocytes present likely alters tumor destiny; hypothetically, cytotoxic cells may promote regression whereas regulatory T-cells may favor immunotolerance.

On the other hand, intermediate and late regression, defined as fibroplasia and other findings as described above, may be associated with poorer prognosis, albeit this point remains controversial (Fig. 2.5) [31]. Only when regression area reaches approximately 75 % has association with metastasis been more clearly demonstrated [27, 32]. Given the discrepancy of prognostic significance between early and intermediate or late regression, the term "tumor-infiltrating lymphocytes" is probably more descriptive and clearer than "early regression." The term "regression" may be best saved for when there are intermediate or late stages of regression, signifying a possible poor prognosis, noting that the interobserver variation and lack of standardized criteria make use of regression as a prognostic factor less reliable.

Radial and Vertical Growth Phases

Melanoma growth phases are mainly described as radial or vertical. The prototype lesions for radial growth phase are the lentigo maligna and the superficial spreading types of melanoma (Fig. 2.1) [33, 34]. Conventionally, a lesion with predominantly radial growth will demonstrate three or more rete ridges of in situ disease "shouldering" the primary focus of melanoma (Fig. 2.6). This feature results in the appearance of a lesion that is much wider than deep. Alternatively, lesions with predominantly vertical growth phase have deeper invasive components. The presence of any mitotic figures in the dermis or the presence of a dermal cluster larger than the largest epidermal cluster of melanoma cells defines a vertical growth phase, with the prototype lesion being nodular melanoma. Vertical growth phase carries an adverse prognostic value for cutaneous melanoma. For instance, a prior study demonstrated that in thin superficial spreading melanomas, the vertical growth phase was the only statistically significant prognostic factor [34].

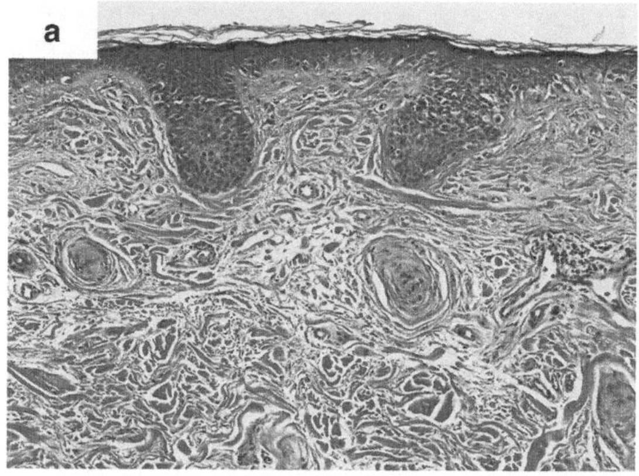

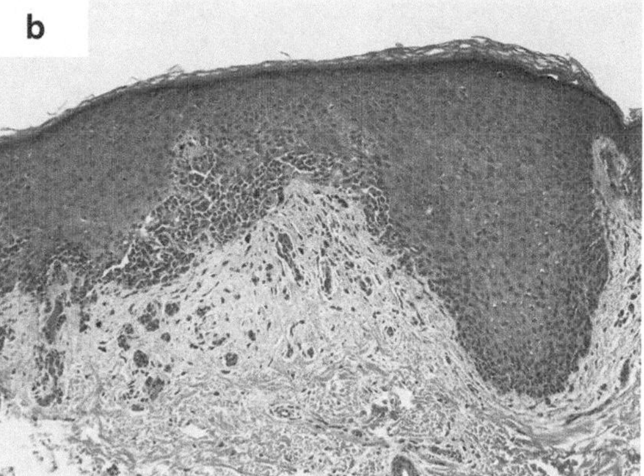

Fig. 2.6 Comparison between melanoma in situ (MIS) and melanoma in radial growth phase. (**a**) MIS demonstrates melanocytic proliferation only affecting the epidermis. (**b**) RGP melanoma with epidermal involvement and microinvasion into the dermis

The background for evaluating the prognostic relevance of growth phases is described in in vitro studies [34–36]. Melanoma cells isolated from vertical growth phase lesions grown in culture demonstrate higher proliferative activity and, when injected into study animals, permanent growth of tumor cells is observed. In immunosuppressed animals, these cells are able to undergo frank melanoma formation, exemplifying an aggressive pattern. Melanoma cells from radial growth phase lesions lack such aggressiveness, as no melanoma formation was observed upon injection of cells into immunosuppressed animals [33–36]. Melanomas in radial growth phase are likely incapable of metastasis.

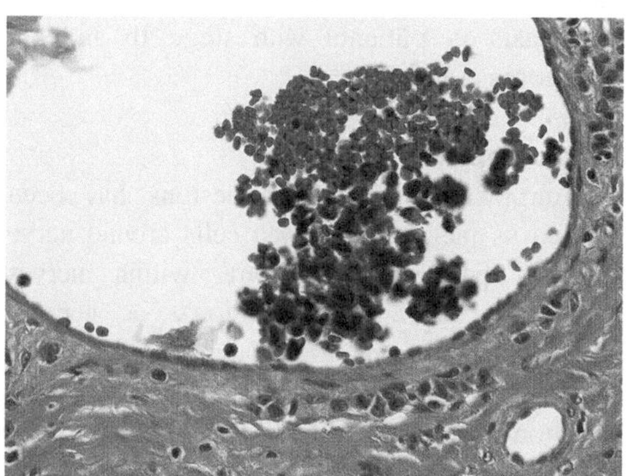

Fig. 2.7 Intravascular invasion. Melanoma tumor cells within a blood vessel

Vascular Invasion

As one might predict, the presence of melanoma cells in vascular spaces is a poor prognostic factor. These cells may indicate in-transit malignant cells and increase the likelihood of metastatic potential. It has been shown in prior studies that vascular invasion defined as tumor within blood or lymphatic vessels, or melanoma cells immediately adjacent to vascular spaces, results in significantly increased risk of relapse and death and reduced the survival associated with melanoma (Fig. 2.7) [37, 38].

In cases of invasive melanoma, lymphovascular invasion may help predict lymph node involvement. In one study, 67 % of cases with lymphovascular invasion had positive lymph node involvement compared to 19 % of cases without invasion [39]. Moreover, in this immunohistochemistry-based study using anti-podoplanin (D2–40) for the detection of lymphatic invasion, patients with invasion had more distant metastases as well as regional recurrence. Lymphovascular invasion resulted in a decrease in overall and disease-specific survival. In addition, specific to lymphatic invasion, studies have also demonstrated that lymphatic invasion alone may be an independent prognostic

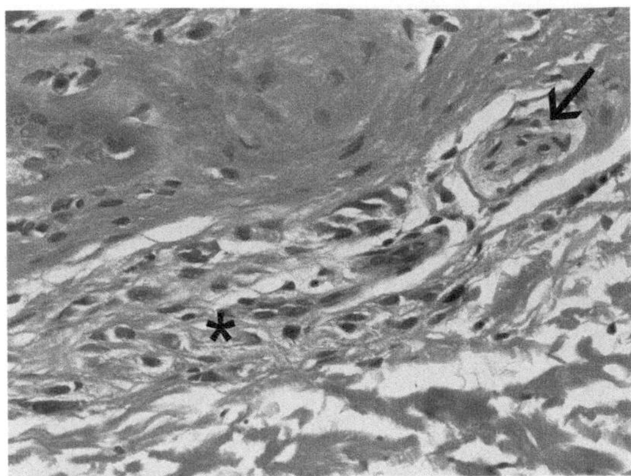

Fig. 2.8 Neurotropism. Melanoma cells (*asterix*) invading nerve tissue (*arrow*) in the dermis

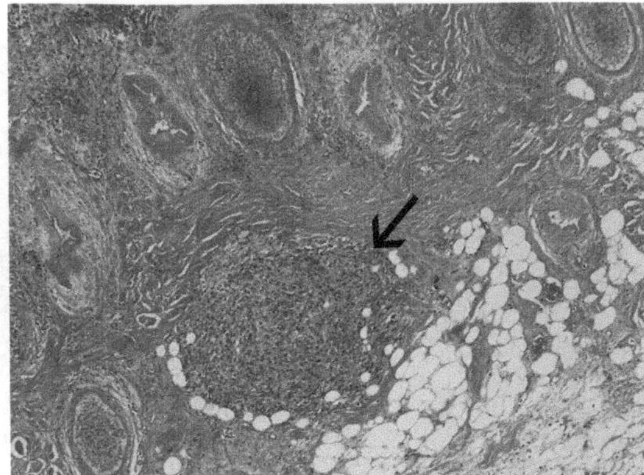

Fig. 2.9 Satellitosis. Satellite of nested melanoma cells (*arrow*) distant from primary tumor and separated by normal intervening tissue

factor and significantly increase the risk of metastasis in patients with stage Ib and IIa melanomas [40].

Neurotropism

Neurotropism in melanoma lesions has been defined as melanoma-derived cells around nerve sheaths (perineural invasion), within nerves themselves (intraneural invasion), or neuroid transformation/morphology of the melanoma itself (neural transformation) (Fig. 2.8) [2, 41]. Most commonly, perineural invasion is seen in desmoplastic-neuroid subtypes, although any melanoma may also show this feature [42]. As with most tumors, perineural invasion is an unfavorable prognostic factor. In melanomas, it may indicate increased risk for local recurrence, and in desmoplastic melanomas, perineural invasion results in statistically significant decrease in survival [42]. Hence, neurotropism may influence management decisions [42]. For instance, if perineural invasion is present, the clinician may opt for wider local excision and/or adding adjuvant therapies.

Caution is advised however, when assessing perineural invasion, as local resident nerves may be entrapped and not invaded by an expanding melanoma tumor. In such cases, perineural invasion should be looked for elsewhere and not reported unless more clearly determined. When in doubt, the pathologist may note the diagnostic uncertainty under the comments section of the report.

Microscopic Satellitosis

Microscopic satellitosis is defined as nests of metastatic tumor cells that are discontinuous from the primary tumor (Fig. 2.9). Satellites are likely foci of local metastasis. Hence, satellitosis is not included in the measurement of primary tumor depth; however, it should be accounted for and reported. Satellites have been demonstrated to be an independent negative prognostic factor for melanomas [43]. It is noteworthy that separation of the apparent satellite nest from the primary tumor by fibrosis or inflammation does not amount to the classification of a satellite; such a nest should be considered a contiguous part of the parent tumor. In general, a satellite is defined as being disconnected from the principal invasive tumor with intervening normal tissue creating a minimum of 0.3 mm of separation. For standardization purposes, microsatellite tumor nests have a minimum diameter of 0.05 mm and are located in the reticular dermis, subcutaneous adipose tissue, or vessels.

The rate of sentinel lymph node positivity in patients with microscopic satellitosis has been shown to be 43 % [44]. The presence of satellitosis is also frequently associated with other adverse histologic features including ulceration, lack of lymphocytic infiltration, and lymphovascular invasion. Given these negative prognostic features, satellitosis is a recommended histopathologic feature to be included in the pathology report.

Associated Melanocytic Nevus

It is currently generally accepted that presence of an associated melanocytic nevus does not directly aid in prognosticating melanomas. However, the report of such associated lesion may provide knowledge regarding the original histologic features of the biopsied specimen and help with the interpretation of re-excisions that show residual tumor. In these cases, the residual tumor may be in fact a recurrent nevus or the so-called pseudomelanoma.

Prior studies have shed some light in the epidemiology of these two concurrent lesions as well as some of their clinical features. Melanomas with associated melanocytic nevi tend to occur at similar rates in males and females, and occur with some higher frequency on the trunk when compared to upper extremities, lower extremities, head, and neck (34.5 %, 24.3 %, 20.3 %, 14.2 %, respectively, in one study) [45]. In addition, melanomas containing associated melanocytic nevi had lower Breslow thickness when compared to melanomas without associated lesions (average of 0.95 mm versus 1.3 mm); however, no prognostic significance was found when data was stratified by tumor thickness.

The distinction between a melanoma and an associated melanocytic nevus with high-grade atypia may be difficult or sometimes impossible. Careful evaluation of cell/nuclear morphology and mitotic figures is critical. At times, one can distinguish a second cell population that clues the pathologist regarding an associated lesion; however, these are often not clearly evident. Care should be taken when assessing these lesions and at this time, no prognostic value should be drawn until new research data comes to light.

Margins

Involvement of the excision margins is a subject of great interest given the inherent concern for increased risk of local and loco-regional recurrence when margins are affected by the tumor. Unfortunately, most assessments of margins are limited given that only few sections are prepared and evaluated during processing and consequently biased by sampling. In addition, genetic abnormalities cannot be visualized in hematoxylin-eosin stained slides and, although a section may appear benign, resident cells may have mutations that could lead to melanoma recurrence. For instance, comparative genomic hybridization and fluorescent in situ hybridization studies of histologically apparent benign excision specimens of "normal" skin surrounding primary melanoma from acral sites demonstrated 84 % of margins affected by abnormal cells [46]. Strikingly, these cells could be observed more than 4 mm away from the margin of the invasive melanoma assessed histologically. This exemplifies that histopathologic assessment may help but is not definitive in establishing a true clear margin. It is therefore important to adequately discuss these limitations with patients so that the risk of recurrence is addressed appropriately.

With these limitations in mind, the pathologist and clinician may use the margin report to guide clinical management [47, 48]. There are multiple margins that must be reported in melanomas. Both peripheral and deep margins must be noted. In addition, both the in situ component and invasive component should have margins described separately. For the in situ component, the peripheral margin is reported. For the invasive component, both deep and peripheral margins are reported [2]. When margins are not involved, the distance (to the nearest 1 mm if >2 mm distance or to the nearest 0.1 mm if <2 mm) from the tumor to the nearest uninvolved margin is reported.

In addition to guidance regarding clinical management, whether the margins are involved by the tumor or not is also of value to the pathologist evaluating re-excision specimens. If the re-excision demonstrates melanoma, prior report of involved margins may help differentiate residual tumor from a metastatic focus. However, as noted before, "clear" margins histopathologically may only suggest complete removal of the tumor. Residual abnormal cells may still be present in "clear" sections, thus, the determination of residual tumor versus metastatic tumor in previously clear margin specimens relies on humble speculation.

Synoptic Report

Synoptic reporting is a checklist-type of reporting. For example, the CAP issues a frequently updated checklist available for the reporting of multiple cancer types in an effort to improve consistency and completeness. For colorectal cancers, a few prior studies have demonstrated that synoptic reporting increased completeness, irrespective of subspecialist interest [49]. When using a standardized, checklist-like report format (typically used by non-subspecialists), the reports were deemed more complete and included features such as circumferential radial margin, lymphovascular invasion, and perineural invasion more often than narrative reports by subspecialists in gastrointestinal pathology.

Similarly, a protocol or checklist is issued by the CAP for melanomas, which may be utilized for reporting. However, it is much more common to find narrative-based formats of reporting, given the heavily subspecialized nature of skin pathology. This non-standardized report type, although possibly more thorough, detailed, and lesion/patient pertinent, leads to wide variations in style. As for gastrointestinal cancers, few studies have evaluated the concordance and differences between synoptic reporting and non-synoptic styles. In a study in Australia, synoptic reporting seemed to lead to more frequent reporting of the main pathological features of melanoma [50]. When synoptic reporting was utilized, there was no significant difference found between reports from a specialist melanoma center and nonspecialist center. A separate study evaluated retrospectively, the concordance of melanoma pathology reports with the necessary features required to stage melanoma [51]. In this report, only half of the initial excision reports included the features required to stage melanoma based on 2002 AJCC guidelines, prompting the conclusion that wider adoption of synoptic reporting may increase the quality of melanoma reports. It remains unknown, however, whether non-standardized, narrative style reporting from dermatopathologists compared to nonspecialized pathologists varies in terms of inclusion of the principal pathological melanoma features.

Pathologic staging using pTNM criteria can also be included as part of a checklist in synoptic reporting in order to increase the accuracy and incidence of reporting key histopathologic findings. First, TNM descriptors can be employed such as "m" for multiple, "r" for recurrent, and "y" for posttreatment. For the primary tumor (pT), pTX, pT0, pTis, pT1a, pT1b, pT2a, pT2b, pT3a, pT3b, pT4a, and pT4b stages can be used to describe the specimen under evaluation given observed features as noted in Table 2.1.

If synoptic reporting is to be used more widely, it is imperative that enough emphasis is placed in an associated narrative when appropriate. This is of critical importance so that the viewpoint of the subspecialist or more experienced pathologist can be reported with his or her indispensable familiarity with the subtle histologic features of melanoma and the individual differences and peculiarities between lesions can be preserved.

References

1. Frishberg DP, Balch C, Balzer BL, Crowson AN, Didolkar M, McNiff JM, et al. Protocol for the examination of specimens from patients with melanoma of the skin. Arch Pathol Lab Med. 2009;133(10):1560–7.
2. Scolyer RA, Judge MJ, Evans A, Frishberg DP, Prieto VG, Thompson JF, et al. Data set for pathology reporting of cutaneous invasive melanoma: recommendations from the international collaboration on cancer reporting (ICCR). Am J Surg Pathol. 2013;37(12):1797–814.
3. Balch CM, Gershenwald JE, Soong SJ, Thompson JF, Atkins MB, Byrd DR, et al. Final version of 2009 AJCC melanoma staging and classification. J Clin Oncol. 2009;27(36):6199–206.
4. Weyers W, Euler M, Diaz-Cascajo C, Schill WB, Bonczkowitz M. Classification of cutaneous malignant melanoma: a reassessment of histopathologic criteria for the distinction of different types. Cancer. 1999;86(2):288–99.
5. Curtin JA, Fridlyand J, Kageshita T, Patel HN, Busam KJ, Kutzner H, et al. Distinct sets of genetic alterations in melanoma. N Engl J Med. 2005;353(20):2135–47.
6. Azzola MF, Shaw HM, Thompson JF, Soong SJ, Scolyer RA, Watson GF, et al. Tumor mitotic rate is a more powerful prognostic indicator than ulceration in patients with primary cutaneous melanoma: an analysis of 3661 patients from a single center. Cancer. 2003;97(6):1488–98.
7. Balch CM, Murad TM, Soong SJ, Ingalls AL, Halpern NB, Maddox WA. A multifactorial analysis of melanoma: prognostic histopathological features comparing Clark's and Breslow's staging methods. Ann Surg. 1978;188(6):732–42.
8. Breslow A. Thickness, cross-sectional areas and depth of invasion in the prognosis of cutaneous melanoma. Ann Surg. 1970;172(5):902–8.

9. Freeman SR, Gibbs BB, Brodland DG, Zitelli JA. Prognostic value of sentinel lymph node biopsy compared with that of Breslow thickness: implications for informed consent in patients with invasive melanoma. Dermatol Surg. 2013;39(12):1800–12.
10. Breslow A. Prognosis in cutaneous melanoma: tumor thickness as a guide to treatment. Pathol Annu. 1980; 15(Pt 1):1–22.
11. McCarty MF, Bielenberg DR, Nilsson MB, Gershenwald JE, Barnhill RL, Ahearne P, et al. Epidermal hyperplasia overlying human melanoma correlates with tumour depth and angiogenesis. Melanoma Res. 2003;13(4):379–87.
12. Edge SB, Compton CC. The American Joint Committee on Cancer: the 7th edition of the AJCC cancer staging manual and the future of TNM. Ann Surg Oncol. 2010;17(6):1471–4.
13. Balch CM, Soong SJ, Gershenwald JE, Thompson JF, Reintgen DS, Cascinelli N, et al. Prognostic factors analysis of 17,600 melanoma patients: validation of the American Joint Committee on Cancer melanoma staging system. J Clin Oncol. 2001;19(16):3622–34.
14. Kelly JW, Sagebiel RW, Blois MS. Regression in malignant melanoma. A histologic feature without independent prognostic significance. Cancer. 1985; 56(9):2287–91.
15. Kelly JW, Sagebiel RW, Clyman S, Blois MS. Thin level IV malignant melanoma. A subset in which level is the major prognostic indicator. Ann Surg. 1985;202(1):98–103.
16. Ross MI, Gershenwald JE. Sentinel lymph node biopsy for melanoma: a critical update for dermatologists after two decades of experience. Clin Dermatol. 2013;31(3):298–310.
17. Mraz-Gernhard S, Sagebiel RW, Kashani-Sabet M, Miller 3rd JR, Leong SP. Prediction of sentinel lymph node micrometastasis by histological features in primary cutaneous malignant melanoma. Arch Dermatol. 1998;134(8):983–7.
18. Hale CS, Qian M, Ma MW, Scanlon P, Berman RS, Shapiro RL, et al. Mitotic rate in melanoma: prognostic value of immunostaining and computer-assisted image analysis. Am J Surg Pathol. 2013;37(6):882–9.
19. Sekula-Gibbs SA, Shearer MA. Sentinel node biopsy should be offered in thin melanoma with mitotic rate greater than one. Dermatol Surg. 2011;37(8):1080–8.
20. Scolyer RA, Shaw HM, Thompson JF, Li LX, Colman MH, Lo SK, et al. Interobserver reproducibility of histopathologic prognostic variables in primary cutaneous melanomas. Am J Surg Pathol. 2003;27(12): 1571–6.
21. Tetzlaff MT, Curry JL, Ivan D, Wang WL, Torres-Cabala CA, Bassett RL, et al. Immunodetection of phosphohistone H3 as a surrogate of mitotic figure count and clinical outcome in cutaneous melanoma. Mod Pathol. 2013;26(9):1153–60.
22. Thareja S, Zager JS, Sadhwani D, Thareja S, Chen R, Marzban S, et al. Analysis of tumor mitotic rate in thin metastatic melanomas compared with thin melanomas without metastasis using both the hematoxylin and eosin and anti-phosphohistone 3 IHC stain. Am J Dermatopathol. 2014;36(1):64–7.
23. Ikenberg K, Pfaltz M, Rakozy C, Kempf W. Immunohistochemical dual staining as an adjunct in assessment of mitotic activity in melanoma. J Cutan Pathol. 2012;39(3):324–30.
24. Ruiter DJ, Spatz A, van den Oord JJ, Cook MG, Pathology Committee of the European Organization Research and Treatment of Cancer Melanoma Group. Pathologic staging of melanoma. Semin Oncol. 2002; 29(4):370–81.
25. In 't Hout FE, Haydu LE, Murali R, Bonenkamp JJ, Thompson JF, Scolyer RA. Prognostic importance of the extent of ulceration in patients with clinically localized cutaneous melanoma. Ann Surg. 2012; 255(6):1165–70.
26. Grande Sarpa H, Reinke K, Shaikh L, Leong SP, Miller 3rd JR, Sagebiel RW, et al. Prognostic significance of extent of ulceration in primary cutaneous melanoma. Am J Surg Pathol. 2006;30(11):1396–400.
27. Crowson AN, Magro CM, Mihm MC. Prognosticators of melanoma, the melanoma report, and the sentinel lymph node. Mod Pathol. 2006;19 Suppl 2:S71–87.
28. Clark Jr WH, Elder DE, Guerry 4th D, Braitman LE, Trock BJ, Schultz D, et al. Model predicting survival in stage I melanoma based on tumor progression. J Natl Cancer Inst. 1989;81(24):1893–904.
29. Clemente CG, Mihm Jr MC, Bufalino R, Zurrida S, Collini P, Cascinelli N. Prognostic value of tumor infiltrating lymphocytes in the vertical growth phase of primary cutaneous melanoma. Cancer. 1996;77(7): 1303–10.
30. Mihm Jr MC, Clemente CG, Cascinelli N. Tumor infiltrating lymphocytes in lymph node melanoma metastases: a histopathologic prognostic indicator and an expression of local immune response. Lab Invest. 1996;74(1):43–7.
31. Cook MG, Spatz A, Brocker EB, Ruiter DJ. Identification of histological features associated with metastatic potential in thin (<1.0 mm) cutaneous melanoma with metastases. A study on behalf of the EORTC Melanoma Group. J Pathol. 2002;197(2):188–93.
32. Ronan SG, Eng AM, Briele HA, Shioura NN, Das Gupta TK. Thin malignant melanomas with regression and metastases. Arch Dermatol. 1987;123(10): 1326–30.
33. Elder DE, Van Belle P, Elenitsas R, Halpern A, Guerry D. Neoplastic progression and prognosis in melanoma. Semin Cutan Med Surg. 1996;15(4):336–48.
34. Lefevre M, Vergier B, Balme B, Thiebault R, Delaunay M, Thomas L, et al. Relevance of vertical growth pattern in thin level II cutaneous superficial spreading melanomas. Am J Surg Pathol. 2003;27(6): 717–24.
35. Herlyn M, Clark WH, Rodeck U, Mancianti ML, Jambrosic J, Koprowski H. Biology of tumor progression in human melanocytes. Lab Invest. 1987;56(5): 461–74.
36. Satyamoorthy K, DeJesus E, Linnenbach AJ, Kraj B, Kornreich DL, Rendle S, et al. Melanoma cell lines

from different stages of progression and their biological and molecular analyses. Melanoma Res. 1997;7 Suppl 2:S35–42.

37. Kashani-Sabet M, Sagebiel RW, Ferreira CM, Nosrati M, Miller 3rd JR. Vascular involvement in the prognosis of primary cutaneous melanoma. Arch Dermatol. 2001;137(9):1169–73.
38. Yun SJ, Gimotty PA, Hwang WT, Dawson P, Van Belle P, Elder DE, et al. High lymphatic vessel density and lymphatic invasion underlie the adverse prognostic effect of radial growth phase regression in melanoma. Am J Surg Pathol. 2011;35(2):235–42.
39. Petersson F, Diwan AH, Ivan D, Gershenwald JE, Johnson MM, Harrell R, et al. Immunohistochemical detection of lymphovascular invasion with D2-40 in melanoma correlates with sentinel lymph node status, metastasis and survival. J Cutan Pathol. 2009;36(11): 1157–63.
40. Xu X, Chen L, Guerry D, Dawson PR, Hwang WT, VanBelle P, et al. Lymphatic invasion is independently prognostic of metastasis in primary cutaneous melanoma. Clin Cancer Res. 2012;18(1):229–37.
41. Smithers BM, McLeod GR, Little JH. Desmoplastic, neural transforming and neurotropic melanoma: a review of 45 cases. Aust N Z J Surg. 1990;60(12): 967–72.
42. Baer SC, Schultz D, Synnestvedt M, Elder DE. Desmoplasia and neurotropism. Prognostic variables in patients with stage I melanoma. Cancer. 1995;76(11):2242–7.
43. Nagore E, Oliver V, Botella-Estrada R, Moreno-Picot S, Insa A, Fortea JM. Prognostic factors in localized invasive cutaneous melanoma: high value of mitotic rate, vascular invasion and microscopic satellitosis. Melanoma Res. 2005;15(3):169–77.
44. Bartlett EK, Gupta M, Datta J, Gimotty PA, Guerry D, Xu X, et al. Prognosis of patients with melanoma and microsatellitosis undergoing sentinel lymph node biopsy. Ann Surg Oncol. 2014;21(3):1016–23.
45. Kaddu S, Smolle J, Zenahlik P, Hofmann-Wellenhof R, Kerl H. Melanoma with benign melanocytic naevus components: reappraisal of clinicopathological features and prognosis. Melanoma Res. 2002;12(3): 271–8.
46. North JP, Kageshita T, Pinkel D, LeBoit PE, Bastian BC. Distribution and significance of occult intraepidermal tumor cells surrounding primary melanoma. J Invest Dermatol. 2008;128(8):2024–30.
47. Pasquali S, Haydu LE, Scolyer RA, Winstanley JB, Spillane AJ, Quinn MJ, et al. The importance of adequate primary tumor excision margins and sentinel node biopsy in achieving optimal locoregional control for patients with thick primary melanomas. Ann Surg. 2013;258(1):152–7.
48. Heenan PJ. Local recurrence of melanoma. Pathology. 2004;36(5):491–5.
49. Messenger DE, McLeod RS, Kirsch R. What impact has the introduction of a synoptic report for rectal cancer had on reporting outcomes for specialist gastrointestinal and nongastrointestinal pathologists? Arch Pathol Lab Med. 2011;135(11):1471–5.
50. Karim RZ, van den Berg KS, Colman MH, McCarthy SW, Thompson JF, Scolyer RA. The advantage of using a synoptic pathology report format for cutaneous melanoma. Histopathology. 2008;52(2):130–8.
51. Haydu LE, Holt PE, Karim RZ, Madronio CM, Thompson JF, Armstrong BK, et al. Quality of histopathological reporting on melanoma and influence of use of a synoptic template. Histopathology. 2010; 56(6):768–74.

3 Clinicopathologic Correlation in Melanocytic Lesions

Juliana L. Basko-Plluska, Victor G. Prieto, Jon A. Reed, and Christopher R. Shea

Age

Benign melanocytic lesions are more common in childhood, whereas malignant melanoma is more characteristic of older age. Although the incidence of melanoma in adolescents and adults has risen dramatically in the past few decades, childhood melanoma remains uncommon. In the United States, only 0.3–0.4 % of melanomas occur before puberty [1]. In contrast, melanocytic nevi are extremely common in children, with more than 98 % of Caucasians developing at least one nevus by early childhood [2]. Even benign melanocytic nevi may sometimes show features worrisome for melanoma and may be easily misdiagnosed if the histopathologic findings are taken out of context. In particular, congenital nevi in neonates and young children as well as nevi of the elderly raise such concerns. Therefore, the age of the patient is an important characteristic which should be considered before a histopathologic diagnosis is rendered.

J.L. Basko-Plluska, M.D. • C.R. Shea (✉)
University of Chicago Medicine,
5841 S. Maryland Ave., MC 5067, L502,
Chicago, IL 60637, USA
e-mail: cshea@medicine.bsd.uchicago.edu

V.G. Prieto
MD Anderson Cancer Center, University of Houston,
1515 Holcombe Blvd., Unit 85, Houston,
TX 77030, USA

J.A. Reed
CellNEtix Pathology & Laboratories, 1124 Columbia St.,
Suite 200, Seattle, WA 98117, USA

Congenital Nevi

Congenital nevi are classically defined as melanocytic nevi present at birth or within the first few months of life. Histopathologically, most congenital nevi are symmetrical, well-circumscribed, and composed of nests and individual melanocytes which mature with progressive depth into the dermis. Classically, nevus cells wrap around the vessels and the adnexal structures, and splay among the collagen bundles in the reticular dermis. An association between giant congenital melanocytic nevi and malignant melanoma has been established, with the risk estimated to be 5–10 % over a lifetime. Whether such an association exists for small congenital nevi remains controversial.

The diagnosis of a congenital nevus is usually straightforward when all the classic histopathologic features are present. However, a small number of congenital nevi may display atypical features including lentiginous growth, suprabasal spread of melanocytes, dermal mitotic figures, and atypical proliferative nodules [3]. Lentiginous (basilar single-cell) growth is one of the most common findings, particularly in individuals less than 10 years of age and especially in the first year of life (Fig. 3.1). Large and pleomorphic single cells may predominate over nests.

C.R. Shea et al. (eds.), *Pathology of Challenging Melanocytic Neoplasms: Diagnosis and Management*,
DOI 10.1007/978-1-4939-1444-9_3, © Springer Science+Business Media New York 2015

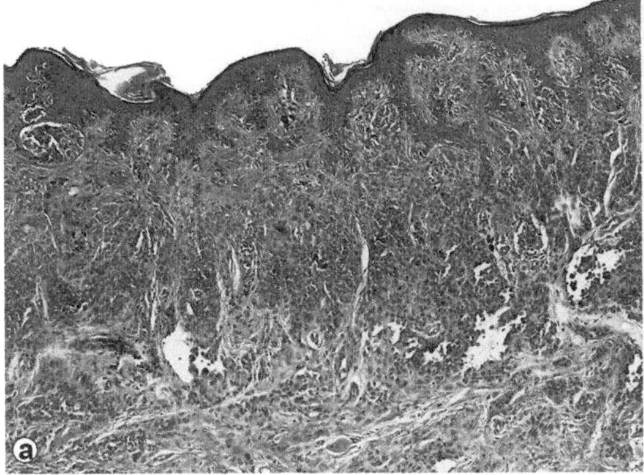

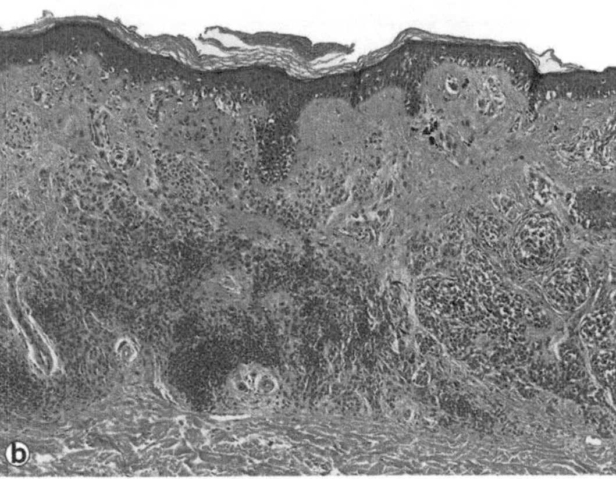

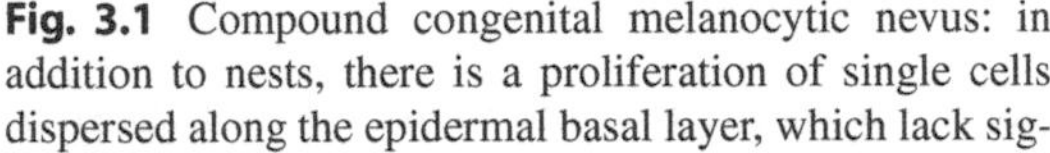

Fig. 3.1 Compound congenital melanocytic nevus: in addition to nests, there is a proliferation of single cells dispersed along the epidermal basal layer, which lack significant cytologic atypia (**a**). Malignant melanoma arising within a congenital nevus for comparison (**b**)

Irregular and abnormally located junctional nests with mitotic activity may also be present. Suprabasal spread of single cells and nests of melanocytes is also common in nevi excised from children during their first year of life, but is usually restricted to the lower half of the epidermis [4]. Suprabasal melanocytes in such nevi, however, usually lack cytologic atypia. While lentiginous growth and suprabasal spread of melanocytes are useful architectural criteria in the diagnosis of malignant melanoma, they are not specific to melanoma and may be misinterpreted if the age of the patient is not accounted for.

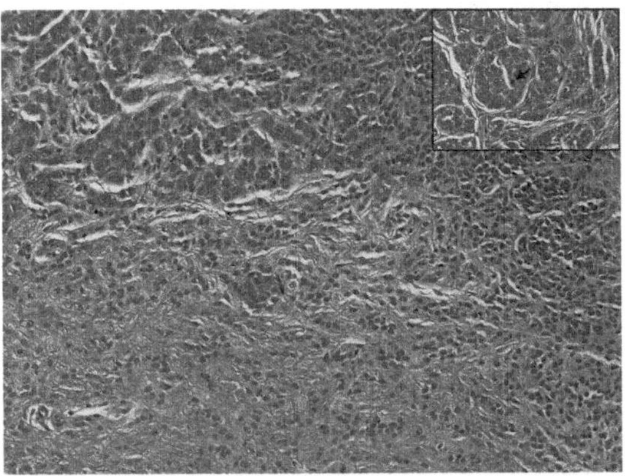

Fig. 3.2 Atypical proliferative nodule arising within a congenital nevus: compare the atypical cells within the proliferative nodule with the small basophilic nevus cells dissecting through the collagen bundles. The proliferative nodule is composed of pleomorphic, epithelioid melanocytes demonstrating severe cytologic atypia. Note the central mitotic figure (*inset*, *arrow*)

Atypical proliferative nodules of congenital nevi may be misconstrued for melanoma arising within the nevus. These nodules frequently present at birth as part of a congenital nevus, but they can also develop later in life. Typically, they occur in the dermis and are composed of large spindled or epithelioid melanocytes (Fig. 3.2). Moderate to severe cytologic atypia is rarely present. The lesional cells usually blend with the surrounding smaller nevus cells; however, this tendency is not invariable and often raises concern for malignancy. Despite their expansile growth and the cytologic atypia, the majority of these proliferative nodules, especially in the neonatal period, behave in a benign fashion. According to Barnhill, melanoma arising in association with a proliferative nodule histopathologically has not been observed in more than 30 years of consultative practice [5, 6]. Therefore, knowledge of the clinical context is extremely important to avoid overdiagnosis of malignant melanoma developing within a congenital nevus. Features that favor the diagnosis of malignancy include high-grade uniform cellular atypia, atypical mitotic figures, and focal necrosis within the nodule.

Prepubertal Nevi

Dysplastic nevi usually become clinically apparent at puberty or adolescence and continue to develop throughout life. True dysplastic nevi have been described in prepubertal children [7, 8]. However, melanoma in prepubertal children is rare, with an incidence of 0.8 per million in the first decade of life [9]. The incidence of melanoma is seven times greater in the second decade of life than in younger children, suggesting that prepubertal children differ from older children and adults [10]. In a study by Evans et al., more than half of the originally diagnosed melanomas in a preadolescent group were considered in retrospect by the experts to be benign nevi [11]. This tendency to overdiagnose prepubertal melanomas may stem from the fact that benign nevi as well as Spitz nevi, which are common in children, frequently have atypical microscopic features that mimic melanoma. However, given the rarity of melanoma in young children, that diagnosis should be rendered with extreme caution.

Nevi of Old Age

While most melanocytic lesions can be unequivocally classified as benign nevi or melanoma, a special type of melanocytic proliferation often encountered in the elderly may pose great diagnostic challenges to the pathologist. Lentiginous dysplastic nevus of the elderly was first described in 1991 by Kossard et al. [12], who observed clinically atypical pigmented lesions with histopathologic features conforming to the pathology of a dysplastic nevus with a lentiginous pattern. This nevus is notable for a lentiginous proliferation of single melanocytes and small nests along the basal layer, with irregular rete ridge pattern of the epidermis. Focal confluence of single melanocytes over the suprapapillary plates is present, as is mild cytologic atypia of melanocytes characterized by large, irregular hyperchromatic nuclei. Suprabasal spread is generally not a feature.

The true biologic potential of this lesion remains debatable. Given the similarities with lentiginous melanoma, some authors have suggested that these two conditions are the same entity [13–17]. Others regard this lesion as a precursor of melanoma-in-situ in the elderly [12, 18, 19]. Kossard et al. observed that 28 out of 78 biopsy cases diagnosed histopathologically as lentiginous dysplastic nevi in individuals over 60 years evolved into melanoma-in-situ [12]. The recognition of a subset of "unstable" atypical nevi in chronic sun-damaged skin, particularly from the seventh decade of life, may be of importance, as these lesions appear to differ from the dysplastic nevi described in younger individuals, which occur particularly in the second to fifth decades. In the elderly, the accumulated sun damage and age-related mutations in the skin, as well as impaired local immunity, may create an aberrant lentiginous nevus pathway that is unstable, leading to progressive growth that can potentiate the development of melanoma [14, 17, 18, 20]. In conclusion, the classification of this lesion as benign or malignant should take into account the patient's age in order to avoid under- or over-treatment and devastating consequences for the patient.

Anatomic Location

A subset of melanocytic nevi shares features with melanoma but are biologically inert and do not appear to portend an increased risk for malignancy transformation to date [21]. These benign nevi with atypical histopathologic features tend to occur on specific anatomic sites and are thus designated "nevi with site-related atypia". Since melanoma may occur at these same sites, it is important for practicing pathologists to recognize the unique features of "nevi of special sites" and avoid misdiagnosis. The benign clinical features contrast with the alarming histopathologic details and can be useful for the correct assessment of the lesion. Anatomic sites that have been implicated in harboring histopathologically atypical but benign nevi include acral sites, genitalia, breast, scalp, ear, and flexural regions.

Acral Nevi

Acral pigmented lesions occur in 4–9 % of the population and consist of nevi (3.9 %), with a minority of lentigines and melanoma [22, 23]. Most acral nevi are symmetrical and lack cytologic atypia or mitotic figures. A small number

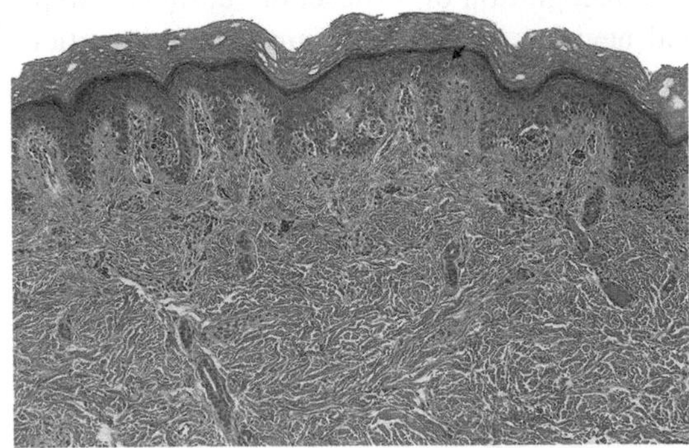

Fig. 3.3 Compound acral nevus: in addition to atypically located junctional nests, this melanocytic nevus also shows a proliferation of single melanocytes along the basal layer. The melanocytes lack significant cytologic atypia. Suprabasal spread of individual melanocytes (*arrow*), particularly over the center of the lesion, is common and should not be misinterpreted as implying malignancy

display atypical histopathologic features, including confluent lentiginous growth, dyshesive nests, variable degrees of cytologic atypia, and suprabasal spread of melanocytes (Fig. 3.3). The two most worrisome features are lentiginous growth and suprabasal spread. Lentiginous growth is usually confined to the center of the lesion; its presence at the margin of the specimen raises concern for a potential melanoma precursor. Suprabasal spread, which sometimes involves the stratum corneum, can be very prominent in up to 40 % of lesions and is usually limited to the center of the lesion [24, 25]. The acronym MANIAC (melanocytic acral nevus with intraepidermal ascent of cells) has been coined to describe these lesions [26]. Cytologic atypia is generally mild, consisting of occasional enlarged melanocytes with hyperchromatic nuclei. The dermal component, if present, consists of small, banal melanocytes showing maturation of the architectural and cytologic features. Because of the aforementioned histopathologic features, the differential diagnosis includes acral lentiginous melanoma; however, knowledge of the site may help the practicing pathologist accept some degree of atypia and avoid overcalling melanoma. There is scant evidence that acral lesions with one or more of the above atypical histopathologic features connote the same increased risk of patient developing melanoma as true nevi with architectural disorder at other sites.

Genital Nevi

Pigmented lesions of the vulva are present in 10–20 % of the general population. Benign vulvar nevi occur in only 2 % of females. A subset of them occurs in young, premenopausal women and children, and has atypical histopathologic features [27–29]. Clinically, they present as pigmented, irregular macules or papules measuring up to 1 cm in diameter. Although benign, histopathologically they may be mistaken for melanoma. Vulvar melanoma, however, is rare, accounting for only 3–7 % of melanoma cases [30, 31]. Taking the relative rarity of vulvar melanoma into consideration, the possibility of a benign lesion should be considered first when evaluating genital pigmented lesions, especially in young patients.

The main histopathologic features of genital nevi are prominent, irregular, and dyshesive junctional nests with some degree of cytologic atypia [27–29]. The junctional nests have marked variability in size and shape and are not confined to the tips of the rete ridges as in nevi at most other anatomic sites. Loss of cellular cohesion and confluence of the nests is present. Suprabasal spread may be noted, but is not a characteristic feature. Many lesions show moderate to severe cytologic atypia. Dermal fibroplasia is prominent. Rare dermal mitotic figures have been observed and cannot be relied upon for distinction from melanoma [28, 29]. When examining nevi from the genital region, the above atypical features may be attributed to the anatomic location and should not be considered diagnostic of melanoma. Distinguishing nevi from melanoma in this region is important to avoid radical and unnecessary disfiguring surgeries for the patient.

Nevi of Special Site (Breast, Scalp, Ear, Flexural Regions)

There has been a recent increase in the number of publications describing atypical melanocytic nevi specific to anatomic sites [32–36]. These sites include the breast, scalp, ear, and flexural regions. Recently, Ronglioletti et al. compared

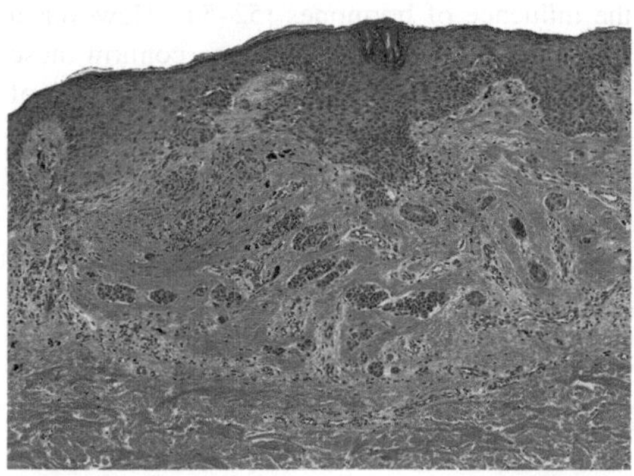

Fig. 3.4 Compound flexural site nevus: peri-umbilical melanocytic nevus showing prominent bridging of the rete ridges and extensive dermal fibrosis

the prevalence of atypical histopathologic features of 101 breast nevi to 97 nevi of the torso and extremities [32]. These authors showed that breast nevi exhibited significantly more atypical features than nevi from other sites. Specifically, suprabasal spread, cytologic atypia, and papillary dermal fibroplasia were more frequently encountered. Fabrizi et al. showed similar atypical histopathologic features in 10 % of scalp nevi, especially in adolescents [35]. A large number of auricular nevi show poor lateral circumscription (93 %), cytologic atypia (62 %), and suprabasal spread (57 %) [34, 36]. Finally, nevi from flexural sites, including the axillary folds, the umbilicus, antecubital and popliteal fossae may show asymmetry, poor lateral circumscription, large and dyshesive nests as well as focal lentiginous proliferation (Fig. 3.4). Recognition of site-related atypia is important given the implications of diagnosing melanoma at these sites and performing radical surgeries.

Nevi in Skin Disease

Nevi in Epidermolysis Bullosa

Large acquired melanocytic nevi occur in patients with epidermolysis bullosa (EB) and are referred to as EB nevi. These unconventional nevi occur in all types of hereditary EB, mostly in childhood, at sites of repeated blisters. They are often eruptive and appear as asymmetrical pigmentary lesions with irregular borders and pigment network intermixed with scarred areas. EB nevi may pose a diagnostic challenge because of their clinical and dermoscopic resemblance to melanoma. These alarming clinical features are thought to be a consequence of repeated disruption of the dermal–epidermal junction, fibrosing inflammation, scar formation, and neovascularization [37]. The histopathologic pattern of the EB nevus ranges from the readily recognizable congenital pattern to a worrisome "pseudomelanoma" pattern [38–43]. In the setting of recessive dystrophic EB, histopathologic examination may show features of recurrent nevus (confluent junctional nests, lentiginous growth, suprabasal spread, nests of melanocytes within dermal fibrosis and inflammation). However, despite the alarming clinical appearance and sometimes even alarming histopathologic features, long-term follow-up has confirmed their benign nature. In a recent 20-year prospective study by Bauer et al., there was no incidence of melanoma arising within an EB nevus [39]. The EB nevus should be considered a distinct diagnostic possibility. Knowledge of the EB nevus phenomenon and its histopathologic resemblance to the recurrent nevus should help the practicing pathologist avoid overdiagnosis of melanoma in young patients.

Nevi in Lichen Sclerosus

Melanocytic proliferations arising in a region of skin affected by lichen sclerosus are rare and difficult to interpret histopathologically as they share features in common with recurrent nevi and may mimic malignant melanoma. Carlson et al. compared the clinicopathologic features of melanocytic proliferations associated with lichen sclerosus to control benign nevi [44]. Lichen sclerosus nevi frequently demonstrated a trizonal pattern similar to that of recurrent nevi, characterized by "melanoma-in-situ" pattern overlying dermal fibrosis and an underlying dermal nevus. In addition, features of confluent junctional nests, lentiginous melanocytic hyperplasia, focal suprabasal spread as well as nests of melanocytes trapped within dermal sclerosis were present (Fig. 3.5).

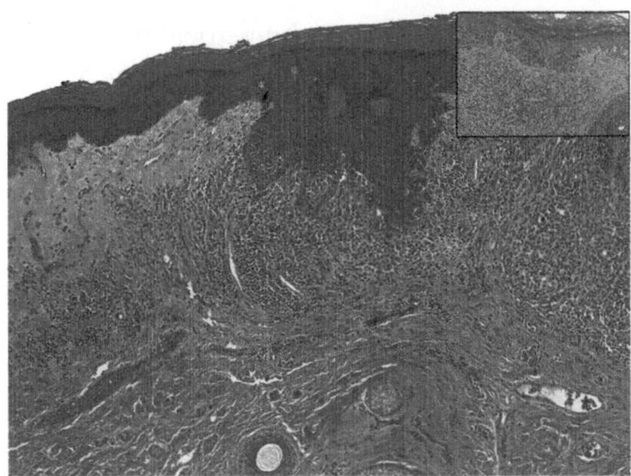

Fig. 3.5 Compound melanocytic nevus in a background of lichen sclerosus demonstrating architectural disorder. Note the marked lentiginous melanocytic hyperplasia (*inset*). Courtesy of Angelica Selim, M.D., Dermatopathology, Duke University

Cytologically, the melanocytes were slightly larger than those in ordinary nevi and had abundant, pale to dusty gray cytoplasm, with oval, vesicular nuclei and prominent nucleoli. Given that similar histopathologic features may be seen in malignant melanoma, melanocytic nevi of genital skin affected by lichen sclerosus may present a diagnostic pitfall and be misdiagnosed as melanoma. Nonetheless, key histopathologic features can distinguish lichen sclerosus nevi from malignant melanoma. Melanoma exhibits poorly circumscribed junctional melanocytes that extend past the dermal changes of fibrosis-sclerosis, dermal mitotic figures, and deep HMB-45 expression. Melanoma also lacks the trizonal pattern and/or a dermal melanocytic nevus underlying the sclerosis found in lichen sclerosus nevi. Furthermore, studies have shown that the coexistence of lichen sclerosus and vulvar malignant melanoma is rare [45–51].

Nevi in Pregnancy

The effect of pregnancy on melanocytic lesions remains extremely controversial. Several studies, most of which were based on patients' observations, have reported pregnancy-related changes to melanocytic nevi, including increase in size and darkening of the lesion, possibly related to the influence of hormones [52–54]. However, a more recent study was unable to confirm these changes [55]. Additionally, only a handful of studies [56, 57] looking at the histopathologic changes in melanocytic nevi in pregnancy existed until recently. The initial studies did not demonstrate any significant histopathologic changes. Chan et al. [58] examined the histopathologic features and Ki-67 proliferation index in dermal nevi excised from pregnant women ($n = 16$) and nevi from location- and aged-matched control patients ($n = 15$). This group found that nevi in pregnancy were more likely to have dermal mitotic figures (62.5 % versus 13.3 %) and higher mitotic rates (1.44 versus 0.20/mm^2) than control nevi; no atypical mitotic figures were identified. The number of dermal mitotic figures ranged from 0 to 4/mm^2 in nevi of pregnancy. In half of the lesions, mitotic figures were present in the deeper aspect of the nevus. The increased number of mitotic figures, especially in the deeper portions of the nevus, may cause potential for misdiagnosis since mitotic figures have long been regarded as a feature concerning for malignancy. An important differential diagnosis of a mitotically active nevus is nevoid melanoma. Nevoid melanoma is known to be a diagnostic pitfall due to its deceptively banal histopathologic appearance, including overall symmetry, circumscription, pseudomaturation, and nevoid morphology of melanocytes. Despite a notable increase in mitotic activity, nevi in pregnancy lack other worrisome atypical features for malignancy, such as asymmetry, pleomorphism, hyperchromatic nuclei, and lack of maturation with depth. Therefore, mitotically active melanocytic lesions should not be overcalled as malignant in the context of pregnancy. However, it is readily apparent how they could be misdiagnosed if the clinical history were omitted. The presence of a lentiginous growth pattern, in conjunction with large, single melanocytes irregularly distributed along the basal layer, has also been described in nevi of pregnancy. While these findings may simulate melanoma-in-situ, in the context of pregnancy, conservative excision and clinical follow-up may be advised. Finally, nevi of pregnancy frequently demonstrate the presence of superficial micronodules of pregnancy (81.3 % versus 26.7 % in banal nevi) [58]. These were recently described as rounded clusters of 3–20 large epithelioid melanocytes with prominent nucleoli, abundant pale eosinophilic cytoplasm, and occasional fine melanosomes. These clusters are distinctive from the deeper, smaller type B and C nevic melanocytes and show consistent immunoreactivity for HMB-45 (anti-gp100). Given such findings, concern for melanoma may rightfully arise if the clinical context is unknown to the practicing pathologist.

Traumatized Nevi

Traumatized melanocytic nevi are usually characterized by changes in the epidermis (parakeratosis, serum crust, ulceration) as well as dermis (fibrosis and melanophages) [59]. Occasionally, they may also display atypical histopathologic features similar to recurrent nevi [59]. Recently, Selim et al. examined the histopathologic features of 92 traumatized nevi [60]. Twenty percent of the lesions demonstrated suprabasal spread of melanocytes limited to the site of trauma, under the areas of parakeratosis (Fig. 3.6), whereas 8 % of the cases had evidence of suprabasal spread away from the traumatized area. Two percent of the lesions showed a single mitotic figure in a dermal melanocyte located adjacent to the site of trauma and mild to moderate cytologic atypia. Severe cytologic atypia, significant suprabasal spread outside of the traumatized area, and dermal mitotic figures were not routinely observed and should be suggestive of malignancy. Adeniran et al. reported two patients with atypical histopathologic and immunohistochemical findings in nevi after cryotherapy with liquid nitrogen [61]. These lesions showed focal suprabasal spread, superficial dermal fibrosis, and paradoxical loss of maturation, both morphologically and with aberrant expression of gp100 (HMB-45) in the dermis, thereby mimicking melanoma. However, the nevus cells outside the regions of trauma did not demonstrate the same features. Laser treatment of nevi has been reported to induce similar changes [62, 63]. Taken together, these data suggest that traumatized nevi may have morphologic and immunohistochemical findings similar to malignant melanoma and can present a diagnostic dilemma. However, such atypical findings limited to the traumatized area are compatible with a benign traumatized nevus.

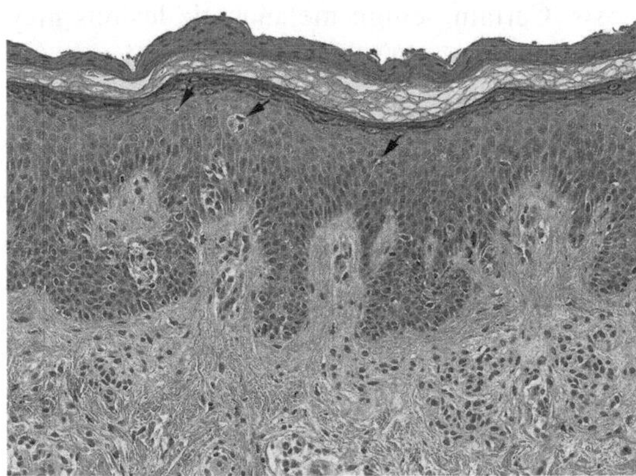

Fig. 3.6 Compound melanocytic nevus, traumatized: marked parakeratosis is seen as a result of cutaneous trauma in the center of this nevus. Suprabasal spread of single cells (*arrow*) and nests of melanocytes are seen in the areas of overlying parakeratosis

Ultraviolet-Irradiated Nevi

Ultraviolet (UV) irradiation of benign nevi has been shown to induce histopathologic changes that may be reminiscent of malignant melanoma. Tronnier and Wolff [64] investigated the short-term effects of UV rays on melanocytic nevi. Specifically, the morphological and immunohistochemical changes after a single UV irradiation (two minimal erythema doses) were studied in 23 nevi and were compared with the non-irradiated part of the same nevus [64]. One week after irradiation, 7 of the 12 nevi showed suprabasal spread of the melanocytes. Significant cytologic atypia of the irradiated melanocytes was not observed. Similar changes were not observed 2–3 weeks after irradiation [65]. The dermal component, if present, did not show any morphological differences. However, a marked increase in the expression of gp100 (HMB-45) was found in all nevi after irradiation, indicating an activation of the melanocytes and active melanosome formation.

The proliferative activity was absent 1 week after treatment. Because of the aforementioned histopathologic changes, UV-irradiated nevus may simulate malignant melanoma. This becomes a diagnostic pitfall especially when a pathologist examines pigmented lesions soon after an intense sun exposure without the appropriate clinical history. Although the presence of parakeratosis above a regular basket-weave stratum corneum and the superficial inflammatory infiltrate in the dermis may be clue to the diagnosis of irritated nevus changes, these are not always present. In this case, the erroneous diagnosis of malignant melanoma may be easily rendered, followed by unnecessary treatment.

Dermoscopic/Photographic-Pathologic Correlation

Over the last several years, there has been a substantial increase in the use of dermoscopy and digital photography in the evaluation of melanocytic lesions by dermatologists. Dermoscopy is a noninvasive in vivo technique that can clinically enhance the ability to accurately diagnose melanocytic lesions. Dermoscopic features of melanocytic lesions result from specific histopathologic changes [66]. For example, the blue-white veil seen on dermoscopy correlates with aggregation of heavily pigmented melanoma cells or melanophages in the dermis combined with overlying compact orthokeratosis. Likewise, radial streaming on dermoscopy corresponds to the radial growth phase of melanoma. In challenging or equivocal cases, the diagnostic accuracy of the histopathologic examination may be enhanced by considering dermoscopic features [67–70]. Dermoscopy is considered as the conceptual and practical link between clinical dermatology (macrocosm) and dermatopathology (microcosm) [71]. Like clinical dermatology, dermoscopy works parallel to the skin surface and provides information on a third dimension—the horizontal spread—which is not evident to the pathologist. However, like histopathology, dermoscopy allows visualization of structures which could not be discernable by the naked eye. Therefore, dermoscopy draws the histopathologist's attention to the suspicious area in a melanocytic lesion, thus orienting the macroscopic sampling and/or suggesting the need of step-sectioning the paraffin block(s) to obtain representative sections. In case of an inconsistency between the dermoscopic and histopathologic diagnoses, it may be advisable to re-evaluate the specimen for the safety of the patient.

In addition to dermoscopy, digital photography can provide the pathologist with additional clues which can assist with a more definite histopathologic diagnosis. Photographic surveillance adds the fourth dimension—time—which can demonstrate subtle changes in lesions which might have otherwise gone unnoticed. Similar to dermoscopy, digital photographs may alert the practicing pathologist to specifically look at the evolving areas and possibly diagnose an early, subtle melanoma [72].

Summary

Clinicopathologic correlation is an important step in the diagnosis of melanocytic lesions. The clinical context, such as the age of the patient, anatomic location of the lesion, presence of an underlying skin disease, history of trauma or ultraviolet irradiation, should be always taken into account in order to make an accurate diagnosis. Certain benign melanocytic lesions may show features that we often associate with malignant melanoma; however, knowledge and recognition of the clinical context may prevent the practicing pathologist from making the wrong diagnosis.

References

1. Huynh PM, Grant-Kels JM, Grin CM. Childhood melanoma: update and treatment. Int J Dermatol. 2005;44:715–23.
2. Dulon M, Weichenthal M, Blettner M, Breibart M, Hetzer M, Greinert R, et al. Sun exposure and number of nevi in 5- to 6-year old European children. J Clin Epidemiol. 2002;55:1075–81.
3. Zayour M, Lazova R. Congenital nevi. Clin Lab Med. 2011;31:267–80.

4. Barnhill RL, Fleischli M. Histopathologic features of congenital melanocytic nevi in infants 1 year of age or younger. J Am Acad Dermatol. 1995;33(5 Pt 1): 780–5.
5. Tannous ZS, Mihm MC, Sober AJ, Duncan LM. Congenital melanocytic nevi: clinical and histopathologic features, risk of melanoma and clinical management. J Am Acad Dermatol. 2005;52:197–203.
6. Barnhill RL. Congenital melanocytic nevi and associated neoplasms, congenital and childhood melanoma. In: Barnhill R, editor. Pathology of melanocytic nevi and malignant melanoma. Boston: Butterworth-Heinemann; 1995. p. 65–96.
7. Clark WH, Reimer RR, Greene MH, Ainsworth AM, Mastrangelo MJ. Origin of familial malignant melanomas from heritable melanocytic lesions: 'the B-K mole syndrome'. Arch Dermatol. 1978;114:732–8.
8. Tucker MA, Greene MH, Clark WH, Kraemer KH, Fraser MC, Elder DE. Dysplastic nevi on the scalp of pre-pubertal children from melanoma-prone families. J Pediatr. 1983;103:65–9.
9. Bonifazi E, Bilancia M, Berloco A, Ciampo L, De Roma MR. Malignant melanoma in children aged 0–12. Review of 289 cases of the literature. Eur J Pediatr Dermatol. 2001;11:157–75.
10. Ferrari A, Bono A, Baldi M, Collini P, Casanova M, Pennacchioli E, Terenziani M, Marcon I, Santinami M, Bartoli C. Does melanoma behave differently in younger children than in adults? A retrospective study of 33 cases of childhood melanoma from a single institution. Pediatrics. 2005;115:649–54.
11. Leman JA, Evans A, Mooi W, MacKie RM. Outcomes and pathological review of a cohort of children with melanoma. Br J Dermatol. 2005;152(6):1321–3.
12. Kossard S, Commens C, Symons M, Doyle J. Lentiginous dysplastic naevi in the elderly: a potential precursor for malignant melanoma. Australas J Dermatol. 1991;32:27–37.
13. Agusti-Mejias A, Badia FM, Ruiz RG, Martinez VO. Alegre de Miquel V. Atypical lentiginous nevus: a clinical and histopathologic study of 14 cases. Actas Dermosifiliogr. 2012;103(5):394–400.
14. King R, Page RN, Googe PB, Mihm Jr MC. Lentiginous melanoma: a histopathologic pattern of melanoma to be distinguished from lentiginous nevus. Mod Pathol. 2005;18:1397–401.
15. Davis T, Zembowicz A. Histopathologic evolution of lentiginous melanoma: a report of five new cases. J Cutan Pathol. 2007;34:296–300.
16. Ferrara G, Zalaudek I, Argenziano G. Lentiginous melanoma: a distinctive clinicopathologic entity. Histopathology. 2008;52:523–5.
17. Weedon D. Lentiginous melanoma. J Cutan Pathol. 2009;36:1232.
18. Kossard S. Atypical lentiginous junctional nevi of the elderly and melanoma. Australas J Dermatol. 2002; 43:93–101.
19. Kossard S, Wilkinson B. Small cell (nevoid) melanoma: a clinicopathologic study of 131 cases. Australas J Dermatol. 1997;38:54–8.
20. King R. Lentiginous melanoma. Arch Pathol Lab Med. 2011;135:337–41.
21. Hosler GA, Moresi JM, Barrett TL. Nevi with site-related atypia: a review of melanocytic nevi with atypical histopathologic features based on anatomic site. J Cutan Pathol. 2008;35:889–98.
22. MacKie RM, English J, Atchison TC, Fitzsimons CP, Wilson P. The number and distribution of benign pigmented moles (melanocytic nevi) in a healthy British population. Br J Dermatol. 1985;113:167.
23. Kopf AW. Pigmented lesions of the palms and soles. Med Rec Ann. 1964;57:511.
24. Cook DL. Melanocytic nevi of special sites. Diagn Histopathol. 2010;16(7):309–16.
25. Boyd A, Rapini R. Acral melanocytic neoplasms: a histopathologic analysis of 158 lesions. J Am Acad Dermatol. 1994;31:740–5.
26. Cheung WL, Smoller BR. Dermatopathology updates on melanocytic lesions. Dermatol Clin. 2012;20: 617–22.
27. Clark WH, Hood AF, Tucker MA, Jampel RM. Atypical melanocytic nevi of the genital type with a discussion of reciprocal parenchymal-stromal interactions in the biology of neoplasia. Hum Pathol. 1998;29:S1.
28. Christensen WN, Friedman KJ, Woodruff JD, Hood AE. Histopathologic characteristics of vulvar nevocellular nevi. J Cutan Pathol. 1987;14:87–91.
29. Gleason BC, Hirsch MS, Nucci MR, Schmidt BA, Zembowicz A, Mihm MC, McKee PH, Brenn T. Atypical genital nevi: a clinicopathologic analysis of 56 cases. Am J Surg Pathol. 2008;32:51–7.
30. Dunton CJ, Kautzy M, Hanau C. Malignant melanoma of the vulva: a review. Obstet Gynecol Surv. 1995;50:739–46.
31. Alexander A, Harris RM, Grossman D, Bruggers CS, Leachman SA. Vulvar melanoma: diffuse melanosis and metastasis to the placenta. J Am Acad Dermatol. 2004;50:293–8.
32. Ronglioletti F, Urso C, Batolo D, Chimenti S, Fanti PA, Filotico R, Gianotti R, Innocenzi D, Lentini M, Tomasini C, Pippione M, Rebora A. Melanocytic nevi of the breast: a histopathologic case-control study. J Cutan Pathol. 2004;31:137–40.
33. Ronglioletti F, Ball RA, Marcus R, Barnhill RL. Histopathological features of flexural melanocytic nevi: a study of 40 cases. J Cutan Pathol. 2000;27:215–7.
34. Saad AG, Patel S, Mutasim DF. Melanocytic nevi of the auricular region: histopathologic characteristics and diagnostic difficulties. Am J Dermatopathol. 2005;27:111–5.
35. Lazova R, Lester B, Glusac RJ, Handerson T, McNiff J. The characteristic histopathologic features of nevi on and around the ear. J Cutan Pathol. 2005;32:40–4.
36. Fabrizi G, Pagliarello C, Parente P, Massi G. Atypical nevi of the scalp in adolescence. J Cutan Pathol. 2007;34:365–9.
37. Lanschuetzer CM, Emberger M, Laimer M, Diem A, Bauer JW, Soyer HP, Hintner H. Epidermolysis

bullosa nevi reveal distinctive dermoscopic pattern. Br J Dermatol. 2005;153(1):97–102.

38. Cash SH, Dever TT, Hyde P, Lee J. Epidermolysis bullosa nevus: an exception to the clinical and dermoscopic criteria for melanoma. Arch Dermatol. 2007;143(9):1164–7.
39. Bauer JW, Schaeppi H, Kaserer C, Hantich B, Hintner H. Large melanocytic nevi in hereditary epidermolysis bullosa. J Am Acad Dermatol. 2001;44(4): 577–84.
40. Soltani K, Pepper MC, Simjee S, Apatoff BR. Large acquired nevocytic nevus induced by the Koebner phenomenon. J Cutan Pathol. 1984;11(4):296–9.
41. Hoss DM, McNutt NS, Carter DM, Rothaus KO, Kenet BJ, Lin AN. Atypical melanocytic lesions in epidermolysis bullosa. J Cutan Pathol. 1994;21(2): 164–9.
42. Stavrianeas NG, Katoulis AC, Moussatou V, Bozi E, Petropoulou H, Limas C, Georgala S. Eruptive large melanocytic nevus in a patient with hereditary epidermolysis bullosa simplex. Dermatology. 2003;207(4): 402–4.
43. Gallardo F, Toll A, Malvehy J, Mascaro-Gally JM, Lloreta J, Barranco C, Pujol R. Large atypical melanocytic nevi in recessive dystrophic epidermolysis bullosa: clinicopathological, ultrastructural, and dermoscopic study. Pediatr Dermatol. 2005;22(4):338–43.
44. Carlson JA, Wu XC, Slominski A, Weismann K, Crowson AN, Malfetano J, Prieto V, Mihm MC. Melanocytic proliferations associated with lichen sclerosus. Arch Dermatol. 2002;138:77–87.
45. Weinstock MA. Malignant melanoma of the vulva and vagina in the United States: patterns of incidence and population-based estimates of survival. Am J Obstet Gynecol. 1994;171:1225–30.
46. Tasseron EW, van der Esch EP, Hart AA, Brutel de la Riviere G, Aatsen EJ. A clinicopathologic study of 30 melanomas of the vulva. Gynecol Oncol. 1992;46: 170–5.
47. Raber G, Mempel V, Jackisch C, Hundeiker M, Heinecke A, Kürzl R, Glaubitz M, Rompel R, Schneider HP. Malignant melanoma of the vulva: report of 89 patients. Cancer. 1996;78:2353–8.
48. Ragnarsson-Olding BK, Kanter-Lewensohn LR, Lagerlof B, Nilsson BR, Ringborg UK. Malignant melanoma of the vulva in a nationwide, 25-year study of 219 Swedish females: clinical observations and histopathologic features. Cancer. 1999;86:1273–84.
49. Creasman WT, Philips JL, Menck HR. A survey of hospital management practices for vulvar melanoma. J Am Coll Surg. 1999;188:670–5.
50. Bragdate MG, Rollason TP, McConkey CC, Powell J. Malignant melanoma of the vulva: a clinicopathological study of 50 women. Br J Obstet Gynaecol. 1990;97:124–33.
51. Piura B, Egan M, Lopes A, Monaghan JM. Malignant melanoma of the vulva: a clinicopathologic study of 18 cases. J Surg Oncol. 1992;50:234–40.
52. Winton GB, Lewis CW. Dermatoses of pregnancy. J Am Acad Dermatol. 1982;6:977–98.
53. Pamley T, O'Brien TJ. Skin changes during pregnancy. Clin Obstet Gynecol. 1990;33:713–7.
54. Pennoyer JW, Grin CM, Driscoll MS, Dry SM, Walsh SJ, Gelineau JP, Grant-Kels JM. Changes in size of melanocytic nevi during pregnancy. J Am Acad Dermatol. 1997;36(3 Pt 1):378–82.
55. Grin CM, Rojas AI, Grant-Kels JM. Does pregnancy alter melanocytic nevi? J Cutan Pathol. 2001;28: 389–92.
56. Sanchez JL, Figueroa LD, Rodriguez E. Behavior of melanocytic nevi during pregnancy. Am J Dermatopathol. 1984;6:89–91.
57. Foucar E, Bentley TJ, Laube DW, Rosai J. A histopathologic evaluation of nevocellular nevi during pregnancy. Arch Dermatol. 1985;121:350–4.
58. Chan MP, Chan MM, Tahan SR. Melanocytic nevi in pregnancy: histopathologic features and Ki-67 proliferation index. J Cutan Pathol. 2010;37:843–51.
59. Leleux TM, Prieto VG, Diwan AH. Aberrant expression of HMB-45 in traumatized melanocytic nevi. J Am Acad Dermatol. 2012;67(3):446–50.
60. Selim MA, Vollmer RT, Herman CM, Pham TTN, Turner JW. Melanocytic nevi with nonsurgical trauma: a histopathologic study. Am J Dermatopathol. 2007;29:134–6.
61. Adeniran AJ, Prieto VG, Chon S, Duvic M, Diwan AH. Atypical histopathologic and immunohistochemical findings in melanocytic nevi after liquid nitrogen cryotherapy. J Am Acad Dermatol. 2009; 61(2):341–5.
62. Dummer R, Kempf W, Burg G. Pseudo-melanoma after laser therapy. Dermatology. 1998;197:71–3.
63. Lee HW, Ahn SJ, Lee MW, Choi JH, Moon KC, Koh JK. Pseudomelanoma following laser therapy. J Eur Acad Dermatol Venereol. 2006;20:342–4.
64. Tronnier M, Wolff HH. UV-irradiated melanocytic nevi simulating melanoma in situ. Am J Dermatopathol. 1995;17(1):1–6.
65. Tronnier M, Smolle J, Wolff HH. Ultraviolet irradiation induces acute changes in melanocytic nevi. J Invest Dermatol. 1995;104:475–8.
66. Crotty KA, Menzies SW. Dermoscopy and its role in diagnosing melanocytic lesions: a guide for pathologists. Pathology. 2004;36(5):470–7.
67. Nardone B, Martini M, Busam K, Marghoob A, West D, Gerami P. Integrating clinical/dermoscopic findings and fluorescence in situ hybridization in diagnosing melanocytic neoplasms with less than definitive histopathologic features. J Am Acad Dermatol. 2012; 66:917–22.
68. Ferrara G, Argenziano G, Giorgio CM, Zalaudek I, Kittler H. Dermoscopic-pathologic correlation: apropos of six equivocal cases. Semin Cutan Med Surg. 2009;28:157–64.
69. Bauer J, Metzler G, Rassner G, Garbe C, Blum A. Dermatoscopy turns histopathologist's attention to

the suspicious area in melanocytic lesions. Arch Dermatol. 2001;137:1338–40.

70. Ferrara G, Argenyi Z, Argenziano G, Cerio R, Cerroni L, Di Blasi A, et al. The influence of clinical information in the histopathologic diagnosis of melanocytic skin neoplasms. PLoS One. 2009;4(4):e5375.
71. Argenziano G, Puig S, Zalaudek I, Sera F, Corona R, Alsina M, et al. Dermoscopy improves accuracy of primary care physicians to triage lesions suggestive of skin cancer. J Clin Oncol. 2006;24:1877–82.
72. Salerni G, Carrera C, Lovatto L, Marti-Laborda RM, Isern G, Palou J, Alos L, Puig S, Malvehy J. Characterization of 1152 lesions excised over 10 years using total-body photography and digital dermatoscopy in the surveillance of patients at high risk for melanoma. J Am Acad Dermatol. 2012;67:836–45.

Anathema or Useful? Application of Immunohistochemistry to the Diagnosis of Melanocytic Lesions

4

Victor G. Prieto, Christopher R. Shea, and Jon A. Reed

Antibodies Commonly Used in Dermatopathology

S-100 protein: S100 proteins constitute a family of acidic calcium-binding proteins that are important in intracellular calcium metabolism but some of them are secreted and thus are likely involved in cell–cell interactions. S100 protein was originally extracted from the brain and contains two polypeptide chains, S100a and S100b. These polypeptides can present in three possible combinations: S100aa, S100ab, and S100bb. S100aa proteins are mostly expressed in macrophages [1] and therefore macrophages are usually nonreactive with the "standard" anti-S100 antibodies (this antibody mainly reacts with cells containing S100B polypeptide chains). Subsequently, monoclonal antibodies were developed that mainly react with several variants of the S100a chains. More than 95 % of melanomas cells in primary cutaneous melanomas react with the standard poly- or monoclonal anti-S100 antibody, and show both a cytoplasmic and nuclear pattern. However, several situations may affect its expression, such as too much or too little fixation time, previously frozen tissue, and excessive enzymatic pretreatment (e.g., with trypsin) [2].

Of the several antigens detected by anti-S100, A6 is expressed in a differential manner by standard nevi, Spitz nevi, and melanoma. Spitz nevi show strong expression of S100 A6 in both junctional and dermal components while standard nevi and melanoma are usually negative in the junctional component and weakly or negative in the dermal component [3]. In addition, detection of S100 A6 is a very helpful marker in the differential diagnosis of neurothekeomas [1, 4].

gp100 (as detected with the antibody HMB-45): This is a fairly specific antibody for melanocytic differentiation. Although other lesions express this marker (angiomyolipoma, sugar cell tumor of the lung, and so-called "pecoma"), they do not usually enter in the differential diagnosis of cutaneous lesions. We use HMB-45 because it is particularly helpful in detecting the pattern of "maturation" of nevi. It is well known that benign melanocytes change their morphology according to their distance from epithelia. Thus, superficial, type-A melanocytes (epithelioid shape, intraepidermal or close to the epithelium, and mostly pigmented) express neuronal markers and gp100 while the deeply located type-C melanocytes

V.G. Prieto, M.D., Ph.D. (✉)
MD Anderson Cancer Center, University of Houston, 1515 Holcombe Blvd., Unit 85, Houston, TX 77030, USA
e-mail: vprieto@mdanderson.org

C.R. Shea
University of Chicago Medicine, 5841 S. Maryland Ave., MC 5067, L502, Chicago, IL 60637, USA

J.A. Reed
CellNEtix Pathology & Laboratories, 1124 Columbia St., Suite 200, Seattle, WA 98117, USA

C.R. Shea et al. (eds.), *Pathology of Challenging Melanocytic Neoplasms: Diagnosis and Management*, DOI 10.1007/978-1-4939-1444-9_4, © Springer Science+Business Media New York 2015

(spindle cells) express schwannian markers [5, 6]. Uncommon exceptions to this rule include blue nevi, related lesions (e.g., deep penetrating nevi), and some Spitz nevi, in which the entire lesion is labeled with HMB-45. Therefore, we may consider that decreased expression of this marker with increasing depth in the dermis or diffuse expression throughout the lesion is suggestive of a benign diagnosis, i.e., nevus.

In contrast to nevi, primary cutaneous melanomas usually express gp100 in a patchy pattern, with isolated or clustered cells throughout the dermis; such pattern is also seen in nevoid melanoma [7]. Furthermore, in addition to analyzing the dermal component, HMB-45 also labels the intraepidermal portion and, in melanoma, will help to highlight the characteristic single-cell pattern of growth or pagetoid upward migration.

MART1 (Melanoma Antigen Recognized by T cells): MART1 is one of the most important melanocytic markers [8]. It is detected by two different antibodies (Melan-A and A-103) and is expressed by most melanocytic lesions, benign and malignant. Therefore, it is very helpful in detecting melanocytic differentiation [9]. Furthermore, the only melanocytic lesion that consistently lacks MART1 expression is spindle cell/desmoplastic melanoma. Conversely, if anti-MART1 strongly and diffusely labels a spindle cell melanocytic lesion, desmoplastic melanoma is unlikely.

In addition to melanocytes, other cells may also express this marker. In particular, steroid-producing tumors may react with A103. Also, and similar to gp100, angiomyolipoma, sugar cell tumor of lung, lymphangioleiomyomatosis, and "pecoma" consistently react with anti-MART1 [10]. As a possible pitfall, since the antibody is so sensitive, the labeling of the cell processes of melanocytes in sun-exposed skin may give the appearance of more numerous-than-normal melanocytes, thus raising the consideration of melanoma in situ [11]. To avoid this problem, when using anti-MART1 to evaluate the numbers of melanocytes in sun-damaged skin, we recommend counting nuclei of the cells labeled with the antibody rather than simply observing the "amount" of epidermis labeled. As another pitfall, on occasion, macrophages (particularly pigmented ones) are labeled with anti-MART1 [12].

MIB1 (anti-Ki67): This is a proliferation marker expressed in the nuclei of non-G0, cycling cells. Its pattern of expression, similar to that of gp100, helps highlight the presence or absence of "maturation". In general, benign melanocytic lesions display rare proliferating cells, which are located close to the epithelia (either epidermal or adnexal). In contrast, melanomas have a random pattern of immunoreactivity, with proliferating cells present even at the deep edge of the lesion. In a study of 384 melanocytic lesions, there were significant differences in the amount and pattern of cell proliferation among various types of nevus and melanoma [13]. Specifically, common nevi and dysplastic nevi exhibited reactivity in <1 % of cells, generally disposed at the dermal–epidermal junction or in the more superficial dermal compartment. In contrast, melanomas did not show this orderly pattern, but instead had a random pattern of immunoreactivity, and a mean growth fraction of 16.4 %, particularly at the deep edge of the lesion. The authors reclassified 112 lesions that had posed diagnostic problems on routine histology; on subsequent clinical review, systemic progression was demonstrated in 70.7 % of the cases finally classified as melanoma but in none of the lesions finally classified as benign. Similarly, desmoplastic melanomas have a much higher proliferation rate as detected with MIB1 than do desmoplastic nevi [14].

Tyrosinase is an enzyme that participates in melanogenesis and is therefore fairly specific for melanocytic differentiation. In our hands, tyrosinase expression is very similar to HMB-45 labeling.

MiTF (Microphthalmia Transcription Factor) is a nuclear protein involved in the development of melanocytes and the regulation of melanin synthesis in melanocytic lesions [15, 16]. It may be expressed by macrophages, lymphocytes, fibroblasts, Schwann cells, and smooth muscle cells. Due to its nuclear pattern of expression, we find that anti-MiTF is very helpful when quantifying the number of intraepidermal melanocytes in areas of pigmented epidermis [2, 17]. MITF is also positive in cellular neurothekeoma.

To increase the sensitivity of immunohistochemistry applied to dermatopathology, several cocktails have been developed to include more than one antibody. A popular combination is designated "pan-melanocytic cocktail" and consists of HMB-45, anti-MART1, and anti-tyrosinase. Analogously, at M.D. Anderson Cancer Center, we have developed two cocktails for the study of melanocytic lesions; one combines anti-MART1 and anti-Ki67, and the other HMB45 and anti-Ki67. MART1 and gp100 are cytoplasmic markers while Ki67 is a nuclear marker; thus they can be differentiated by using two different detection systems (e.g., avidin biotin complex and alkaline phosphatase) with two different chromogens (e.g., diaminobenzidine [brown] and Vulcan Red [red]). In this way, it is relatively easy to identify which cells express both markers, thus highlighting the fraction of melanocytes that are proliferating.

p16 (also called p16INK4 and CDKN2) is a protein expressed in most benign melanocytes and only a fraction of melanoma cells [18–20]. The p16 gene maps to 9p21 and its protein inhibits CDK4 thus impeding the transition past the G1 phase of the cell cycle. Up-regulation of p16 inhibits melanocyte growth in culture and loss of replicative potential in melanocytic nevi. Oncogene-induced senescence seems to inhibit further nevus growth and formation of cutaneous melanoma.

Soluble Adenylyl Cyclase (sAC) is an enzyme that generates cyclic adenosine monophosphate, a molecule involved in regulating melanocyte functions [21]. R21, a mouse monoclonal antibody against sAC, shows nuclear expression in melanoma in situ, lentigo maligna type, while being mostly negative in benign melanocytes. Thus it may be helpful in distinguishing melanoma in situ from melanocytic hyperplasia in sun-damaged skin.

SOX10 is a neural crest transcription factor involved in maturation and maintenance of Schwann cells and melanocytes. Sox10 nuclear expression has been found in a majority of melanomas and nevi, in benign neural lesions and approximately half of malignant peripheral nerve sheath tumors. Sox10 was diffusely expressed in schwannomas and neurofibromas [22]. Interestingly, SOX10 appears to be strongly and diffusely expressed in spindle cell/desmoplastic melanoma and is helpful in distinguishing melanoma from scar [23].

Other antibodies/antigens that may become more popular in the future include NKI-C3 [24], galactin-3 [25], COX-2 [26], TRP [27], survivin [28], and claudin1 [29].

Practical Application of Immunohistochemical Analysis to the Diagnosis of Melanocytic Lesions

To illustrate an example on how immunohistochemistry may be applied to the distinction between benign and malignant melanocytic lesions, here we will describe the differential diagnosis between standard melanoma and nevus.

As mentioned above, the immense majority of nevi show a pattern of maturation, i.e., a change in expression of several immunohistochemical markers from the top to the bottom of the lesion (with the exception of some Spitz nevi and the group of blue nevi and related lesions). In our experience, the two most helpful markers to detect a pattern of maturation are the HMB-45 antigen (gp100) and Ki67. Both markers are predominantly expressed in those melanocytes located either within the epidermis/adnexa or in the periepithelial dermis (papillary and adventitial). Therefore, a pattern in which HMB-45 antigen and Ki67 are expressed in the intraepithelial and periepithelial components, but are almost completely absent from the deep areas of the lesion, is more consistent with a nevus than with a melanoma (Fig. 4.1). Regarding Ki67, it has been suggested to count the number of positive cells for Ki67 [13]. However, rather than performing an actual count of the number of melanocytes expressing this marker, we prefer comparing the patterns of expression at the top and the bottom of the lesion. Regardless of the absolute number of positive cells, nevi should have many fewer labeled cells at the base of the lesion than in the superficial areas (intraepithelial and periepithelial). A possible exception to the rule of minimal dermal proliferation is seen in nevi from pregnant women, since such lesions

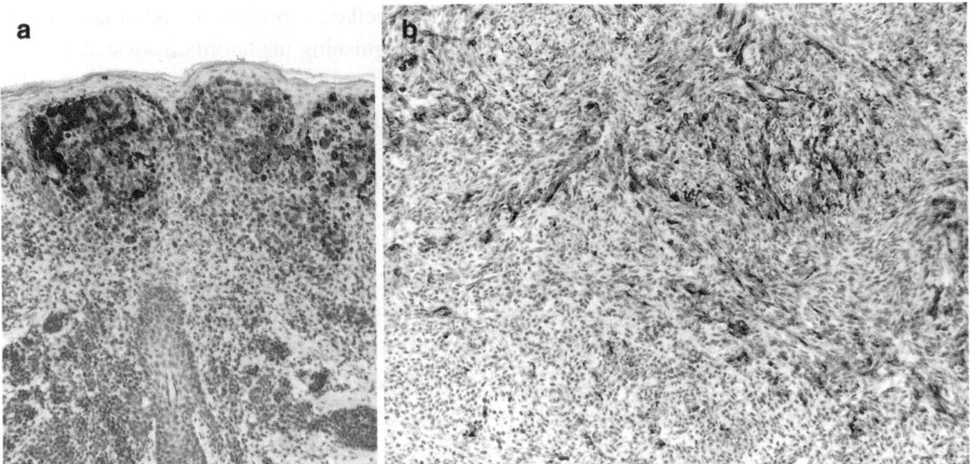

Fig. 4.1 Distinction between nevus and melanoma. (**a**) HMB45 labels the intraepidermal and upper dermal components of this large compound nevus. In contrast (**b**) melanoma cells show strong, but patchy labeling with HMB45, without showing the zonation change typical of nevi (HMB45, diaminobenzidine with light hematoxylin)

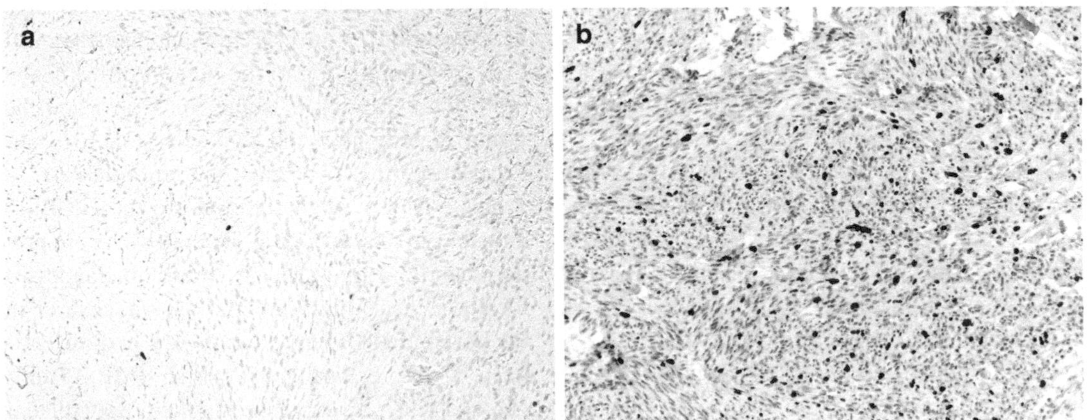

Fig. 4.2 Comparison of degree of proliferation between a large intradermal nevus and a melanoma. (**a**) The former has very rare cells in the dermis expressing Ki67. In contrast (**b**) melanoma cells typically have high rates of proliferation (anti-Ki67, diaminobencidine, with light hematoxylin)

may show occasionally dermal mitotic figures and slightly increased numbers of dermal cells positive for Ki67 [30].

The two types of nevi that diverge from this pattern of maturation with HMB-45 are blue nevi (including cellular blue, plexiform, and "deep penetrating" nevi) and Spitz nevi, since both may show diffuse labeling with HMB-45 throughout the lesion. However, as with common nevi, these lesions show a very low proliferation rate as assessed with Ki67 expression (Fig. 4.2).

The use of these two immunohistochemical markers may help also in the distinction between combined nevi and melanomas arising in association with a nevus. The most common scenario of a combined nevus is probably intradermal and blue. These combined nevi show low proliferation rates with anti-Ki67 (in both components) and display strong and diffuse labeling with HMB-45 in the blue nevus area only, while the standard intradermal nevus is negative. Similarly, immunohistochemistry may be helpful in delimiting the

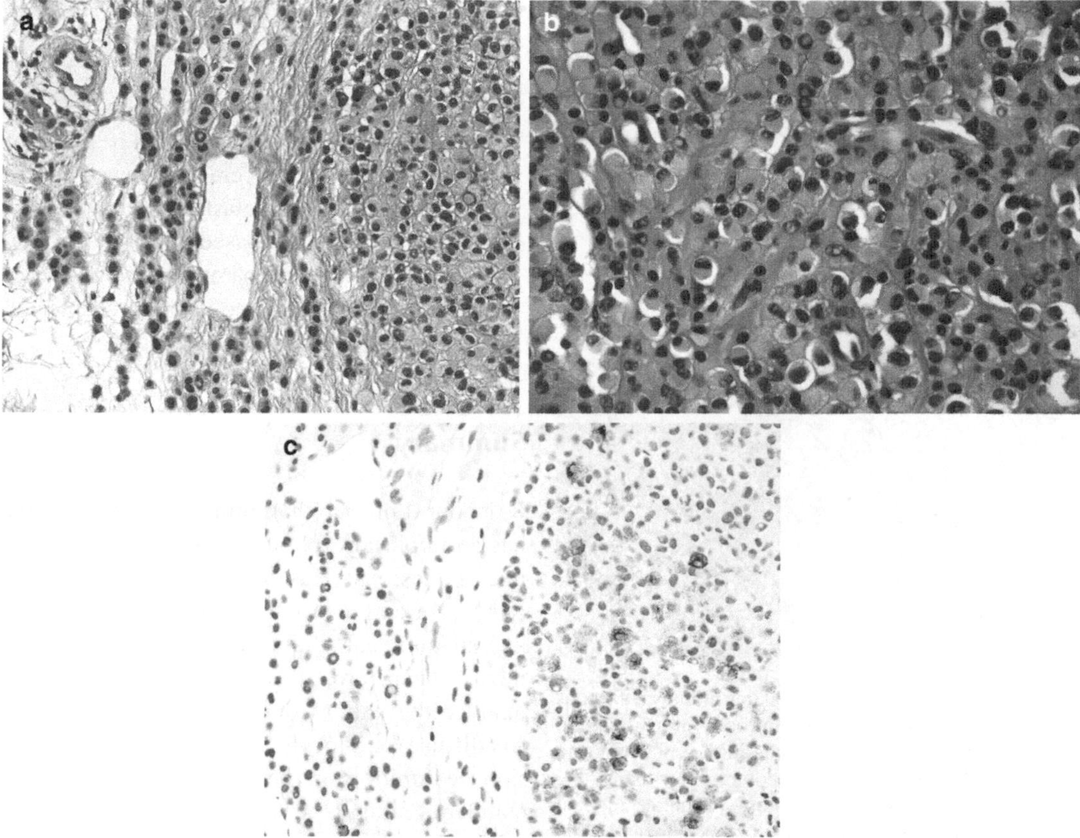

Fig. 4.3 Melanoma arising in association with a nevus; note the two different areas within the lesion. (**a**) This area shows benign-appearing melanocytes without significant cytologic atypia. (**b**) Other areas show atypical melanocytes. (**c**) HMB45 labels the atypical melanocytes (to the right) but not the benign melanocytes of the associated nevus (to the left) (HMB45, Diaminobenzidine and light hematoxylin as counterstain)

depth of invasion of melanomas arising in association with nevi (Fig. 4.3). In contrast with the associated dermal nevus, the invasive component of melanoma is usually positive with HMB-45 and has a higher percentage of Ki67-positive cells. Furthermore, by examining the pattern of expression of gp100 in a blue-nevus-type lesion it may be possible to distinguish primary blue-nevus-type melanoma from metastatic melanoma. A number of these melanomas resembling blue nevus (so-called malignant blue nevus) arise in association with a blue nevus. In such lesions, gp100 is strongly and diffusely expressed in the benign, preexistent blue nevus, while its expression becomes patchy in the malignant areas, along with increased Ki67 (see Chap. 10).

Possible Pitfalls of Immunohistochemistry Applied to the Diagnosis of Melanocytic Lesions

Some of the pitfalls to be included in this section also apply to other fields in pathology. Thus it is very important to determine that there is appropriate immunoreaction on the slide by observing the presence of both positive and negative internal controls. For instance, when examining a lesion for possible expression of MART1, it is necessary to examine the overlying epidermis and confirm that normal melanocytes are positive while keratinocytes are negative.

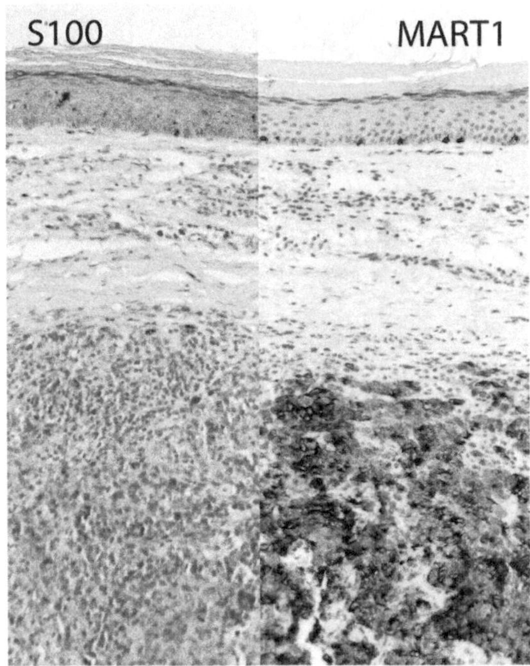

Fig. 4.4 Weak expression of S100 in a primary cutaneous melanoma likely due to fixation/processing reasons. To the left S100 only labels rare cells in the epidermis and dermis, likely dendritic cells. In contrast, note the strong expression of MART1 highlighting the intraepidermal melanocytes as well as the invasive component (anti-S100 protein and andi-MART1, DAB with light hematoxylin as counterstain)

Possible immunohistochemical pitfalls that we have observed are:

- Decreased or absent expression of S100 protein [31]. As mentioned above, the antibody anti-S100 detects S100 protein in formalin-fixed tissue (since it requires cross-linkage). Therefore, it may not work in frozen sections. Also the antibody may not highlight consistently melanocytes in formalin-fixed, paraffin-embedded sections of previously frozen tissue. Furthermore, if the tissue is over- or underfixed, S100 expression may be impaired (Fig. 4.4). Also, it has been suggested that S100 expression may be decreased in sun-damaged melanocytes [32].
- Labeling of macrophages by anti-MART1 (and less frequently HMB-45) [12]. It is possible that current detection systems are more sensitive and may detect melanocytic antigens that have been phagocytized by macrophages.
- Increased expression of gp100 (HMB-45 antigen) in benign melanocytic lesions. We have observed that the latest clones of HMB-45 appear to be more sensitive than the older ones. Dermatopathologists should be aware of this possibility; we recently reviewed a case that had been called metastatic melanoma to a sentinel lymph node, based upon the location (subcapsular and intraparenchymal) and reactivity with HMB-45 (see also the chapter on sentinel lymph nodes).

Summary

It is our opinion that immunohistochemistry has an important role in the diagnosis of melanocytic lesions. However, there is no single marker, or combination thereof, that establishes an unequivocal diagnosis of melanoma or nevus. Therefore, it is necessary to carefully analyze the pattern of expression (patchy versus diffuse) and localization/pattern of distribution (maturation) in the context of morphologic standard features.

References

1. McNutt NS. The S100 family of multipurpose calcium-binding proteins. J Cutan Pathol. 1998;25(10):521–9.
2. Prieto VG, Shea CR. Immunohistochemistry of melanocytic proliferations. Arch Pathol Lab Med. 2011; 135(7):853–9.
3. Ribe A, McNutt NS. S100A6 protein expression is different in Spitz nevi and melanomas. Mod Pathol. 2003;16(5):505–11.
4. Fullen DR, Lowe L, Su LD. Antibody to S100a6 protein is a sensitive immunohistochemical marker for neurothekeoma. J Cutan Pathol. 2003;30(2):118–22.
5. Prieto VG, McNutt NS, Lugo J, Reed JA. The intermediate filament peripherin is expressed in cutaneous melanocytic lesions. J Cutan Pathol. 1997;24(3): 145–50.
6. Huttenbach Y, Prieto VG, Reed JA. Desmoplastic and spindle cell melanomas express protein markers of the neural crest but not of later committed stages of Schwann cell differentiation. J Cutan Pathol. 2002; 29(9):562–8.
7. McNutt NS, Urmacher C, Hakimian J, Hoss DM, Lugo J. Nevoid malignant melanoma: morphologic patterns and immunohistochemical reactivity. J Cutan Pathol. 1995;22:502–17.

8. Busam KJ, Chen YT, Old LJ, et al. Expression of melan-A (MART1) in benign melanocytic nevi and primary cutaneous malignant melanoma. Am J Surg Pathol. 1998;22(8):976–82.
9. Jungbluth AA, Busam KJ, Gerald WL, et al. A103: An anti-melan-a monoclonal antibody for the detection of malignant melanoma in paraffin-embedded tissues. Am J Surg Pathol. 1998;22(5):595–602.
10. Fetsch PA, Fetsch JF, Marincola FM, Travis W, Batts KP, Abati A. Comparison of melanoma antigen recognized by T cells (MART-1) to HMB-45: additional evidence to support a common lineage for angiomyolipoma, lymphangiomyomatosis, and clear cell sugar tumor. Mod Pathol. 1998;11(8):699–703.
11. El Shabrawi-Caelen L, Kerl H, Cerroni L. Melan-A: not a helpful marker in distinction between melanoma in situ on sun-damaged skin and pigmented actinic keratosis. Am J Dermatopathol. 2004;26(5):364–6.
12. Trejo O, Reed JA, Prieto VG. Atypical cells in human cutaneous re-excision scars for melanoma express p75NGFR, C56/N-CAM and GAP-43: evidence of early Schwann cell differentiation. J Cutan Pathol. 2002;29(7):397–406.
13. Rudolph P, Schubert C, Schubert B, Parwaresch R. Proliferation marker Ki-S5 as a diagnostic tool in melanocytic lesions. J Am Acad Dermatol. 1997;37(2 Pt 1):169–78.
14. Harris GR, Shea CR, Horenstein MG, Reed JA, Burchette Jr JL, Prieto VG. Desmoplastic (sclerotic) nevus: an underrecognized entity that resembles dermatofibroma and desmoplastic melanoma. Am J Surg Pathol. 1999;23(7):786–94.
15. King R, Googe PB, Weilbaecher KN, Mihm Jr MC, Fisher DE. Microphthalmia transcription factor expression in cutaneous benign, malignant melanocytic, and nonmelanocytic tumors. Am J Surg Pathol. 2001;25(1):51–7.
16. Koch MB, Shih IM, Weiss SW, Folpe AL. Microphthalmia transcription factor and melanoma cell adhesion molecule expression distinguish desmoplastic/spindle cell melanoma from morphologic mimics. Am J Surg Pathol. 2001;25(1):58–64.
17. Ivan D, Prieto VG. Use of immunohistochemistry in the diagnosis of melanocytic lesions: applications and pitfalls. Future Oncol. 2010;6(7):1163–75.
18. Reed JA, Loganzo Jr F, Shea CR, et al. Loss of expression of the p16/cyclin-dependent kinase inhibitor 2 tumor suppressor gene in melanocytic lesions correlates with invasive stage of tumor progression. Cancer Res. 1995;55(13):2713–8.
19. Stefanaki C, Stefanaki K, Antoniou C, et al. G1 cell cycle regulators in congenital melanocytic nevi. Comparison with acquired nevi and melanomas. J Cutan Pathol. 2008;35(9):799–808.
20. Alonso SR, Ortiz P, Pollan M, et al. Progression in cutaneous malignant melanoma is associated with distinct expression profiles: a tissue microarray-based study. Am J Pathol. 2004;164(1):193–203.
21. Magro CM, Yang SE, Zippin JH, Zembowicz A. Expression of soluble adenylyl cyclase in lentigo maligna. Arch Pathol Lab Med. 2012;136(12): 1558–64.
22. Nonaka D, Chiriboga L, Rubin BP. Sox10: a pan-schwannian and melanocytic marker. Am J Surg Pathol. 2008;32(9):1291–8.
23. Ramos-Herberth FI, Karamchandani J, Kim J, Dadras SS. SOX10 immunostaining distinguishes desmoplastic melanoma from excision scar. J Cutan Pathol. 2010;37(9):944–52.
24. Paul E, Cochran AJ, Wen DR. Immunohistochemical demonstration of S-100 protein and melanoma-associated antigens in melanocytic nevi. J Cutan Pathol. 1988;15(3):161–5.
25. Prieto VG, Mourad-Zeidan AA, Melnikova V, et al. Galectin-3 expression is associated with tumor progression and pattern of sun exposure in melanoma. Clin Cancer Res. 2006;12(22):6709–15.
26. Chwirot BW, Kuzbicki L. Cyclooxygenase-2 (COX-2): first immunohistochemical marker distinguishing early cutaneous melanomas from benign melanocytic skin tumours. Melanoma Res. 2007;17(3):139–45.
27. Hashimoto Y, Ito Y, Kato T, Motokawa T, Katagiri T, Itoh M. Expression profiles of melanogenesis-related genes and proteins in acquired melanocytic nevus. J Cutan Pathol. 2006;33(3):207–15.
28. Ding Y, Prieto VG, Zhang PS, et al. Nuclear expression of the antiapoptotic protein survivin in malignant melanoma. Cancer. 2006;106(5):1123–9.
29. Cohn ML, Goncharuk VN, Diwan AH, Zhang PS, Shen SS, Prieto VG. Loss of claudin-1 expression in tumor-associated vessels correlates with acquisition of metastatic phenotype in melanocytic neoplasms. J Cutan Pathol. 2005;32(8):533–6.
30. Chan MP, Chan MM, Tahan SR. Melanocytic nevi in pregnancy: histologic features and Ki-67 proliferation index. J Cutan Pathol. 2010;37(8):843–51.
31. Prieto VG, Shea CR. Use of immunohistochemistry in melanocytic lesions. J Cutan Pathol. 2008;35 Suppl 2:1–10.
32. Sigal AC, Keenan M, Lazova R. P75 nerve growth factor receptor as a useful marker to distinguish spindle cell melanoma from other spindle cell neoplasms of sun-damaged skin. Am J Dermatopathol. 2012; 34(2):145–50.

5 Applications of Additional Techniques to Melanocytic Pathology

Victor G. Prieto, Christopher R. Shea, and Jon A. Reed

The application of molecular techniques has much improved our knowledge of molecular abnormalities in melanocytic lesions. It is accepted that there are three cell signaling pathways in melanocytes critical for their survival and proliferation, including (A) mitogen-activated protein kinase (MAPK)/extracellular regulated kinase (ERK), (B) phosphoinositide-3 kinase (PI3K)-AKT/PTEN, and (C) receptors such as KIT, melanocortin-1 receptor, (MC1R) and glutamate receptor metabotropic (GRM3) receptor [1]. The most commonly detected mutations in melanoma include alteration in RAF. Of the three isoforms (A, B, and C), BRAF is the primary isoform in the RAS/MAPK pathway and the isoform most susceptible for mutation in several solid tumors. Mutation in the *BRAF* gene located on chromosome 7 accounts for approximately 80 % of activation mutations in benign nevi and 50–60 % in primary cutaneous melanoma [2–4]. The majority of mutations occur in exon 15 as a single point mutation with substitution from thymine to adenine (T to A) that converts valine to glutamic acid at the 600 position (*BRAF V600E*) and less frequently other including *V600K* and *V600R* [5]. When compared to the wild form, melanoma cells containing the mutation *BRAF* V600E demonstrate an almost 500-fold increase in activity.

A second group of genes with mutations detected in melanoma is the *RAS* oncogene family (*NRAS*, *HRAS*, and *KRAS*). Activated RAS recruits RAF, which activates MEK and ERK and promotes cell proliferation, differentiation, and survival. *NRAS* mutations in melanocytic nevi and melanoma most commonly occur in exons 2 and 3. *NRAS* mutations occur in 14–20 % of cutaneous melanoma (particularly nodular and lentigo maligna histologic subtypes) [6–8]. Alterations in *HRAS* are seen in nearly 30 % of Spitz nevi [9, 10]. Increased copy number of chromosome 11p (site of *HRAS* gene by CGH or FISH)/mutations in *HRAS* have been reported in over 20 % of Spitz nevi [11]. In contrast, spitzoid melanomas usually lack detectable mutations in *HRAS* [10].

NRAS and *BRAF* mutations are mostly exclusive; however, there are small percentages of melanomas which may harbor both *NRAS* and *BRAF* mutations (around 1 %) [8, 12, 13].

KIT is a tyrosine kinase growth factor receptor and *KIT* mutations and or increased copy numbers are seen in 15–20 % of acral-lentiginous/mucosal

V.G. Prieto, M.D., Ph.D. (✉)
MD Anderson Cancer Center, University of Houston, 1515 Holcombe Blvd., Unit 85, Houston, TX 77030, USA
e-mail: vprieto@mdanderson.org

C.R. Shea
University of Chicago Medicine, 5841 S. Maryland Ave., MC 5067, L502, Chicago, IL 60637, USA

J.A. Reed
CellNEtix Pathology & Laboratories, 1124 Columbia St., Suite 200, Seattle, WA 98117, USA

C.R. Shea et al. (eds.), *Pathology of Challenging Melanocytic Neoplasms: Diagnosis and Management*, DOI 10.1007/978-1-4939-1444-9_5, © Springer Science+Business Media New York 2015

melanomas and lentigo maligna melanomas (chronic sun damage) [14, 15]. Most mutations in *KIT* in melanomas occur not only in exon 11, but also in exons 13 and 17 [16, 17].

GNAQ and *GNA11* encode for the α-subunit of G-protein-coupled receptor. Benign and malignant melanocytic lesions show mutations at codon 209 with change of glutamine to leucine or proline (Q209L or Q209P). This results in constitutive activation of this G-protein. Such mutations have been detected in 83 % of blue nevi, 50 % of melanoma with blue nevus features, 46 % of uveal melanoma, and in 4 % of lentigo maligna [18].

Another gene mutated in melanocytic lesions is *CDKN2A/INK4A* in chromosome 9p21 which codes p16INK4a [19]. It is associated with familial melanoma and dysplastic nevus syndrome [20–22]. Within the last 10 years there have been descriptions of application of additional techniques applied to the detection of genetic abnormalities, particularly those described in this paragraph, that seem helpful in the diagnosis and treatment of melanocytic lesions.

In comparative genomic hybridization (CGH), DNA derived from a tumor of interest is labeled with a fluorochrome and mixed with a reference DNA labeled with a different fluorochrome. Chromosomal gains and losses are represented by relative changes of color. Bastian and colleagues initially described the use of CGH to detect multiple discrete gains and losses in primary melanomas [23]. In contrast, only rare nevi (mostly of the Spitz type) showed single isolated gains of the entire short arm of chromosome 11 [24]. Furthermore, in those rare nevi with alterations, these typically involved whole chromosomes or whole chromosomal arms. CGH also confirmed that the histologic subtypes of melanoma (superficial spreading type, acral-lentiginous, lentigo maligna) have different patterns of chromosomal aberrations.

As a drawback, CGH requires a relatively large amount of pure tumor cells. Thus small lesions or those with admixed inflammatory or stromal cells are less amenable to CGH analysis.

Fluorescence in situ hybridization (FISH) has been used as an alternative to CGH. It uses fluorescently labeled probes to be hybridized to formalin-fixed, paraffin-embedded sections. By counting the number of signals per nucleus, aberrations are described as a percentage of tumor nuclei with more or less than two signals. The current FISH assay for melanoma originated from studies of Bastian and colleagues [25]. The original four probes were: centromere 6 (CEN6) as a surrogate of the number of chromosomes, RREB1 (6p25), MYB (6q23), and CCND1 (11q13) (see also below). The cutoffs to determine gains or losses are different depending on the authors. Depending on the studies, the overall sensitivity of FISH in distinguishing between melanomas and nevi is around 80 % with an overall specificity of 90 % [25].

Some other studies have concentrated in ambiguous lesions to try to determine the feasibility of FISH when applied to the diagnosis of "difficult" cases [26, 27]. Gaiser et al. compared the FISH results with histopathologic assessment, array CGH, and clinical follow up. Overall, when comparing FISH results with clinical outcome there was a sensitivity of 60 % and a specificity of 50 % [26]. Vergier et al. characterized 113 ambiguous tumors according to clinical outcome [27]. Expert histopathologic review yielded a sensitivity and specificity of 95 % and 52 %, compared to 43 % and 80 % for FISH. Tetzlaff et al. [28] reported a specificity of 87.5 %, positive predictive value of 62.5 %, and negative predictive value of 80.7 %. Overall, these studies indicated that the combination of expert histopathologic review and FISH generated the best results. Also important is to consider a possible pitfall of FISH: the presence of polyploidy yields potentially false positive FISH results [29]. This is important because a number of Spitz nevi, with benign behavior, display polyploidy, so if the FISH results are misinterpreted the lesion may be labeled as "malignant" (we have encountered several such cases referred to our institution as melanoma). Therefore, whoever analyzes the FISH studies should make every effort to remove from the final counts those cells with increased copy numbers on all probes (including the centromere one) thus consistent with polyploidy. A newer set includes p16 (9p21) instead of MYB and, sometimes, an added MYC (8q24). Analysis of 9p21 appears to provide better distinction between Spitz nevi and spitzoid melanoma, since spitzoid lesions with aggressive behavior (i.e., malignant) show homozygous deletion of 9p21 [30]. Regarding 8q24, it seems that gains of this gene result in an amelanotic phenotype due to downregulation of MITF and tyrosinase [31], and may be associated with poor prognosis [30].

Regarding FISH, in summary, we believe that: (1) FISH is insufficient as an isolated diagnostic assay in the differential diagnosis between melanoma and nevus, (2) a positive FISH should not modify treatment in the absence of histopathologic confirmation, (3) a negative FISH test does not exclude melanoma, and (4) FISH should be applied with caution in desmoplastic/sclerotic (because it may be difficult to collect pure enough DNA from the tumor cells) and spitzoid lesions (for the possibility of polyploidy).

Another technique that may be helpful in the distinction between nevus and melanoma is mass spectroscopy to determine differences in the protein components of melanocytic lesions. The group of Dr. Lazova has applied this technique to spitzoid lesions and has determined that there is a different spectrum of proteins present either in the lesional cells or in the stroma of Spitz nevi and spitzoid melanomas [32]. Interestingly, of the 12 proteins that are differentially expressed between these two types of lesions, two of them are the almost ubiquitous vimentin and actin. Other studies are ongoing to study other types of melanocytic lesions, such as ocular melanoma [33].

Molecular studies may also be used to help determining prognosis in patients with cutaneous melanoma. There is a trend to shorter melanoma-specific survival and disease-free survival in *NRAS* mutant melanomas [34]. The presence of mutant *BRAF* does not appear to have an effect on disease-free interval (DFI) or overall survival (OS) in primary melanomas [35] but it appears to lower OS in stage IV patients [13, 35]. Furthermore, patients with *BRAF* or *NRAS* mutations develop more frequently than the average patient metastasis to the central nervous system metastasis.

In summary, molecular studies have revolutionized the study of melanocytic lesions. Further studies are needed to determine the appropriate role of such techniques to the diagnosis of melanocytic lesions.

References

1. Prickett TD, Wei X, Cardenas-Navia I, et al. Exon capture analysis of G protein-coupled receptors identifies activating mutations in GRM3 in melanoma. Nat Genet. 2011;43(11):1119–26.
2. Davies H, Bignell GR, Cox C, et al. Mutations of the BRAF gene in human cancer. Nature. 2002; 417(6892):949–54.
3. Pollock PM, Harper UL, Hansen KS, et al. High frequency of BRAF mutations in nevi. Nat Genet. 2003;33(1):19–20.
4. Hocker T, Tsao H. Ultraviolet radiation and melanoma: a systematic review and analysis of reported sequence variants. Hum Mutat. 2007;28(6):578–88.
5. Beadling C, Jacobson-Dunlop E, Hodi FS, et al. KIT gene mutations and copy number in melanoma subtypes. Clin Cancer Res. 2008;14(21):6821–8.
6. Curtin JA, Fridlyand J, Kageshita T, et al. Distinct sets of genetic alterations in melanoma. N Engl J Med. 2005;353(20):2135–47.
7. Lee JH, Choi JW, Kim YS. Frequencies of BRAF and NRAS mutations are different in histological types and sites of origin of cutaneous melanoma: a meta-analysis. Br J Dermatol. 2011;164(4):776–84.
8. Goel VK, Lazar AJ, Warneke CL, Redston MS, Haluska FG. Examination of mutations in BRAF, NRAS, and PTEN in primary cutaneous melanoma. J Invest Dermatol. 2006;126(1):154–60.
9. Bastian BC, LeBoit PE, Pinkel D. Mutations and copy number increase of HRAS in Spitz nevi with distinctive histopathological features. Am J Pathol. 2000; 157(3):967–72.
10. Da Forno PD, Pringle JH, Fletcher A, et al. BRAF, NRAS and HRAS mutations in spitzoid tumours and their possible pathogenetic significance. Br J Dermatol. 2009;161(2):364–72.
11. van Dijk MC, Bernsen MR, Ruiter DJ. Analysis of mutations in B-RAF, N-RAS, and H-RAS genes in the differential diagnosis of Spitz nevus and spitzoid melanoma. Am J Surg Pathol. 2005;29(9):1145–51.
12. Ellerhorst JA, Greene VR, Ekmekcioglu S, et al. Clinical correlates of NRAS and BRAF mutations in primary human melanoma. Clin Cancer Res. 2011; 17(2):229–35.
13. Jakob JA, Bassett RL, Ng CS, Lazar AF, Joseph RW, Alvarado GC, Rohlfs ML, Richard J, Curry JL, Gershenwald JE, Hwu P, Kim KB, Davies MA. NRAS mutation status is an independent prognostic factor in metastatic melanoma. Cancer. 2012;118(16): 4014–23.

14. Curtin JA, Busam K, Pinkel D, Bastian BC. Somatic activation of KIT in distinct subtypes of melanoma. J Clin Oncol. 2006;24(26):4340–6.
15. Torres-Cabala CA, Wang WL, Trent J, et al. Correlation between KIT expression and KIT mutation in melanoma: a study of 173 cases with emphasis on the acral-lentiginous/mucosal type. Mod Pathol. 2009;22(11):1446–56.
16. Hornick JL, Fletcher CD. The role of KIT in the management of patients with gastrointestinal stromal tumors. Hum Pathol. 2007;38(5):679–87.
17. Corless CL, Heinrich MC. Molecular pathobiology of gastrointestinal stromal sarcomas. Annu Rev Pathol. 2008;3:557–86.
18. Van Raamsdonk CD, Bezrookove V, Green G, et al. Frequent somatic mutations of GNAQ in uveal melanoma and blue naevi. Nature. 2009;457(7229):599–602.
19. Haluska FG, Housman DE. Recent advances in the molecular genetics of malignant melanoma. Cancer Surv. 1995;25:277–92.
20. Czajkowski R, Placek W, Drewa G, Czajkowska A, Uchanska G. FAMMM syndrome: pathogenesis and management. Dermatol Surg. 2004;30(2 Pt 2):291–6.
21. Piepkorn M. Melanoma genetics: an update with focus on the CDKN2A(p16)/ARF tumor suppressors. J Am Acad Dermatol. 2000;42(5 Pt 1):705–22. quiz 723–706.
22. Ranade K, Hussussian CJ, Sikorski RS, et al. Mutations associated with familial melanoma impair p16INK4 function. Nat Genet. 1995;10(1):114–6.
23. Bastian BC, LeBoit PE, Hamm H, Brocker EB, Pinkel D. Chromosomal gains and losses in primary cutaneous melanomas detected by comparative genomic hybridization. Cancer Res. 1998;58(10):2170–5.
24. Bastian BC, Olshen AB, LeBoit PE, Pinkel D. Classifying melanocytic tumors based on DNA copy number changes. Am J Pathol. 2003;163(5):1765–70.
25. Gerami P, Jewell SS, Morrison LE, et al. Fluorescence in situ hybridization (FISH) as an ancillary diagnostic tool in the diagnosis of melanoma. Am J Surg Pathol. 2009;33(8):1146–56.
26. Gaiser T, Kutzner H, Palmedo G, et al. Classifying ambiguous melanocytic lesions with FISH and correlation with clinical long-term follow up. Mod Pathol. 2010;23(3):413–9.
27. Vergier B, Prochazkova-Carlotti M, de la Fouchardiere A, et al. Fluorescence in situ hybridization, a diagnostic aid in ambiguous melanocytic tumors: European study of 113 cases. Mod Pathol. 2011;24(5):613–23.
28. Tetzlaff MT, Wang WL, Milless TL, et al. Ambiguous melanocytic tumors in a tertiary referral center: the contribution of fluorescence in situ hybridization (FISH) to conventional histopathologic and immunophenotypic analyses. Am J Surg Pathol. 2013;37(12):1783–96.
29. Isaac AK, Lertsburapa T, Pathria Mundi J, Martini M, Guitart J, Gerami P. Polyploidy in spitz nevi: a not uncommon karyotypic abnormality identifiable by fluorescence in situ hybridization. Am J Dermatopathol. 2010;32(2):144–8.
30. Gerami P, Cooper C, Bajaj S, et al. Outcomes of atypical spitz tumors with chromosomal copy number aberrations and conventional melanomas in children. Am J Surg Pathol. 2013;37(9):1387–94.
31. Pouryazdanparast P, Brenner A, Haghighat Z, Guitart J, Rademaker A, Gerami P. The role of 8q24 copy number gains and c-MYC expression in amelanotic cutaneous melanoma. Mod Pathol. 2012;25(9):1221–6.
32. Lazova R, Seeley EH, Keenan M, Gueorguieva R, Caprioli RM. Imaging mass spectrometry—a new and promising method to differentiate Spitz nevi from Spitzoid malignant melanomas. Am J Dermatopathol. 2012;34(1):82–90.
33. Daniels AB, Lee JE, MacConaill LE, et al. High throughput mass spectrometry-based mutation profiling of primary uveal melanoma. Invest Ophthalmol Vis Sci. 2012;53(11):6991–6.
34. Devitt B, Liu W, Salemi R, et al. Clinical outcome and pathological features associated with NRAS mutation in cutaneous melanoma. Pigment Cell Melanoma Res. 2011;24(4):666–72.
35. Long GV, Menzies AM, Nagrial AM, et al. Prognostic and clinicopathologic associations of oncogenic BRAF in metastatic melanoma. J Clin Oncol. 2011;29(10):1239–46.

Part II

Diagnostic Challenges

6 Spitz Nevus Versus Spitzoid Melanoma

Victor G. Prieto, Christopher R. Shea, and Jon A. Reed

Spitz nevus is a biologically benign nevus associated with a good prognosis, but sometimes it can cause diagnostic concern since it can be difficult to distinguish from atypical melanocytic lesions and melanoma on histological grounds. Originally designated as "juvenile melanoma", it presents as a solitary rapidly growing, red or flesh-colored papule arising on the face, trunk, or extremities of children and adolescents. Most Spitz nevi are compounds although they can be junctional or intradermal. The lesions tend to show lateral circumscription and are symmetric. The junctional nests, when present, are cohesive and vertically oriented, surrounded by retraction artifact, sometimes referred to as "hanging bananas" [1, 2] (Fig. 6.1). Adjacent rete ridges are usually elongated, sometimes showing pseudoepitheliomatous hyperplasia. Cells are epithelioid or spindled. There may be pagetoid upward migration but this is circumscribed to the center of the lesion and not at the periphery. Adjacent to melanocytes there are eosinophilic globules (Kamino bodies), PAS positive and composed of laminin, type IV collagen, and fibronectin.

In the dermis, the cells are arranged in fascicles and have a large ample eosinophilic cytoplasm with eosinophilic nucleoli. Some of the epithelioid cells can show bizarre shapes but the degree of cytologic atypia is mostly uniform throughout the entire lesion. Commonly there is maturation with descent in the dermis and cells infiltrate among collagen bundles. The upper dermis may show edema and superficial telangiectases. There are features that appear to be different in Spitz nevi depending on the patient's age. There may be mitotic figures in the superficial dermal portion of the nevus, especially in younger patients. Pagetoid growth and/or melanin deposits in the keratin layer are more common in little children. Ulceration is statistically more frequent in peripuberty patients than in adults. In adults, isolated cells within the lateral edges of the lesion are more common in Spitz nevus than in spitzoid melanoma [3].

Pigmented spindle cell nevus of Reed is considered by most authors to be a pigmented variant of Spitz nevus, more common in young women, in the extremities (particularly on the thigh). The desmoplastic variant presents as a brown papule on the extremities of young adults. It is wedge-shaped, with pleomorphic spindle and epithelioid cells with abundant eosinophilic cytoplasm arranged among thick collagen fibers [4].

V.G. Prieto, M.D., Ph.D. (✉)
MD Anderson Cancer Center, University of Houston, 1515 Holcombe Blvd., Unit 85, Houston, TX 77030, USA
e-mail: vprieto@mdanderson.org

C.R. Shea
University of Chicago Medicine, 5841 S. Maryland Ave., MC 5067, L502, Chicago, IL 60637, USA

J.A. Reed
CellNEtix Pathology & Laboratories, 1124 Columbia St., Suite 200, Seattle, WA 98117, USA

C.R. Shea et al. (eds.), *Pathology of Challenging Melanocytic Neoplasms: Diagnosis and Management*, DOI 10.1007/978-1-4939-1444-9_6,

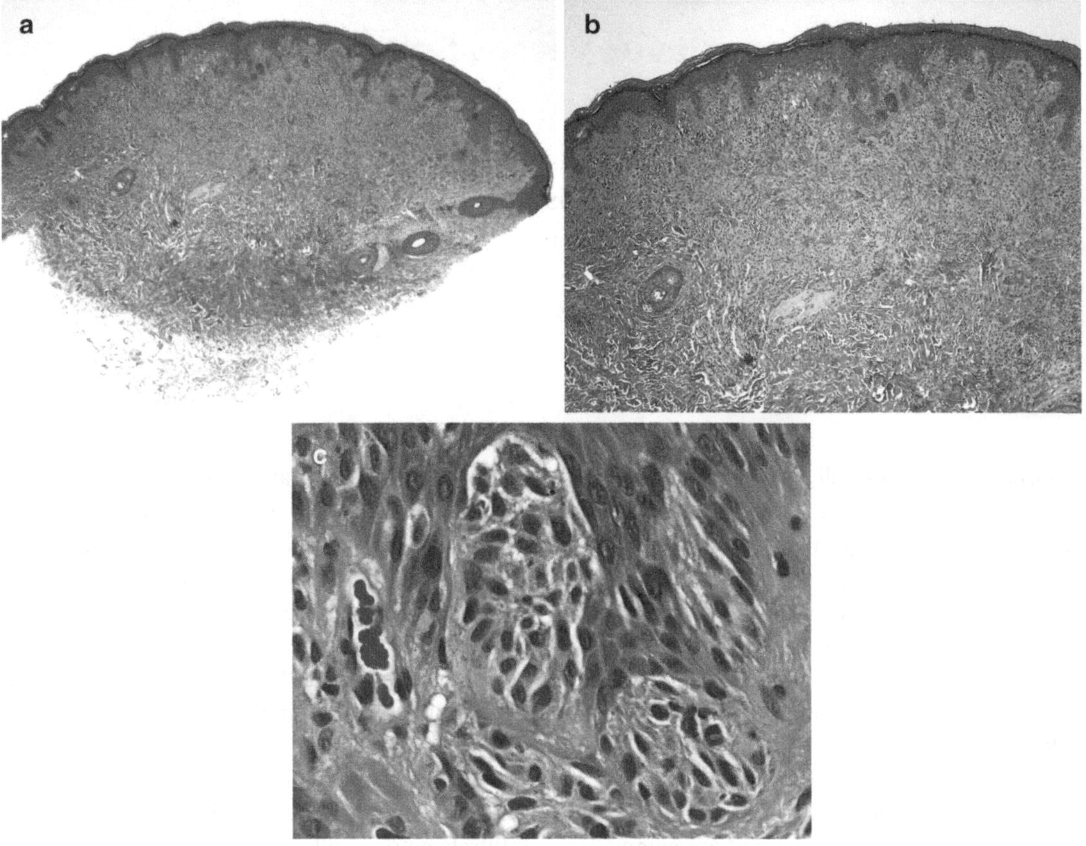

Fig. 6.1 Compound Spitz nevus: (**a** and **b**) note the regular elongation of rete ridges and the wedge-shape of the lesion in the dermis. (**c**) Large epithelioid cells in the epidermis. Note the similarity shape and chromatin among the cells

The differential diagnosis includes other cutaneous epithelioid and spindle cell lesions. Epithelioid fibrous histiocytoma [5] presents as a raised, nonpigmented or light brown papule on the extremities of adults. Histologically it is a dermal lesion, composed of clusters of epithelioid, bland-looking cells, with abundant eosinophilic cytoplasm and scattered mitotic figures. Precisely due to the last feature, epithelioid fibrous histiocytoma may be confused with either Spitz nevus or spitzoid melanoma. In contrast with either one, epithelioid fibrous histiocytoma does not express melanocytic markers such as MART1, gp100, or MiTF. The lesional cells are typically positive for FXIIIa, CD68, and CD163. Anti-S100 may be a pitfall since it labels dendritic cells and thus it may be incorrectly interpreted as positive in the lesional cells.

Junctional Spitz nevi may resemble dysplastic nevi; furthermore, some authors have suggested the term "Spark" nevus for lesions that have features common to "Clark" (dysplastic) and "Spitz" nevi [6]. In general, dysplastic nevi occur in patients at any age, are symmetrical, and show irregular elongation of rete ridges with "bridging". Dermis is irregularly fibrous, with lamellar fibrosis, vascular proliferation, and a lymphocytic infiltrate containing melanophages [7]. In general, for such cases with mixed features between Spitz and dysplastic, the differential diagnosis may not be so important, since in both cases a complete excision is probably the recommended management (see also Chap. 9).

Spitzoid melanoma is the preferred term for those malignant melanocytic lesions showing large, epithelioid melanocytes with prominent

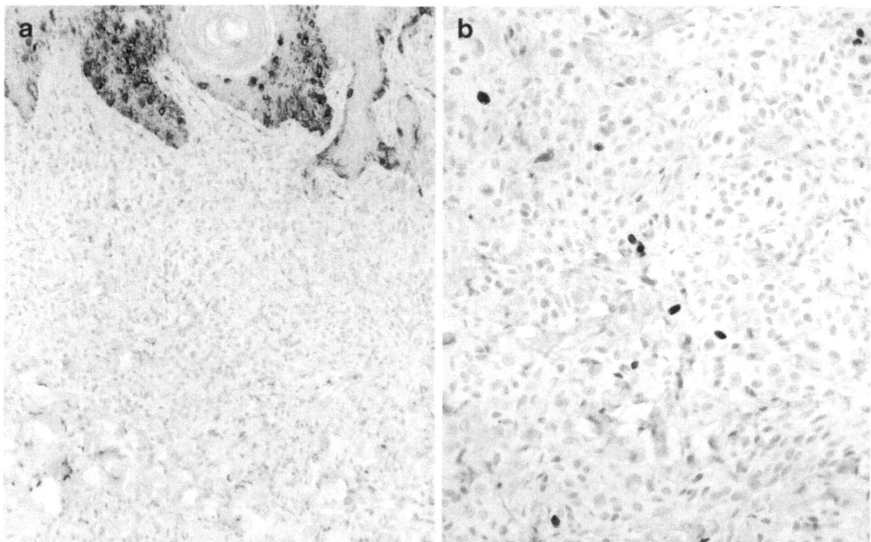

Fig. 6.2 Compound Spitz nevus: (**a**) HMB45 shows decreased expression with depth. (**b**) A double immunostudy shows very low proliferation (HMB45/anti-MART1 and anti-Ki67; light hematoxylin as the counterstain)

nucleoli, and predominantly arranged in clusters and nests in the dermis. Those lesions have at least some of the features of standard melanomas: irregular junctional component (variably sized nests), dermal mitotic figures (located in the lower half of the lesion), possibly of atypical shapes, pagetoid upward migration prominent or else at the periphery of the lesion, expansile pattern of growth in the dermis, pushing border in the deep dermis.

Immunohistochemistry may be helpful in the diagnosis of spitz lesions. As it is the case in most nevi, there is a pattern of maturation in Spitz nevi, i.e., with change in expression of several immunohistochemical markers from the top to the bottom of the lesion, particularly HMB-45 antigen (gp100) and Ki67. A pattern in which HMB-45 antigen and Ki67 are expressed in the intraepithelial and periepithelial components, but are almost completely absent from the deep areas of the lesion, is more consistent with a Spitz nevus than with a spitzoid melanoma (Fig. 6.2). As mentioned in Chap. 4, rather than performing an actual count of the number of melanocytes expressing this marker, we prefer comparing the patterns of expression at the top and the bottom of the lesion. Regardless of the absolute number of positive cells, nevi should have many fewer labeled cells at the base of the lesion than in the superficial areas (intraepithelial and periepithelial). It is important to remember that nevi from pregnant women may show dermal mitotic figures and slightly increased numbers of dermal cells positive for Ki67 [8].

Regarding HMB-45 some Spitz nevi may show diffuse labeling with HMB-45 throughout the lesion, similar to the pattern seen in blue nevi.

Another marker that has been suggested for the differential diagnosis between Spitz nevus and spitzoid melanoma is p16, since it is expressed in most benign melanocytes and only a fraction of melanoma cells [9–11]. However, other studies have not supported its usefulness [12].

Expression of neuropilin-2 has been reported in spitzoid melanoma but not in Spitz nevus [13].

Recently, there has been recognition of a subtype of spitzoid lesions that lack BAP1 (BRCA Associated Protein 1). In addition to a mutation resulting in loss of BAP1, these lesions commonly have BRAF V600E mutations.

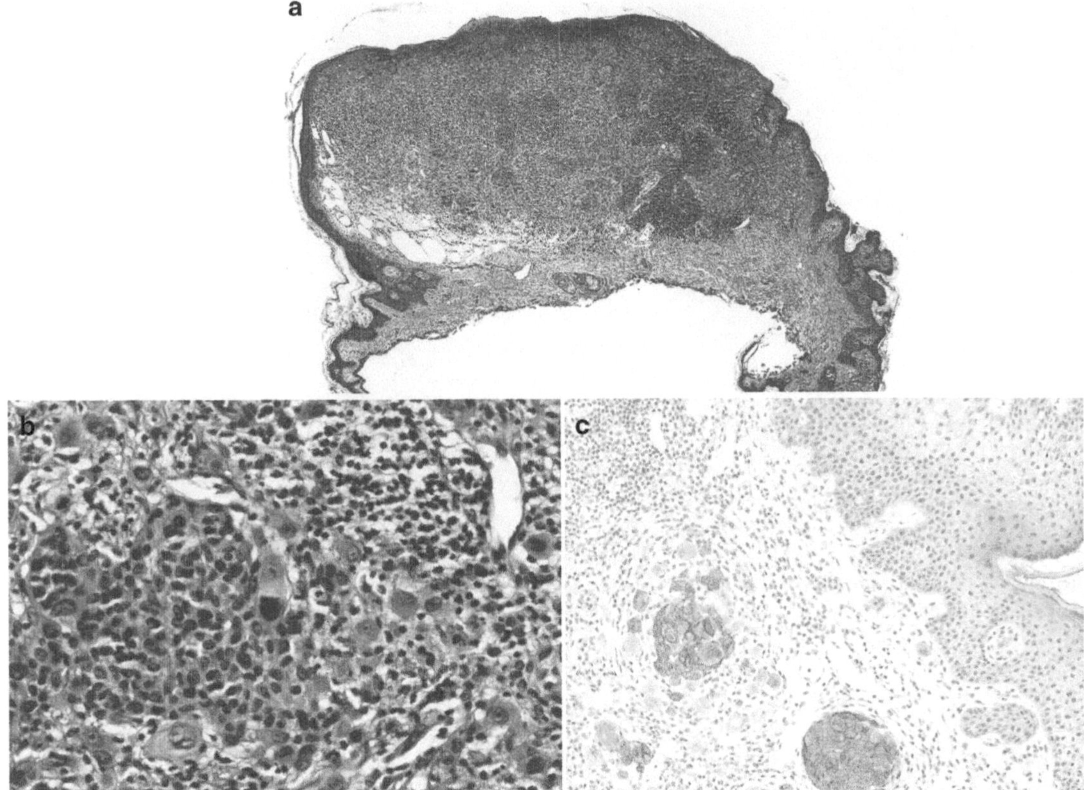

Fig. 6.3 Spitz lesion with loss of BAP1. (**a**) Large dermal nodule. (**b**) Large epithelioid cells with prominent nucleoli. (**c**) Loss of nuclear expression of BAP1

Such lesions are primarily located in the dermis, with epithelioid melanocytes with abundant amphophilic cytoplasm and defined cytoplasmic borders. Nuclei are pleomorphic and vesicular, with prominent nucleoli [14] (Fig. 6.3). It is important to recognize this type of lesions since they can be a marker of patients with increased risk for cutaneous and ocular melanoma (including relatives).

In summary, Spitz nevi occur in relatively young patients (although they can be seen in any age), and show a symmetrical, wedge-shaped contour, with pagetoid migration limited to the center of the lesion, very rare (superficial) mitotic figures, and features of maturation with H&E and immunohistochemistry. Additional techniques show gains of 11p and tetraploidy in the benign lesions and homozygous deletion of 9p21 in the malignant lesions associated with recurrence, metastasis, or death.

References

1. Weedon D, Little JH. Spindle and epithelioid cell nevi in children and adults. A review of 211 cases of the Spitz nevus. Cancer. 1977;40(1):217–25.
2. Crotty KA. Spitz naevus: histological features and distinction from malignant melanoma. Australas J Dermatol. 1997;38 Suppl 1:S49–53.
3. Diaconeasa A, Boda D, Solovan C, Enescu DM, Vilcea AM, Zurac S. Histopathologic features of Spitzoid lesions in different age groups. Rom J Morphol Embryol. 2013;54(1):51–62.
4. Paredes B, Hardmeier T. Spitz nevus and Reed nevus: simulating melanoma in adults. Pathologe. 1998; 19(6):403–11.
5. Glusac EJ, McNiff JM. Epithelioid cell histiocytoma: a simulant of vascular and melanocytic neoplasms. Am J Dermatopathol. 1999;21(1):1–7.
6. Ko CJ, McNiff JM, Glusac EJ. Melanocytic nevi with features of Spitz nevi and Clark's/dysplastic nevi ("Spark's" nevi). J Cutan Pathol. 2009;36(10):1063–8.
7. Shea CR, Vollmer RT, Prieto VG. Correlating architectural disorder and cytologic atypia in Clark (dysplastic) melanocytic nevi. Hum Pathol. 1999;30(5):500–5.

8. Chan MP, Chan MM, Tahan SR. Melanocytic nevi in pregnancy: histologic features and Ki-67 proliferation index. J Cutan Pathol. 2010;37(8):843–51.
9. Reed JA, Loganzo Jr F, Shea CR, et al. Loss of expression of the p16/cyclin-dependent kinase inhibitor 2 tumor suppressor gene in melanocytic lesions correlates with invasive stage of tumor progression. Cancer Res. 1995;55(13):2713–8.
10. Stefanaki C, Stefanaki K, Antoniou C, et al. G1 cell cycle regulators in congenital melanocytic nevi. Comparison with acquired nevi and melanomas. J Cutan Pathol. 2008;35(9):799–808.
11. Alonso SR, Ortiz P, Pollan M, et al. Progression in cutaneous malignant melanoma is associated with distinct expression profiles: a tissue microarray-based study. Am J Pathol. 2004;164(1):193–203.
12. Mason A, Wititsuwannakul J, Klump VR, Lott J, Lazova R. Expression of p16 alone does not differentiate between Spitz nevi and Spitzoid melanoma. J Cutan Pathol. 2012;39(12):1062–74.
13. Wititsuwannakul J, Mason AR, Klump VR, Lazova R. Neuropilin-2 as a useful marker in the differentiation between Spitzoid malignant melanoma and Spitz nevus. J Am Acad Dermatol. 2013;68(1):129–37.
14. Wiesner T, Murali R, Fried I, et al. A distinct subset of atypical Spitz tumors is characterized by BRAF mutation and loss of BAP1 expression. Am J Surg Pathol. 2012;36(6):818–30.

7 Halo Nevus Versus Melanoma with Regression

Penvadee Pattanaprichakul, Christopher R. Shea, Jon A. Reed, and Victor G. Prieto

Halo nevus (Sutton nevus, leukoderma acquisitum centrifugum) is a melanocytic nevus surrounded by a rim of depigmentation that occurs in approximately 1 % of the population (mainly in children and young adults) without sex or race predilection. The back is the most commonly affected site [1]. The clinical appearance of a halo correlates with focal histologic regression, which may lead to complete disappearance of the nevus. Such lesions leave behind a depigmented macule and in a majority of cases the repigmentation return after months to years. In halo nevus, this immunologic reaction produces progressive regression of the nevus cells [1–3]. Cell-mediated immunity with predominant cytotoxic T-cell response is likely to play a role in this process [4]. The halo phenomenon can be associated with several melanocytic lesions including banal melanocytic nevi, dysplastic nevi, congenital nevi, Spitz nevi, balloon cell nevi, other atypical nevi, as well as melanoma. Depending on the time when the biopsy is taken, there may not be a significant lymphocytic infiltrate [5–9]. The sudden change in appearance of a halo nevus may cause patients' concern of a changing mole and thus suspicion of melanoma.

The histopathologic changes in halo nevus typically comprise of a dense inflammatory infiltrate predominantly of lymphocytes, sharply demarcated, surrounding and infiltrating the small, centrally placed nevus cells. Melanocytic nests located in dermoepidermal junction and dermis can be obscured by this infiltrate; there may be mild to moderate cellular atypia of melanocytes as characterized by slightly enlarged, ovoid and round melanocytes with vesicular nuclei. Markedly atypical melanocytes or, very rarely, superficial mitotic figures can be seen in halo nevi, thus raising the differential diagnosis of melanoma. However, the markedly atypical cells are only scattered in a background of benign-looking typical nevus cells. The density of the infiltrate should be uniform throughout the lesion rather than irregular distribution and poor circumscription as commonly seen in melanoma. Beside lymphocytes, the infiltrate of halo nevus can be admixed with histiocytes, Langerhans cells and only a few or no plasma cells. Granulomatous inflammation with multinucleated giant cells has been report in halo nevus [10]. There may also be colloid bodies and melanophages,

P. Pattanaprichakul
Faculty of Medicine Siriraj Hospital, Mahidol University, 2 Prannok Rd., Bangkoknoi, Bangkok 10700, Thailand

C.R. Shea (✉)
University of Chicago Medicine, 5841 S. Maryland Ave., MC 5067, L502, Chicago, IL 60637, USA
e-mail: cshea@medicine.bsd.uchicago.edu

J.A. Reed
CellNEtix Pathology & Laboratories, 1124 Columbia St., Suite 200, Seattle, WA 98117, USA

V.G. Prieto, M.D., Ph.D. (✉)
MD Anderson Cancer Center, University of Houston, 1515 Holcombe Blvd., Unit 85, Houston, TX 77030, USA
e-mail: vprieto@mdanderson.org

C.R. Shea et al. (eds.), *Pathology of Challenging Melanocytic Neoplasms: Diagnosis and Management*, DOI 10.1007/978-1-4939-1444-9_7,

also from destruction of keratinocytes (innocent bystander). There is decrease of cell size with maturation along with descent in the dermis. The overlying epidermis of the halo nevus can be effaced over the junctional nests and there may be "consumption" of the epidermis, similar to melanoma [11, 12]. The depigmented areas may show a decreased number of lesional melanocytes (as detected by anti-MART-1 or anti-tyrosinase) as well as less melanin pigment in the basal keratinocytes (as detected by Fontana Masson stain). In later stages, there may be histologic features of complete dermal regression [3], with some viable single or ill-defined clusters of intraepidermal melanocytes with mild atypia; inflammatory infiltrate, markedly increased number of S100-positive intraepidermal Langerhans cells and a dermal inflammatory infiltrate without viable nevus cells. The papillary dermis is usually expanded and edematous without prominent fibrosis, and with overlying normal or elongated epidermis in contrast to a regressed melanoma where the epidermal junction and rete ridges appear flattened and there is marked fibroplasia of the dermis.

Differential Diagnosis of Halo Nevus

The most challenging differential diagnosis of the halo nevus and other benign melanocytic lesions with halo phenomenon is the malignant melanoma with regression [13, 14]. Although the association of a clinical halo with melanoma is rare, primary cutaneous melanoma can develop areas of irregular depigmentation, and complete regression can also be found in 4–8 % of patients [2, 15]. Distinguishing between halo nevus and regressed melanoma in the later stages of disease progression is not as diagnostically challenging due to the presence of dense fibrosis, telangiectasia, and varying number of melanophages in regressed melanoma. Late stage halo nevus usually lack dense fibrosis, probably related to the lack of expression of some cytokines associated with dermal fibrosis (IL-6, platelet-derived growth factor, and transforming growth factor-β (TGF-β)) and higher expression of the antifibrotic cytokine tumor necrosis factor-α (TNF-α) [16]. Some features that are useful to help distinguish between halo nevus and melanoma with regression are: (1) Clinically, the lesion of halo nevus is small, symmetrical, circumscribed and usually lacks ulceration. It is more common in young adults; (2) The inflammatory infiltrate in halo nevus is evenly distributed at both sides and at the base of the lesion. In melanoma, the infiltrate is scattered and irregular at the base of lesion (Fig. 7.1a, b); (3) The infiltrate in halo nevus is typically composed of small mature lymphocytes with a small number of macrophages, Langerhans cells, and occasional plasma cells, in contrast with melanoma, which may have numerous plasma cells [17]; (4) In halo nevus, if there are cells with hyperchromatic, irregular nuclei they are located in the junctional nests and upper portion of the nevus with a pattern of maturation toward the base of the lesion. There may be rare, superficial, mitotic figures, compared to deep-

Fig. 7.1 (continued) There is focal effacement of rete ridges. Scattered melanophages are located in papillary and superficial reticular dermis (**a**). Superficial spreading melanoma, low magnification, can mimic of halo dysplastic nevus with asymmetrical feature and irregular elongation of rete ridges and variable junctional melanocytic nests extended to the periphery of the lesion with bridging pattern, focally prominent fibrosis of subjacent papillary dermis in the center of the lesion suggestive of focal regression. The lichenoid infiltrate is unevenly distributed along the lower portion of the tumor without infiltrate into the melanocytic nests (**b**). Halo nevus, compound type: predominantly dermal melanocytic nests admix with lymphocytes throughout the lesion; minimal pagetoid upward migration is observed in the center of lesion. Scattered small lymphocytes are present in dermal melanocytic nests with mild cytological atypia. Mitotic figures are not identified in this halo nevus (**c**). Contiguous single cell proliferation and irregular junctional nests in in situ melanoma. Fibrosis, increase dermal vasculature, and scatter lymphocytes with reduced dermal invasive component are suggestive of melanoma with focal regression. There may be marked cytologic atypia with pagetoid upward migration of individual atypical melanocytes (**d, e**). Nodal metastatic melanoma demonstrating the same tumor phenotypes of epithelioid cells with markedly atypia and increased mitotic figures in the same patient (**f**)

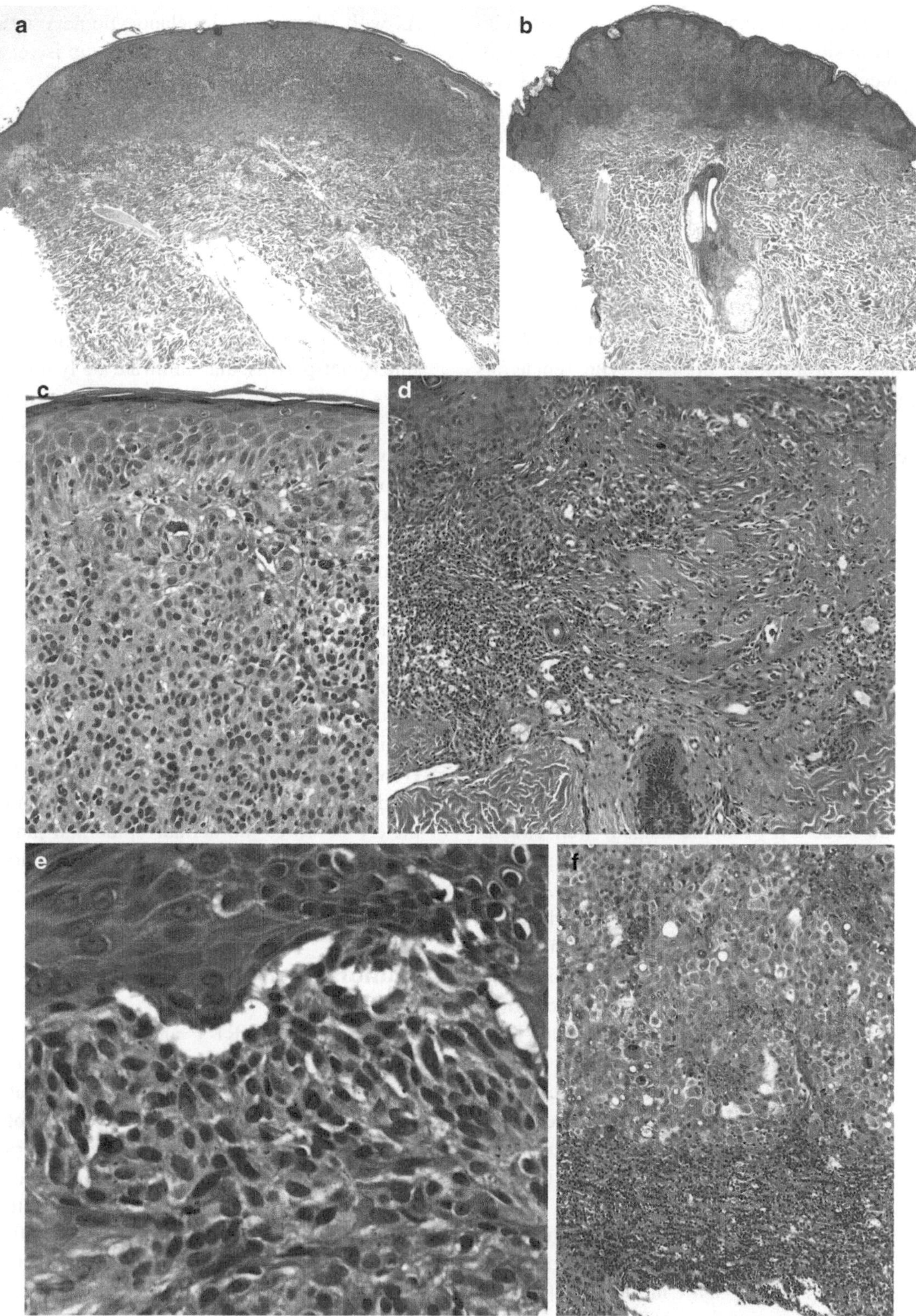

Fig. 7.1 Comparison of halo nevus (**a**) and superficial spreading melanoma with focal regression (**b**). Low magnification; exophytic, symmetrical melanocytic lesion with a dense, regularly distributed, lichenoid infiltrate that obscures the dermal–epidermal junction and infiltrates among dermal melanocytic nests and nevus cells.

dermal ones in melanoma. The presence of melanoma in situ with pagetoid upward migration of atypical melanocytes at the edges of the lesion is more consistent with melanoma (Fig. 7.1c–e); (5) Melanoma with regression may show complete absence of tumor cells and is replaced by a dense fibrotic tissue with increased vasculature and scattered melanophages. The overlying epidermis appears flattened. Halo nevus with the feature of complete regression shows decreased or diminished number of nevus cells, decreased epidermal pigmentation, and dermal melanophages without prominent fibrosis. The epidermis appears intact with normal rete ridges.

Other differential diagnosis of halo nevus includes:

- Dysplastic nevus with halo phenomenon (halo dysplastic nevus): characteristic features include remnants of a compound dysplastic melanocytic nevus with some degree of architectural disorder and cytological atypia. There may be a superposition of the features of host response typical of dysplastic nevus (lamellar and concentric fibroplasia, and concentric fibroplasia, and melanophages) (Fig. 7.2). Clinically, there may be well-defined, hypopigmented or depigmented halo.
- Spitz nevus with halo phenomenon preserves the structure of dome-shaped, well circumscribed, nested, symmetrical, with epidermal hyperplasia, compact orthokeratosis, eosinophilic globules (Kamino bodies), and clefting between junctional nests and adjacent epidermis. Nevus cells are spindled or epithelioid, with decreased size with depth in the dermis. Mitotic figures are usually superficial. There may be either diffuse labeling or loss of labeling with HMB45 as opposed to patchy positivity in the dermal component of melanoma. Molecular study may be helpful, since Spitz nevi only exceptionally may show homozygous deletion of 9p21.
- Congenital melanocytic nevus with halo phenomenon is very rare and has infrequently been associated with melanoma [18–20]. As with all congenital melanocytic nevi with unusual features, long-term follow-up is very important.
- Meyerson nevus [21, 22] is a nevus with eczematous halo reaction. This nevus is different, clinically and histologically, from halo nevi. Clinically, there is erythema (eczematous halo) surrounding the nevus without area of depigmentation. Histologic findings include epidermal acanthosis with eosinophilic spongiosis and occasional intraepidermal vesicle formation. The dermis contains a superficial perivascular infiltrate of lymphocytes, histiocytes, and eosinophils surrounding the nevus. There may be occasional cytologic atypia of melanocytes, e.g., hyperchromatic, irregular nuclei.
- Halo reaction or band-like lichenoid infiltrate has been described in other non-melanocytic lesions, such as seborrheic keratosis, lichen planus, benign lichenoid keratosis, keratoacanthoma, keloid, insect bites, dermatofibroma, basal cell carcinoma, and squamous cell carcinoma [4, 23, 24]. In all these lesions, examination of histologic features is usually sufficient to establish the correct diagnosis. However, immunohistochemistry may be needed in cases in which the infiltrate completely obscures the dermal–epidermal junction and it is unclear if there is a proliferation of melanocytes (see below).

Immunohistochemistry

In general, anti-MART-1 and HMB-45 will highlight intraepidermal and dermal melanocytes. However, it has been described that both antibodies may label keratinocytes, presumable due to transfer of melanosome antigens to keratinocytes [25]. In such cases, nuclear markers such as microphthalmia transcription factor (MiTF) or SOX-10 may be more specific. Anti-S100 antibody labels both melanocytes and Langerhans cells; the latter may be inter-

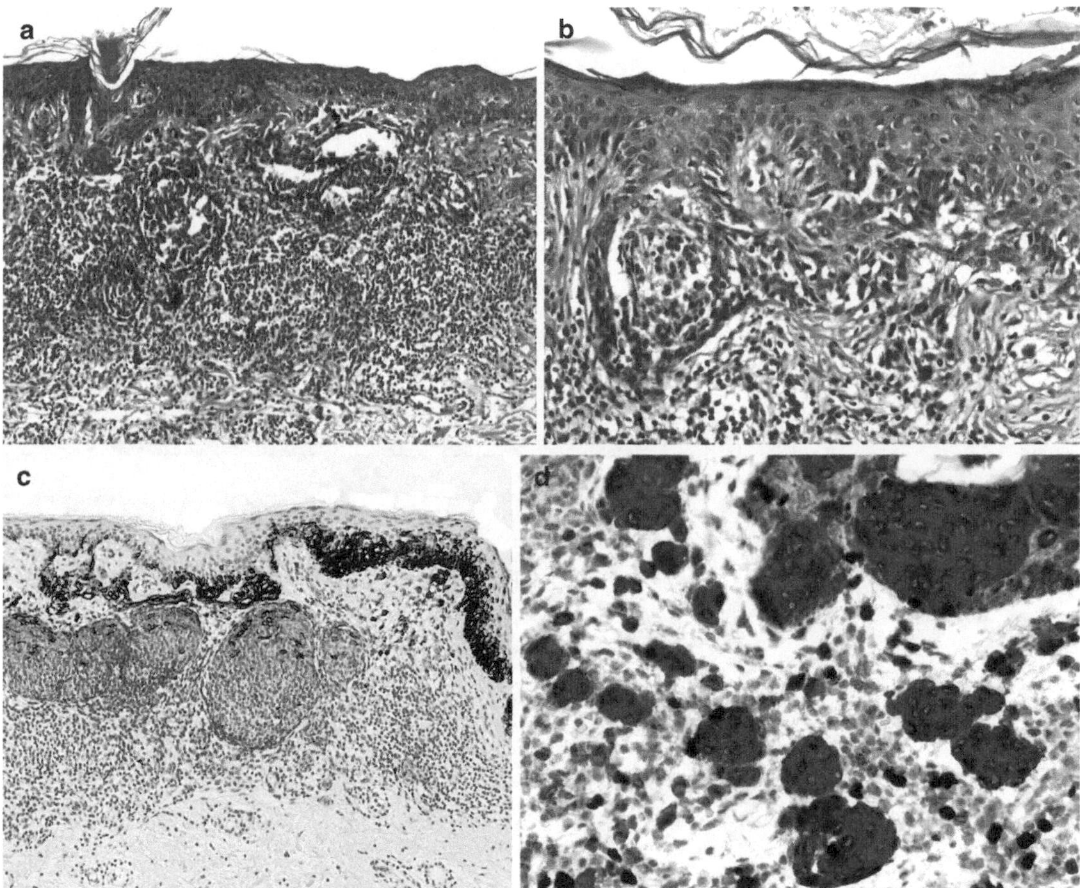

Fig. 7.2 Halo dysplastic nevus with a dense lichenoid infiltrate that obscures the dermal–epidermal junction (**a**). Features of lentiginous pattern and bridging junctional nests with mild cytological atypia and lamella fibrosis at subjacent papillary dermis are observed (**b**). HMB-45 is strongly positive in junctional melanocytic nests and intraepidermal single melanocytes, and much weaker in dermal melanocytic nests and dermal nevus cells (pattern of maturation with HMB-45 in benign nevus) (**c**). High-power; Ki67/MART-1 double immunostudy highlights minimal dermal proliferation in dermal melanocytic components (**d**)

preted to be pagetoid melanocytes (the presence of dendritic cytoplasmic processes would be unusual in pagetoid melanocytes). Loss of HMB-45 labeling with depth in the dermis suggests a pattern of maturation of the nevus cells, thus supportive of a diagnosis of nevus. The proliferative marker Ki67 (MIB-1) can be slightly increased in intradermal/junctional component of the lesion but should be negative in deep-dermal located melanocytic nests in benign nevi. The use of a double immunoreaction (anti-Ki67 and anti-MART-1) will help distinguish proliferating melanocytes from intermixed lymphocytes (Fig. 7.3).

In summary, a dense lymphocytic infiltrate at both sides of a melanocytic lesion, "halo-phenomenon" can be seen in a number of melanocytic lesions, both benign and malignant, and may or may not be associated with a clinical appearance of halo. Careful interpretation of the histologic and immunohistochemical features will allow the correct diagnosis in a vast majority of cases.

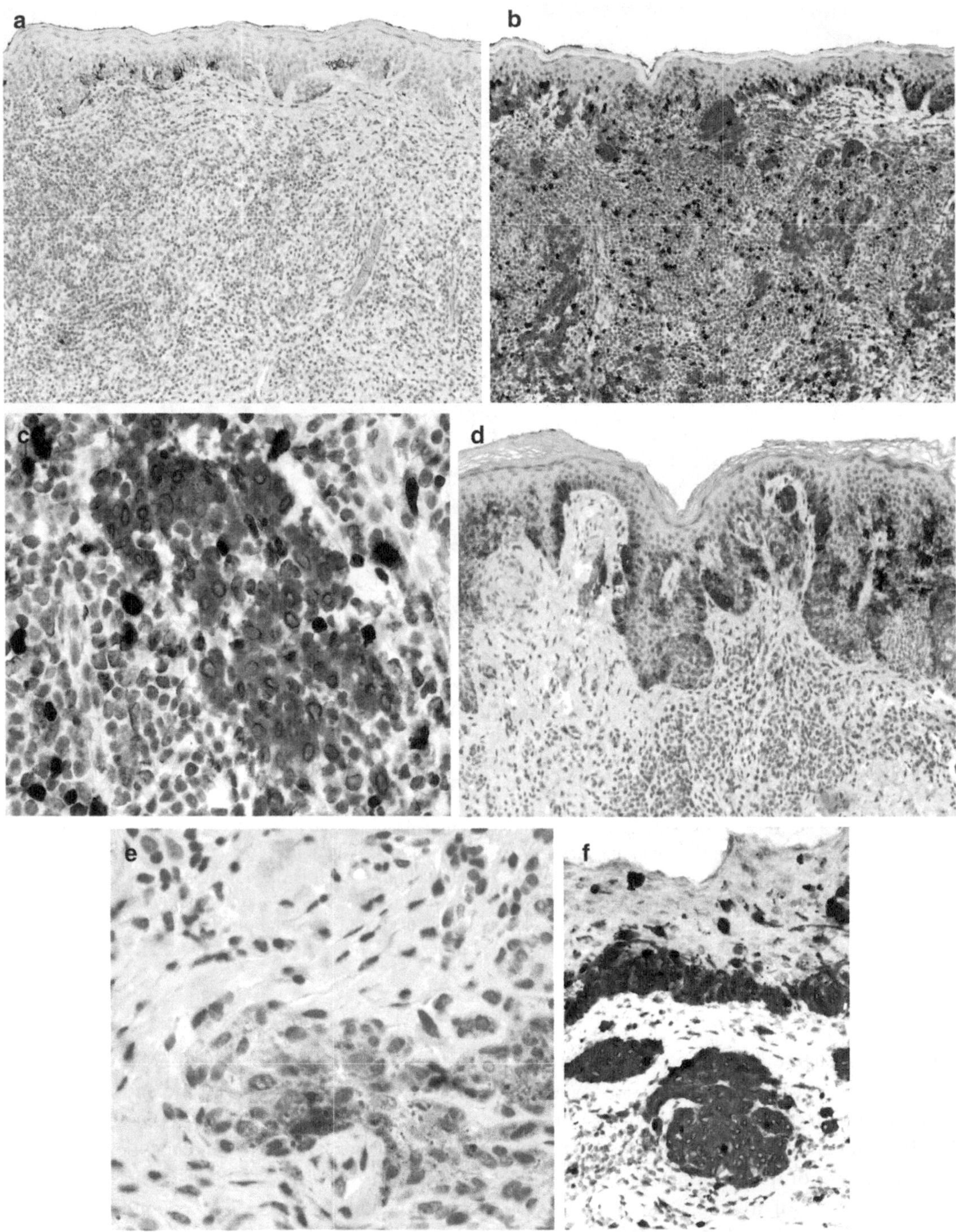

Fig. 7.3 Use of HMB-45 and Ki67/MART-1 double stain to differentiate between benign melanocytic nevi with halo reaction and melanoma with regression. HMB-45 is strongly expressed in intraepidermal nests but lost in the dermal component of halo nevus, thus consistent with maturation (**a**). In contrast, it shows patchy and irregular labeling pattern in dermal nests of melanoma (**b**, **c**), Ki67/MART-1 double stain; melanocytic component in both intraepidermal and dermal location are detected by cytoplasmic stain pattern of MART-1 without increased proliferative index in lesional melanocytes. Nuclear pattern of expression by Ki67 is detected with increased expression in basal keratinocytes and lymphocytic infiltrate but not melanocytic cells (**d**, **e**), in contrast to increased proliferative index in dermal melanocytic cells of melanoma (**f**)

References

1. Zeff RA, Freitag A, Grin CM, Grant-Kels JM. The immune response in halo nevi. J Am Acad Dermatol. 1997;37(4):620–4.
2. Rados J, Pastar Z, Lipozencic J, Ilic I, Stulhofer BD. Halo phenomenon with regression of acquired melanocytic nevi: a case report. Acta Dermatovenerol Croat. 2009;17(2):139–43.
3. Akasu R, From L, Kahn HJ. Characterization of the mononuclear infiltrate involved in regression of halo nevi. J Cutan Pathol. 1994;21(4):302–11.
4. Bayer-Garner IB, Ivan D, Schwartz MR, Tschen JA. The immunopathology of regression in benign lichenoid keratosis, keratoacanthoma and halo nevus. Clin Med Res. 2004;2(2):89–97.
5. Langer K, Konrad K. Congenital melanocytic nevi with halo phenomenon: report of two cases and a review of the literature. J Dermatol Surg Oncol. 1990; 16(4):377–80.
6. Harvell JD, Meehan SA, LeBoit PE. Spitz's nevi with halo reaction: a histopathologic study of 17 cases. J Cutan Pathol. 1997;24(10):611–9.
7. Yasaka N, Furue M, Tamaki K. Histopathological evaluation of halo phenomenon in Spitz nevus. Am J Dermatopathol. 1995;17(5):484–6.
8. Cote J, Watters AK, O'Brien EA. Halo balloon cell nevus. J Cutan Pathol. 1986;13(2):123–7.
9. Mooney MA, Barr RJ, Buxton MG. Halo nevus or halo phenomenon? A study of 142 cases. J Cutan Pathol. 1995;22(4):342–8.
10. Denianke KS, Gottlieb GJ. Granulomatous inflammation in nevi undergoing regression (halo phenomenon): a report of 6 cases. Am J Dermatopathol. 2008; 30(3):233–5.
11. Hantschke M, Bastian BC, LeBoit PE. Consumption of the epidermis: a diagnostic criterion for the differential diagnosis of melanoma and Spitz nevus. Am J Surg Pathol. 2004;28(12):1621–5.
12. Walters RF, Groben PA, Busam K, et al. Consumption of the epidermis: a criterion in the differential diagnosis of melanoma and dysplastic nevi that is associated with increasing breslow depth and ulceration. Am J Dermatopathol. 2007;29(6):527–33.
13. Berger AC, McClay EF, Toporcer M, Wolchok JD, Morris GJ. Completely regressed cutaneous melanocytic lesion: was it benign or was it malignant? Semin Oncol. 2009;36(5):375–9.
14. McCardle TW, Messina JL, Sondak VK. Completely regressed cutaneous melanocytic lesion revisited. Semin Oncol. 2009;36(6):498–503.
15. High WA, Stewart D, Wilbers CR, Cockerell CJ, Hoang MP, Fitzpatrick JE. Completely regressed primary cutaneous malignant melanoma with nodal and/or visceral metastases: a report of 5 cases and assessment of the literature and diagnostic criteria. J Am Acad Dermatol. 2005;53(1):89–100.
16. Moretti S, Spallanzani A, Pinzi C, Prignano F, Fabbri P. Fibrosis in regressing melanoma versus nonfibrosis in halo nevus upon melanocyte disappearance: could it be related to a different cytokine microenvironment? J Cutan Pathol. 2007;34(4):301–8.
17. Mascaro JM, Molgo M, Castel T, Castro J. Plasmacells within the infiltrate of primary cutaneous malignant-melanoma of the skin—a confirmation of its histoprognostic value. Am J Dermatopathol. 1987; 9(6):497–9.
18. Itin PH, Lautenschlager S. Acquired leukoderma in congenital pigmented nevus associated with vitiligo-like depigmentation. Pediatr Dermatol. 2002;19(1):73–5.
19. Garcia RL, Gano SE. Halo congenital nevus. Cutis. 1979;23(3):338–9.
20. Epstein WL, Sagebeil R, Spitler L, Wybran J, Reed WB, Blois MS. Halo nevi and melanoma. JAMA. 1973;225(4):373–7.
21. Nicholls DS, Mason GH. Halo dermatitis around a melanocytic naevus: Meyerson's naevus. Br J Dermatol. 1988;118(1):125–9.
22. Elenitsas R, Halpern AC. Eczematous halo reaction in atypical nevi. J Am Acad Dermatol. 1996;34(2 Pt 2): 357–61.
23. Tegner E, Bjornberg A, Jonsson N. Halo dermatitis around tumours. Acta Derm Venereol. 1990;70(1): 31–4.
24. Schofield C, Weedon D, Kumar S. Dermatofibroma and halo dermatitis. Australas J Dermatol. 2012; 53(2):145–7.
25. Arumi-Uria M, McNutt NS, Finnerty B. Grading of atypia in nevi: correlation with melanoma risk. Mod Pathol. 2003;16(8):764–71.

8 Nevoid Malignant Melanoma vs. Melanocytic Nevus

Jon A. Reed, Victor G. Prieto, and Christopher R. Shea

Nevoid malignant melanoma is one of the most challenging diagnoses among cutaneous melanocytic lesions. As its name implies, this form of melanoma resembles a melanocytic nevus. Unlike the almost ubiquitous melanocytic nevus, however, nevoid melanoma is uncommon, representing approximately 1 % of all cutaneous primary invasive melanomas [1]. The low rate of occurrence and the microscopic similarity to ordinary nevi make diagnosis of nevoid melanoma even more challenging for those who evaluate few biopsies of cutaneous melanocytic lesions. This chapter will focus on the clinical, microscopic, and immunohistochemical features that help to distinguish nevoid malignant melanomas from benign melanocytic nevi. Discussion will follow including an expanded differential diagnosis with several rare variants of benign nevi with histological changes that render their distinction from nevoid melanoma even more difficult.

J.A. Reed, M.S., M.D. (✉)
Baylor College of Medicine,
1 Baylor Plaza, Houston, TX 77030, USA

CellNetix Pathology & Laboratories,
1124 Columbia St., Suite 200, Seattle,
WA 98117, USA
e-mail: jreed@bcm.edu; jreed@cellnetix.com

V.G. Prieto, M.D., Ph.D.
MD Anderson Cancer Center, University of Houston,
1515 Holcombe Blvd., Unit 85, Houston,
TX 77030, USA

C.R. Shea, M.D.
University of Chicago Medicine,
5841 S. Maryland Ave., MC 5067, L502,
Chicago, IL 60637, USA

Nevoid Malignant Melanoma

Clinical Features

Nevoid malignant melanoma appears to affect both males and females of any age, although most patients are in their fourth or fifth decade. Nevoid melanoma usually presents as a slowly enlarging papule or nodule involving the trunk, proximal extremities, or less commonly the face. Individual lesions are well circumscribed, but the degree of pigmentation is inconsistent and may be uniform, variable, or absent for a given patient. In many cases, the lesion is amelanotic and a melanocytic lesion is not suspected clinically.

Initial studies suggested that this form of melanoma had a somewhat better prognosis compared to other more common histological subtypes, but subsequent authors have disputed this point [1–5]. Long-term clinical follow-up data are scarce given the low prevalence of these lesions. Comparisons between studies of nevoid melanoma are further confounded by the variable diagnostic terminology used in the literature. For example, lesions called "minimal deviation melanoma" [3] were further subcategorized based upon their histological resemblance to specific variant nevi (Spitz, halo, cellular blue, etc.) [6, 7].

C.R. Shea et al. (eds.), *Pathology of Challenging Melanocytic Neoplasms: Diagnosis and Management*,
DOI 10.1007/978-1-4939-1444-9_8, © Springer Science+Business Media New York 2015

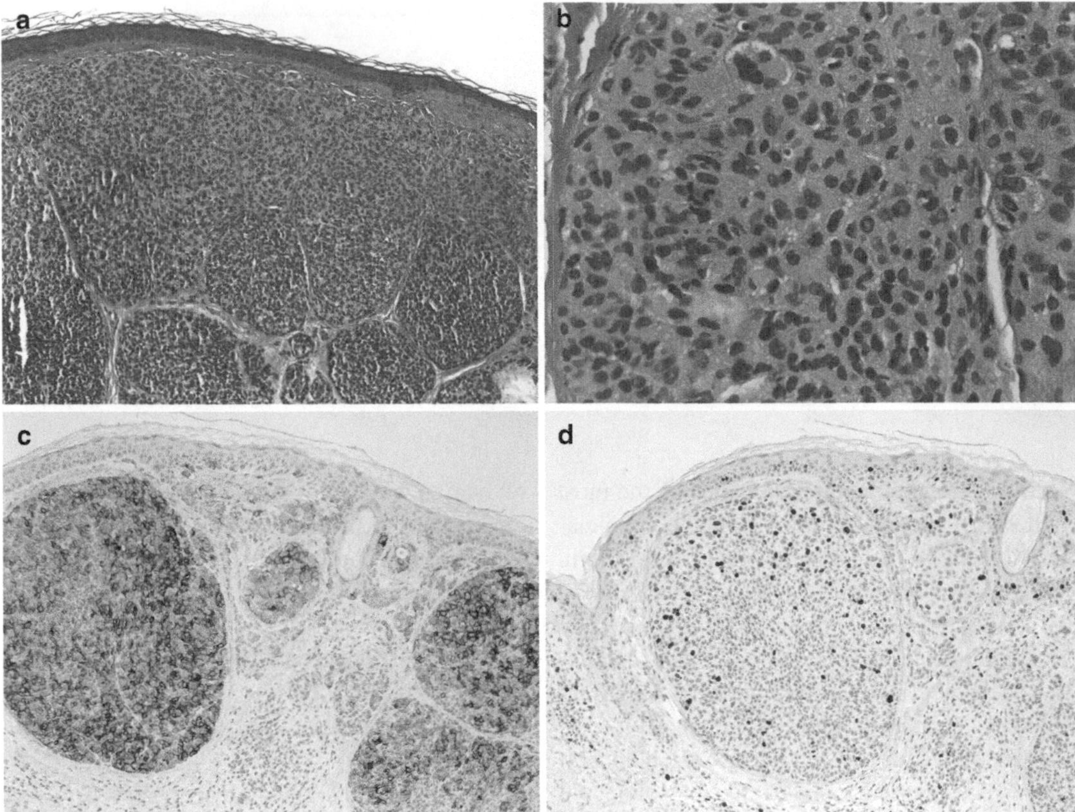

Fig. 8.1 Nevoid malignant melanoma. (**a**) The lesion displays circumscription, but cellular crowding (×10). (**b**) Note nuclear pleomorphism. Mitotic figures are scattered in the lesion including its base (×40). (**c**) Expression of gp100 in a patchy pattern (×20). (**d**) Increased Ki-67 expression toward the base of the lesion (×20)

Others use the term "nevoid melanoma" to refer to lesions that resemble ordinary compound or predominantly intradermal nevi (the subject of this chapter) and/or Spitz nevi [5, 8–10]. The terms "Spitzoid melanoma" and "atypical Spitz tumor" also have been used and their relationship to, and differentiation from, Spitz nevus are more thoroughly discussed in Chap. 7 [11]. Furthermore, it is impossible to glean from the data presented in many studies of malignant melanoma whether the nevoid type was excluded or unrecognized and grouped together with other histological subtypes. Given the lack of consensus on the biological behavior of these lesions, treatment recommendations have largely remained the same as those for other histological types of primary invasive melanoma of the same clinical stage.

Microscopic Features

As stated above, this form of malignant melanoma histologically resembles an ordinary melanocytic nevus. Compound and purely intradermal variants have been described. The lesions are usually well circumscribed and the intraepidermal component may be quite small, rendering it practically indistinguishable from a predominantly intradermal melanocytic nevus at low magnification (Fig. 8.1a). These features have led some to suggest that nevoid melanoma may be a variant or precursor of the nodular subtype of melanoma, another form that often lacks an identifiable intraepidermal portion [12].

Dermal nevoid melanoma cells may be predominantly nested or may form larger confluent sheets, the latter feature providing a valuable clue

Table 8.1 Microscopic features that help to distinguish nevoid malignant melanoma from ordinary melanocytic nevus

Diagnosis	Maturation	Hypercellular	Atypical	Mitoses
Nevoid melanoma	+ (Paradoxical)/–	+	+	+ (Including base)
Ordinary nevus	+	–	–	+ (Rare, superficial)/–
Ancient nevus	+	–	+	+ (Rare, superficial)/–
Nevus in pregnancy	+	+	–	+
Invasive melanoma associated with a nevus	+ (Nevus) – (Melanoma)	– (Nevus) + (Melanoma)	– (Nevus) + (Melanoma)	– (Nevus) + (Melanoma)

to the true diagnosis even at low magnification. In some cases, superficial nests of melanocytes may transition to smaller nests and more widely dispersed single cells in the deeper dermis [13]. This so-called "paradoxical maturation" pattern closely resembles the dermal architectural pattern typical of ordinary acquired melanocytic nevi (see below) and is perhaps the most misleading microscopic feature in these lesions. An associated dermal inflammatory cell infiltrate may or may not be present.

Fortunately, several important microscopic features help to distinguish nevoid melanoma from ordinary melanocytic nevi (summarized in Table 8.1). Most of these features become more apparent upon observation of the lesion at higher magnifications (Fig. 8.1b). First, nests of dermal melanocytes appear to be hypercellular compared to those of ordinary nevi. Unlike ordinary nevi, nevoid melanoma cells are typically tightly apposed (cellular crowding). This characteristic may be present throughout the lesion, but is lost toward the base of the lesion in tumors with paradoxical maturation. Second, nevoid melanoma cells display a greater degree of nuclear pleomorphism compared to melanocytic nevus cells. Nevoid melanoma cells often contain enlarged, hyperchromatic nuclei with irregular contours and variably prominent nucleoli. Third, nevoid melanoma cells display an increased proliferation rate, with mitotic figures scattered throughout the lesion, including the base. Nevoid melanomas may contain atypical mitotic figures, but their presence is not required for diagnosis. The presence of deep mitotic figures in a melanocytic lesion is of considerable importance since ordinary nevi lack this feature. Despite each of these important histological differences, nevoid melanomas may escape detection without the aid of additional studies.

Immunohistochemical Features

As discussed in Chap. 4, evaluation of the dermal component of a melanocytic lesion for evidence of maturation and for proliferative activity may be useful for histologically challenging lesions. These considerations are especially true for nevoid melanoma [12].

Immunohistochemical labeling for the melanosomal glycoprotein gp100 (using antibody clone HMB-45) often shows an altered pattern in nevoid melanoma, even in lesions that display paradoxical maturation (Fig. 8.1c). Labeling may be completely absent, uniformly present throughout the lesion, or limited to a subpopulation of cells scattered in a haphazard or patchy pattern. Intensity of immunolabeling may be uniform, but often is variable in different areas of the lesion. The intraepidermal component (if present) may be labeled, thereby highlighting melanocytes in more superficial layers and making the diagnosis of melanoma more straightforward [14].

Labeling for the cell cycle marker Ki-67 (using antibody clone MIB-1) often is notably increased, highlighting the nuclei of cells throughout the lesion including its base (Fig. 8.1d). The percentage of labeled cells may be highly variable among lesions, but the distribution of labeling usually is haphazard and not limited to cells in the superficial dermis. Areas with increased numbers of labeled cells (hot spots) are common. As such, the pattern or distribution of labeling seems to be more important than the actual percentage of cells labeled. Similar observations have been made using another marker of cellular proliferation, proliferating cell nuclear antigen (PCNA) [12].

Melanocytic Nevus

Clinical Features

Ordinary melanocytic nevi are acquired lesions that typically appear early in life. Nevi may occur at any anatomic site affecting males and females alike. One epidemiologic study found an average of 36 ordinary nevi (2 mm in diameter or greater) on Caucasian patients who visited a dermatology clinic, but acknowledged that the number is highly variable among individuals [15]. Nevi may present as pigmented macules and papules that over time may become less pigmented. Most ordinary nevi are small, symmetrical, have a smooth border, and are evenly pigmented.

It is generally accepted that ordinary acquired nevi undergo a process of growth first within the epidermis (junctional nevus), followed by penetration into the dermis (compound nevus) [16]. Over time, the intraepidermal portion is lost and the lesion resides wholly in the dermis (intradermal nevus). This process usually is accompanied by gradual loss of pigmentation and by elevation of the lesion as melanocytes expand the dermis. Over the course of many years, some nevi undergo complete involution.

Microscopic Features

The clinical evolution of an ordinary nevus is associated with changes in its microscopic appearance as well. Junctional nevi contain melanocytes disposed singly and/or grouped into nests within the epidermis. The melanocytes have either an epithelioid or dendritic appearance. Many cells contain abundant cytoplasmic melanin. Nuclei may be enlarged and contain nucleoli, but are uniform in appearance and do not display significant pleomorphism or hyperchromasia. Compound and intradermal nevi display characteristic features of so-called "maturation" in the dermis. Nests of epithelioid melanocytes in the superficial dermis transition into areas with smaller nests and more dispersed smaller epithelioid or fusiform cells in the deeper dermis (Fig. 8.2a). Individual nest do not exhibit cellular crowding, and larger, confluent sheets of cells are uncommon. The change in architecture and cytologic morphology with progressive descent into the dermis is accompanied by visible loss of cytoplasmic melanin and by reduction in cellular size (Fig. 8.2b). Although a few mitotic figures may be present in the superficial dermal component of a nevus, few if any are present in the deeper portion. One study found that the nevi of younger patients were more likely to contain superficial dermal mitotic figures [17]. Ordinary benign melanocytic nevi are thus distinguished from nevoid melanomas by their lack of a sheet-like growth pattern, and by their cellular crowding, significant nuclear pleomorphism, and low mitotic rate. The only possible exception is that of nevi occurring in pregnant women, since they may have mitotic figures in the lesion (please see below).

Immunohistochemical Features

In comparison to nevoid melanoma, ordinary nevi display an immunophenotype of maturation and low proliferative activity in their dermal component. Labeling for gp100 is limited to the intraepidermal (if present) and superficial nested, more pigmented dermal portions of the lesion (Fig. 8.2c). Patchy labeling throughout the lesion or labeling of cells toward the base is not observed. Importantly, any labeling present toward the base of a nevus should be interpreted with extreme caution since some melanophages may display immunoreactivity for gp100 as well as other melanosomal glycoproteins [18]. Similarly, labeling for Ki-67 is largely restricted to melanocytes in the epidermis and in the superficial dermal nests. Labeling (if present) is symmetrically distributed across the superficial portion. Very few, if any, melanocytes toward the base of a nevus are labeled (Fig. 8.2d) [14].

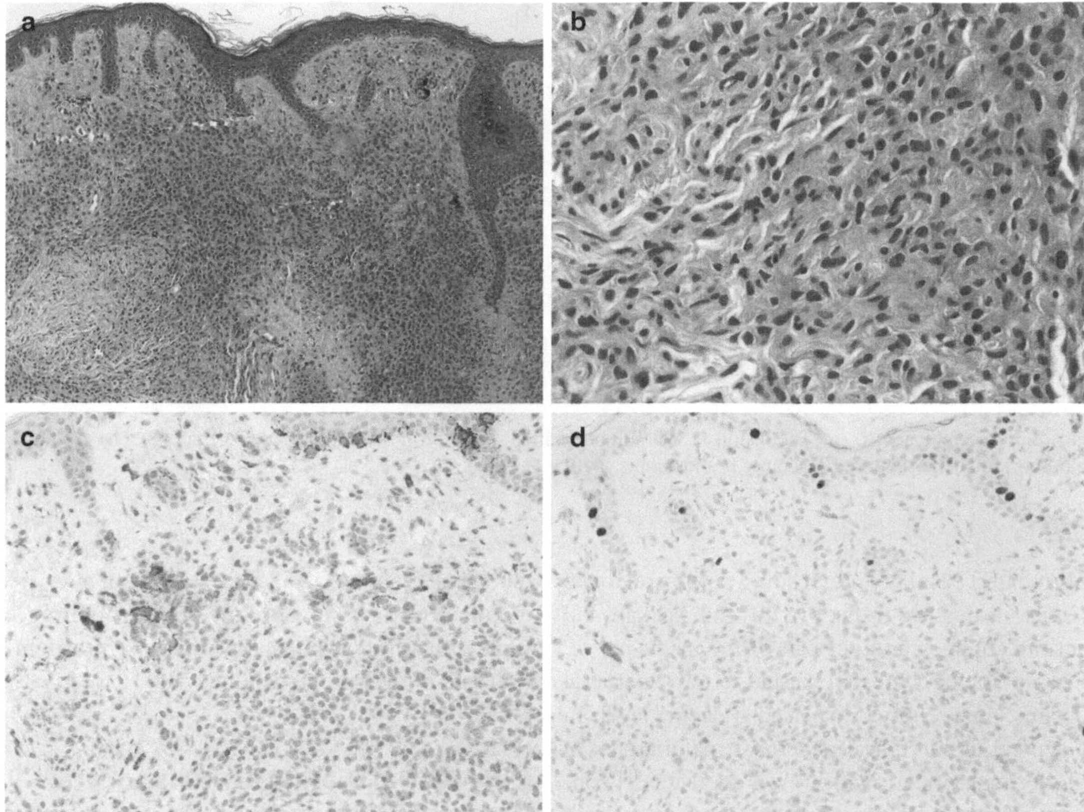

Fig. 8.2 Ordinary benign melanocytic nevus. (**a**) The lesion displays circumscription and maturation, and lacks cellular crowding (×10). (**b**) Maturation with progressive descent into the dermis (×20). (**c**) Expression of gp100 is seen only in the superficial dermis (×20). (**d**) Ki-67 expression is limited to only a few cells (×20)

Differential Diagnosis: Melanocytic Nevus with "Ancient" Change

Clinical Features

Over time, ordinary melanocytic nevi may undergo changes that make their distinction from nevoid melanoma even more difficult. One example of this phenomenon is the so-called "ancient nevus" named for its histological similarities to ancient schwannoma [19, 20]. These nevi are almost exclusively long-standing papules on chronically sun-damaged skin. Head and neck are the most frequent sites of involvement. Based upon the usual clinical presentation and biological behavior of these lesions, most consider this histological change to be the result of cellular senescence within an otherwise ordinary benign melanocytic nevus.

Microscopic Features

Observation at low magnification usually reveals the architectural features typical of a predominantly intradermal nevus in a background related to chronic sun exposure. These background actinic changes include variable degrees of epidermal atrophy, increased basal layer pigmentation, venous telangiectasia, perilesional collagen sclerosis, and solar elastosis (Fig. 8.3a). Intraepidermal melanocytes may be increased in number and uniformly distributed along the

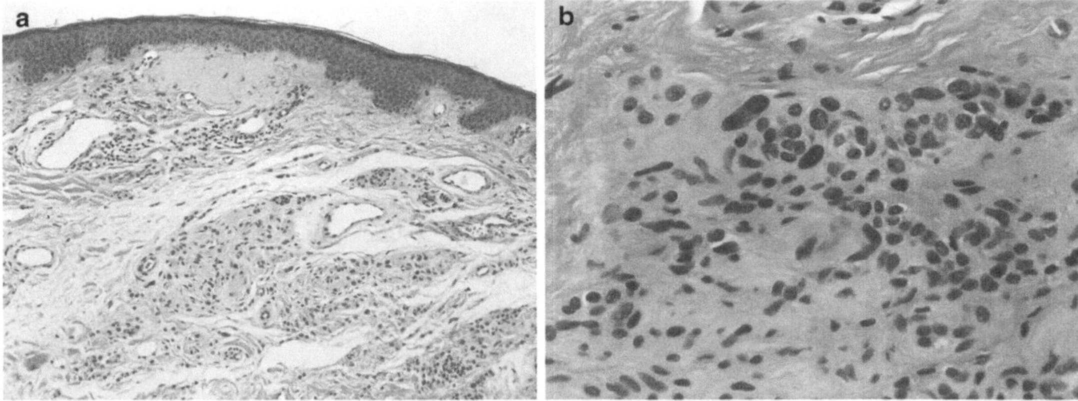

Fig. 8.3 Ancient nevus. (**a**) The lesion is well circumscribed. Note prominent actinic changes (×10). (**b**) Atypical, pleomorphic cells scattered randomly in the dermis (×40)

pigmented basal layer extending peripheral to the nevus, a feature reflective of the background actinic changes and not part of the nevus per se. Dermal melanocytes are nested in the superficial dermis, but are more dispersed at deeper levels in a typical architectural pattern of maturation. On higher magnification; however, ancient nevi contain scattered enlarged pleomorphic cells with hyperchromatic nuclei similar to those seen in nevoid melanoma (Fig. 8.3b). Nucleoli and/or nuclear pseudo-inclusions may be present in the atypical cells. The atypical melanocytes are haphazardly distributed in the lesion, giving the appearance of an altered pattern of maturation. However, unlike nevoid melanoma, ancient/senescent nevi are less cellular, and the atypical cells fewer in number. Few if any mitotic figures are present in the lesion, and those present are located in the upper regions of the lesion, a feature compatible with the theory that these lesions are in a state of cellular senescence.

Immunohistochemical Features

Although ancient/senescent nevi are less cellular and contain fewer atypical cells, their degree of cytologic atypia may be so severe as to warrant serious consideration of a nevoid melanoma or of a melanoma arising in association with a preexisting benign melanocytic nevus (see below). Fortunately, the gp100 and Ki-67 immunohistochemical features of ancient/senescent nevi are identical to those of ordinary nevi, exhibiting a typical maturation phenotype and low proliferation rate in the dermal melanocytes.

Differential Diagnosis: Melanocytic Nevus in Pregnancy

Clinical Features

Numerous studies have documented that long-standing ordinary melanocytic nevi may undergo dramatic clinical changes during pregnancy [21]. Nevi in pregnancy may grow rapidly, develop irregular borders, and/or display irregularities of pigmentation [22]. These changes are particularly concerning given that malignant melanoma during pregnancy is often biologically more aggressive. Many believe that these clinical and biological features are related to hormonal fluctuations associated with normal pregnancy. Identification of estrogen receptor-beta expression by melanocytes and melanoma cells has given support to this theory [23].

Microscopic Features

These lesions present perhaps the most significant challenge in the differential diagnosis of nevoid melanoma. Pregnancy-associated melanocytic

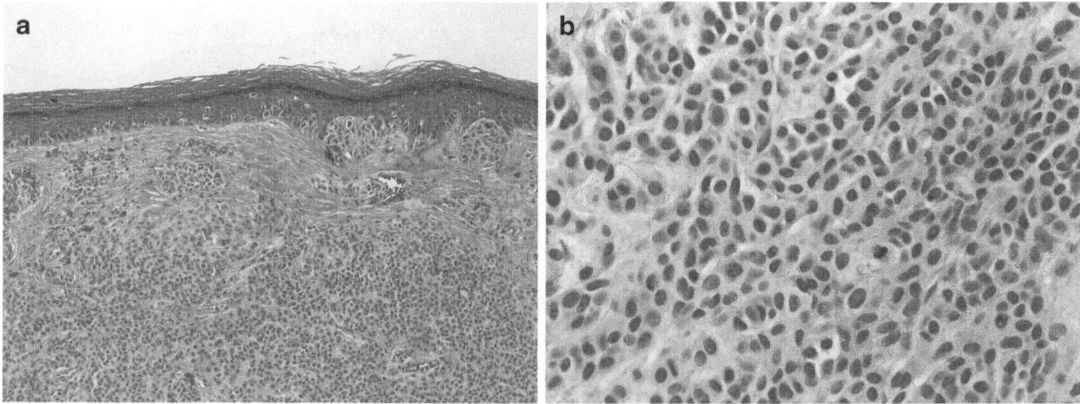

Fig. 8.4 Nevus associated with pregnancy. (**a**) The lesion is asymmetrical and hypercellular (×10). (**b**) Cells do not display significant cytologic atypia or pleomorphism, but mitotic figures are present (×40)

nevi may display some of the aforementioned microscopic features of both ordinary nevus and of nevoid melanoma. Specifically, these lesions may show significant cellular crowding having an appearance very similar to nevoid melanoma at low magnification (Fig. 8.4a). On higher magnification; however, melanocytes usually do not show the degree of nuclear pleomorphism found in nevoid melanoma. Hyperchromasia and irregular contours are not pronounced in these lesions. Unfortunately, mitotic figures may be scattered throughout the lesion (Fig. 8.4b), but atypical mitotic figures should not be present.

Immunohistochemical Features

Labeling for gp100 typically has the pattern of an ordinary nevus with labeling restricted to the intraepidermal and superficial dermal components. Labeling for Ki-67; however, is more reflective of the increased mitotic rate seen in these nevi [24]. An increased percentage of melanocytes are labeled and, more importantly, hot spots may be present making the distinction from nevoid melanoma on this basis alone practically impossible. In such cases, some authors have advocated that these lesions be considered to have indeterminate biological potential and be treated like an invasive melanoma reporting histological attributes important for pathological staging.

Differential Diagnosis: Malignant Melanoma Associated with a Melanocytic Nevus

Clinical Features

Another important differential diagnosis for nevoid melanoma is malignant melanoma arising in association with a pre-existing nevus. A large, multi-institutional study found that approximately 30 % of all sporadic, cutaneous primary invasive melanomas are associated with a pre-existing nevus [25]. The pre-existing nevi are equally distributed between ordinary and atypical (dysplastic) types. Melanoma that develops in association with a pre-existing acquired nevus often presents as a changing pigmented lesion. In many cases, the lesion had been present for many years before a change in clinical appearance. These lesions may present as a nevus that has increased in size, developed an irregular border, asymmetry, and/or variation in color including focal loss of pigmentation.

Microscopic Features

Melanomas that arise in association with pre-existing melanocytic nevi usually have one of two architectural patterns. Both of these patterns differ from the microscopic features of nevoid melanoma.

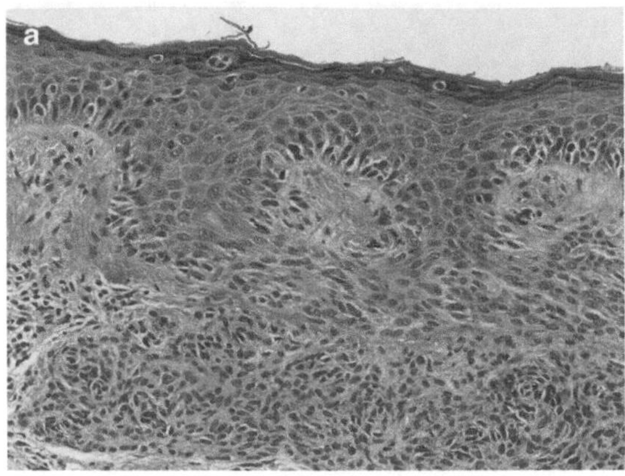

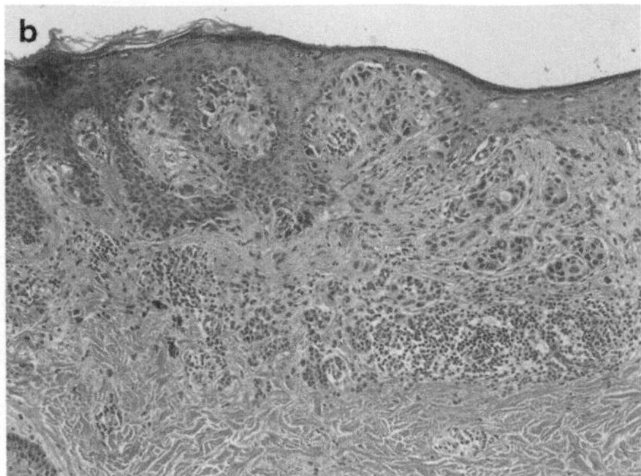

Fig. 8.5 Malignant melanoma associated with a pre-existing melanocytic nevus. (**a**) Melanoma in situ overlying benign nevus. Note the atypical melanocytes in superficial epidermal layers. Dermal melanocytes lack significant cytologic atypia (×20). (**b**) Invasive melanoma associated with a nevus. Note the biphenotypic melanocytes in the dermis. Clusters of pleomorphic, large, cytologically atypical cells (*) are present adjacent to clusters of smaller, less atypical nevus cells that display features associated with maturation with progressive descent (×20)

In the first pattern, atypical melanocytes are restricted to the epidermis and display architectural features typical of malignant melanoma in situ (Fig. 8.5a). The dermal portion of the lesion; however, has features of an ordinary melanocytic nevus. Dermal melanocytes lack significant cytologic atypia and display maturation pattern typical of a nevus. Mitotic figures are not present in the dermal component.

The second pattern represents acquisition of invasive melanoma within a pre-existing nevus and may be considered progression from the first architectural pattern. In this case the dermal component of the lesion appears biphenotypic, having areas with cytologically atypical invasive melanoma cells surrounded by residual ordinary nevus cells (Fig. 8.5b). In this pattern, invasive melanoma usually can be distinguished from the associated nevus by its difference in cytomorphology. If this distinction is clear, the depth of invasion is measured to the base of the more cytologically atypical component. Occasionally, the invasive component may display a more subtle degree of cytologic atypia or be partially obscured by an associated inflammatory cell infiltrate. In this case, immunohistochemistry may allow better distinction of the boundary between the invasive melanoma and the nevus.

Melanomas that arise in association with congenital nevi may exhibit a third architectural pattern. These rare lesions may arise entirely within the dermal portion of the nevus and are characterized by an expanding nodule having atypical cells with high mitotic rate and foci of cellular necrosis. The degree of cytologic atypia and the presence of necrosis help to distinguish this form of melanoma from a benign proliferative nodule within an otherwise ordinary benign congenital nevus [26–30].

Immunohistochemical Features

Immunohistochemistry may be useful to better delineate melanoma from an associated melanocytic nevus. Certainly this distinction has important implications for determining the depth of invasion and thus the pathologic staging of the lesion. For the first architectural pattern (melanoma in situ overlying a nevus), expression of gp100 and of Ki-67 in the dermis is identical to that observed in ordinary nevi. Labeling for gp100 also will highlight atypical melanocytes scattered in the superficial layers of the epidermis facilitating the diagnosis of overlying melanoma in situ.

In the second architectural pattern, labeling for gp100 and for Ki-67 may help to better define the boundary between the invasive melanoma and the residual nevus. In theory, the lesion should exhibit the two distinct labeling patterns for areas containing melanoma cells and those with nevus cells. In practice; however, labeling for gp100 may have less value if the invasive component is limited to the superficial dermis where nevus cells also may be immunoreactive. Similarly, labeling for Ki-67 should be interpreted with caution in inflamed areas that have a significant number of labeled lymphocytes. Given these limitations, several studies have focused on other markers that may better delineate the boundary between the melanoma and nevus with promising results [31–33]. Recently, fluorescence in situ hybridization (FISH) has been used to better define the invasive component within these diagnostically challenging transitional lesions [34, 35].

Conclusions

The diagnosis of nevoid malignant melanoma may be quite difficult, especially for those unaccustomed to interpreting pigmented lesions. Careful consideration of the detailed clinical information, microscopic features at low and high magnifications, and the selective use of immunohistochemistry may help to obviate some of the diagnostic pitfalls presented by this rare form of melanoma. Despite all of these efforts; however, some lesions cannot be definitively classified as a nevoid melanoma or as a benign melanocytic nevus. In such cases, it should be acknowledged that some melanocytic lesions currently defy classification and are best considered as biologically indeterminate [11, 36, 37]. In these rare cases, molecular cytogenetic testing may provide valuable information favoring one diagnosis over the other. To date, such analyses have not been widely performed specifically on nevoid melanomas. Recently, two small series of nevoid melanomas were shown to harbor cytogenetic abnormalities typical of other melanomas using FISH, but these lesions were not considered to be ambiguous on routine histological evaluation [34, 38]. Clearly, larger series of nevoid melanomas need to be studied to determine if a specific set of chromosomal aberrations could serve as a diagnostic marker in lesions that are indeterminate by routine histology and by immunohistochemistry.

References

1. Stas M, van den Oord JJ, Garmyn M, Degreef H, De Wever I, De Wolf-Peeters C. Minimal deviation and/or naevoid melanoma: is recognition worthwhile? A clinicopathological study of nine cases. Melanoma Res. 2000;10:371–80.
2. Muhlbauer JE, Margolis RJ, Mihm MCJ, Reed RJ. Minimal deviation melanoma: a histologic variant of cutaneous malignant melanoma in its vertical growth phase. J Invest Dermatol. 1983;80(Suppl):63s–5s.
3. Barr LH, Goldman LI, Solomon JA, Sanusi DI, Reed RJ. Minimal deviation melanoma. Surg Gynecol Obstet. 1984;159:546–8.
4. Schmoeckel C, Castro CE, Braun-Falco O. Nevoid malignant melanoma. Arch Dermatol Res. 1985;277: 362–9.
5. Wong TY, Suster S, Duncan LM, Mihm MCJ. Nevoid melanoma: a clinicopathological study of seven cases of malignant melanoma mimicking spindle and epithelioid cell nevus and verrucous dermal nevus. Hum Pathol. 1995;26:171–9.
6. Reed RJ, Martin P. Variants of melanoma. Semin Cutan Med Surg. 1997;16:137–58.
7. Reed RJ, Webb SV, Clark WHJ. Minimal deviation melanoma (halo nevus variant). Am J Surg Pathol. 1990;14:53–68.
8. Zembowicz A, McCusker M, Chiarelli C, et al. Morphological analysis of nevoid melanoma: a study of 20 cases with a review of the literature. Am J Dermatopathol. 2001;23:167–75.
9. McNutt NS. "Triggered trap": nevoid malignant melanoma. Semin Diagn Pathol. 1998;15:203–9.
10. Wong TY, Duncan LM, Mihm MCJ. Melanoma mimicking dermal and Spitz's nevus ("nevoid" melanoma). Semin Surg Oncol. 1993;9:188–93.
11. Barnhill RL, Cerroni L, Cook M, et al. State of the art, nomenclature, and points of consensus and controversy concerning benign melanocytic lesions: outcome of an international workshop. Adv Anat Pathol. 2010;17:73–90.
12. McNutt NS, Urmacher C, Hakimian J, Hoss DM, Lugo J. Nevoid malignant melanoma: morphologic patterns and immunohistochemical reactivity. J Cutan Pathol. 1995;22:502–17.
13. Ruhoy SM, Prieto VG, Eliason SL, Grichnik JM, Burchette JLJ, Shea CR. Malignant melanoma with paradoxical maturation. Am J Surg Pathol. 2000;24: 1600–14.

14. Prieto VG, Shea CR. Immunohistochemistry of melanocytic proliferations. Arch Pathol Lab Med. 2011;135:853–9.
15. Holly EA, Kelly JW, Shpall SN, Chiu SH. Number of melanocytic nevi as a major risk factor for malignant melanoma. J Am Acad Dermatol. 1987;17:459–68.
16. Lund HZ, Stobbe GD. The natural history of the pigmented nevus; factors of age and anatomic location. Am J Pathol. 1949;25:1117–55. incl 4 pl.
17. Ruhoy SM, Kolker SE, Murry TC. Mitotic activity within dermal melanocytes of benign melanocytic nevi: a study of 100 cases with clinical follow-up. Am J Dermatopathol. 2011;33:167–72.
18. Trejo O, Reed JA, Prieto VG. Atypical cells in human cutaneous re-excision scars for melanoma express p75NGFR, C56/N-CAM and GAP-43: evidence of early Schwann cell differentiation. J Cutan Pathol. 2002;29:397–406.
19. Kerl H, Soyer HP, Cerroni L, Wolf IH, Ackerman AB. Ancient melanocytic nevus. Semin Diagn Pathol. 1998;15:210–5.
20. Kerl H, Wolf IH, Kerl K, Cerroni L, Kutzner H, Argenyi ZB. Ancient melanocytic nevus: a simulator of malignant melanoma. Am J Dermatopathol. 2011; 33:127–30.
21. Driscoll MS, Grant-Kels JM. Nevi and melanoma in the pregnant woman. Clin Dermatol. 2009;27: 116–21.
22. Zampino MR, Corazza M, Costantino D, Mollica G, Virgili A. Are melanocytic nevi influenced by pregnancy? A dermoscopic evaluation. Dermatol Surg. 2006;32:1497–504.
23. Nading MA, Nanney LB, Boyd AS, Ellis DL. Estrogen receptor beta expression in nevi during pregnancy. Exp Dermatol. 2008;17:489–97.
24. Chan MP, Chan MM, Tahan SR. Melanocytic nevi in pregnancy: histologic features and Ki-67 proliferation index. J Cutan Pathol. 2010;37:843–51.
25. Gruber SB, Barnhill RL, Stenn KS, Roush GC. Nevomelanocytic proliferations in association with cutaneous malignant melanoma: a multivariate analysis. J Am Acad Dermatol. 1989;21:773–80.
26. Hendrickson MR, Ross JC. Neoplasms arising in congenital giant nevi: morphologic study of seven cases and a review of the literature. Am J Surg Pathol. 1981;5:109–35.
27. Kiyohara T, Sawai T, Kumakiri M. Proliferative nodule in small congenital melanocytic naevus after childhood. Acta Derm Venereol. 2012;92(1):96–7.
28. Mancianti ML, Clark WH, Hayes FA, Herlyn M. Malignant melanoma simulants arising in congenital melanocytic nevi do not show experimental evidence for a malignant phenotype. Am J Pathol. 1990; 136:817–29.
29. Lowes MA, Norris D, Whitfeld M. Benign melanocytic proliferative nodule within a congenital naevus. Australas J Dermatol. 2000;41:109–11.
30. Xu X, Bellucci KS, Elenitsas R, Elder DE. Cellular nodules in congenital pattern nevi. J Cutan Pathol. 2004;31:153–9.
31. Skelton HG, Smith KJ, Barrett TL, Graham JH. HMB-45 staining in benign and malignant melanocytic lesions. A reflection of cellular activation. Am J Dermatopathol. 1991;13:543–50.
32. Kossard S, Wilkinson B. Nucleolar organizer regions and image analysis nuclear morphometry of small cell (nevoid) melanoma. J Cutan Pathol. 1995;22:132–6.
33. Saenz-Santamaria MC, Reed JA, McNutt NS, Shea CR. Immunohistochemical expression of BCL-2 in melanomas and intradermal nevi. J Cutan Pathol. 1994;21:393–7.
34. Newman MD, Lertsburapa T, Mirzabeigi M, Mafee M, Guitart J, Gerami P. Fluorescence in situ hybridization as a tool for microstaging in malignant melanoma. Mod Pathol. 2009;22:989–95.
35. Gerami P, Jewell SS, Morrison LE, et al. Fluorescence in situ hybridization (FISH) as an ancillary diagnostic tool in the diagnosis of melanoma. Am J Surg Pathol. 2009;33:1146–56.
36. Scolyer RA, Murali R, McCarthy SW, Thompson JF. Histologically ambiguous ("borderline") primary cutaneous melanocytic tumors: approaches to patient management including the roles of molecular testing and sentinel lymph node biopsy. Arch Pathol Lab Med. 2010;134:1770–7.
37. Elder DE, Xu X. The approach to the patient with a difficult melanocytic lesion. Pathology. 2004;36: 428–34.
38. Gerami P, Wass A, Mafee M, Fang Y, Pulitzer MP, Busam KJ. Fluorescence in situ hybridization for distinguishing nevoid melanomas from mitotically active nevi. Am J Surg Pathol. 2009;33:1783–8.

9 Dysplastic Nevi Versus Melanoma

Adaobi I. Nwaneshiudu, Jon A. Reed,
Victor G. Prieto, and Christopher R. Shea

The Dysplastic Nevus

Historical Perspective

The concept of an abnormal melanocytic proliferation falling short of histologic features diagnostic of frank melanoma, with a tendency for occurrence within melanoma-prone families, was insinuated as early as the 1950s. E. Cawley and colleagues are to be credited with the first description of a genetic aspect to melanoma [1]. In 1978, W. Clark and colleagues described a distinctive type of nevus ("B-K mole"), arising in melanoma-prone families and clinically exhibiting size >5 mm, with variability in color and border. Histopathologically, Dr. Clark described the presence of atypical melanocytic hyperplasia with stromal changes in the papillary dermis and lymphocytic infiltrates [2]. The term "Clark nevus," in recognition of Dr. Clark's seminal contribution, is used synonymously with "dysplastic nevus" (DN). H. Lynch, months later, reported very similar findings and coined the term "Familial Atypical Multiple Mole and Melanoma syndrome (FAMMM)" based on study of five generations of a single cancer-prone family [3].

Subsequently, D. Elder et al. coined the term "dysplastic nevus syndrome" (DNS), including both familial and sporadic variants of the DN [4]. In the initial description, this group considered the DN to be melanoma precursors, based on the presence of histopathologic dysplasia. They described histopathologic congruence with the B-K mole, but expanded on the features, including nuclear pleomorphism and hyperchromatism, as well as a lymphocytic infiltrate and associated fibroplasia. Two types of dysplasia were described. *Epithelioid cell dysplasia* consisted of cells with dusty pigment within abundant cytoplasm, prominent nucleoli, and an architecture characterized by lateral fusion (bridging) of rete ridges, pleomorphism of nests, and nevus cells located in the papillary dermis having small, hyperchromatic nuclei. *Lentiginous melanocytic dysplasia* was defined as melanocytes having prominent cytoplasmic retraction artifact, and an irregular (non-nested) pattern of growth along the epidermal basal layer [4]. The DNS is now considered to be an autosomal dominant condition due to mutation in the *CDKN2A* gene, which

A.I. Nwaneshiudu • C.R. Shea, M.D. (✉)
University of Chicago Medicine, 5841 S. Maryland Ave., MC 5067, L502, Chicago, IL 60637, USA
e-mail: cshea@medicine.bsd.uchicago.edu

J.A. Reed
CellNEtix Pathology & Laboratories, 1124 Columbia St., Suite 200, Seattle, WA 98117, USA

V.G. Prieto
MD Anderson Cancer Center, University of Houston, 1515 Holcombe Blvd., Unit 85, Houston, TX 77030, USA

C.R. Shea et al. (eds.), *Pathology of Challenging Melanocytic Neoplasms: Diagnosis and Management*, DOI 10.1007/978-1-4939-1444-9_9, © Springer Science+Business Media New York 2015

Table 9.1 Summary of histopathologic features of common acquired nevi, dysplastic nevi, and melanoma

Common acquired nevi	Dysplastic nevi	Melanoma
Well nested at peripheral junctional component (circumscribed)	Mild–moderate: circumscribed Moderate–severe: poorly circumscribed	Single-cell, non-nested melanocytes predominate
Maturation (senescence) transition from pigmented nested melanocytes in superficial dermis to singly dispersed small melanocytes at base	Maturation preserved	Minimal maturation; presence of nests, pigment, or mitotic figures at base of lesion
Symmetric	Mild–moderate: symmetric Moderate–severe: asymmetric	Asymmetric
Nests equidistant with round-oval shape and similar size	Mild–moderate: equidistant, uniform nests Moderate–severe: extensive bridging, variability in nest size and distance	Elongated nests with irregular shapes in random, haphazard distribution
Nests usually at rete tips	Mild–moderate: nests usually at rete tips Moderate–severe: nests at arch of dermal papillae, and sides of rete	Nests at arch of dermal papillae, and sides of rete
Nests in dermis cohesive and smaller than junctional nests (if nevus is compound)	Discohesion and confluence to varied degrees depending on severity	Confluence of melanocytes at DEJ and down adnexae, and discohesion of nests
Absent pigment deep in neoplasm	Absent pigment deep in neoplasm	Presence of pigmented and large nests deep in neoplasm
Minimal mitotic figures	Variable mitotic figures; minimal involvement of depth	Notable mitotic figures including the deepest aspect
Minimal cycling cells (quiescence)	Variable cycling cells	Numerous cells active in cell cycle
Minimal suprabasal (pagetoid) spread (except special sites)	Focal suprabasal (pagetoid) spread in center of lesion	Extensive suprabasal (pagetoid) spread
Minimal inflammatory infiltration (except in halo nevi)	Variable inflammatory cells	Inflammatory infiltrate, sometimes with numerous plasma cells; however, lesions can have minimal inflammation
gp100 (HMB-45) expression top-heavy, with loss of signal at increased depth	gp100 (HMB-45) expression top-heavy, with loss of signal at increased depth	gp100 (HMB-45) expression is patchy

encodes two tumor suppressor proteins expressed by alternative exon splicing, specifically p16-INK2A and p14-ARF, on chromosome 9p [5, 6]. Rare activating mutations in CDK4, a proto-oncogene, have also been noted. Diagnostic criteria for the DNS include: (1) melanoma in one or more first or second degree relatives; (2) presence of a large number of nevi (>50); and (3) nevi with distinctive histopathologic features [7]. However, sporadic DN are much more common than those occurring in the setting of the DNS, and the biologic behavior of sporadic DN, including their risk of exhibiting aggressive behavior or undergoing transformation to melanoma, is not currently clarified.

Histopathologic Features of Dysplastic Nevi

The term "dysplasia" is derived from the Greek "dys-" meaning "bad" or "malfunction" and "-plasia" meaning "growth." Thus, the dysplastic nevus is characterized histopathologically by the presence of nested melanocytic hyperplasia, similar to that of a banal or common acquired nevus, but with variable degrees of architectural disorder and cytologic atypia, as well as stromal changes (Table 9.1). These features, while reminiscent of the changes seen in melanoma, lack the severity or extent diagnostic of outright malignancy. The DN generally may

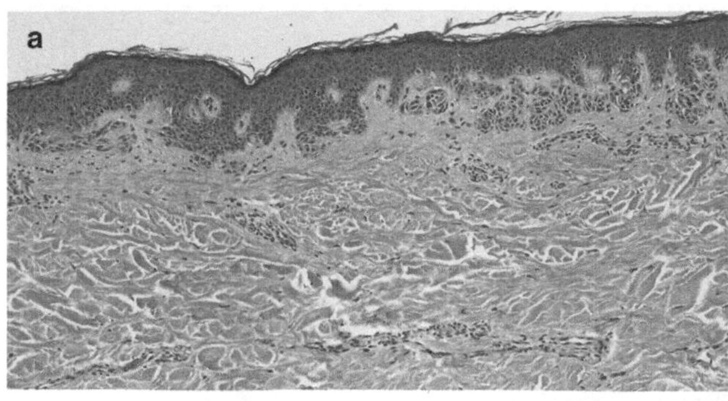

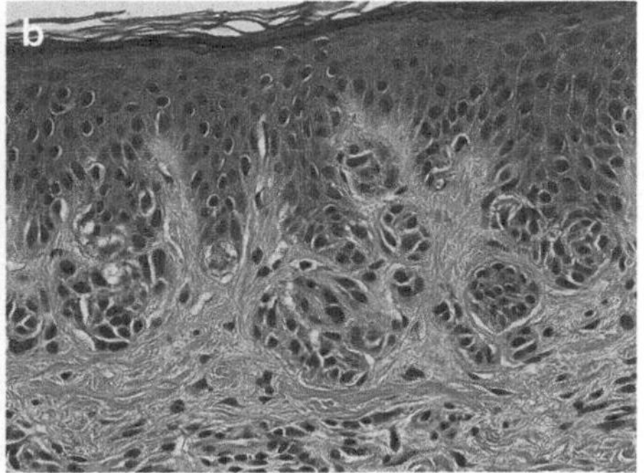

Fig. 9.1 Compound mild dysplastic nevus histology. (**a**)×10 magnification—Proliferation of melanocytes along the dermal–epidermal junction and as dermal nests, with minimal cytologic atypia. Mild architectural disorder with shouldering focal bridging of nests, elongated rete ridges, lamellar and concentric fibrosis around rete and a mild dermal inflammatory infiltrate. (**b**) at ×40 magnification—mild pleomorphism with scattered hyperchromatic cells

be "junctional," with proliferation of melanocytes at the dermoepidermal junction without a dermal component, or "compound," with both epidermal and dermal components (Fig. 9.1); purely intradermal DN are rare. Uncommonly, the dermal component of DN may sometimes have features characteristic of other nevi, including Spitz, halo, blue, or congenital types. DN are characterized by three main features:

- *Architectural disorder*: There is a crowded, lentiginous proliferation of spindled or epithelioid melanocytes in a horizontal arrangement within the epidermis. These cells have finely granular melanin in the cytoplasm, and are arranged either in nests or as single cells, sometimes reaching confluence. The nests can vary in size and are dispersed haphazardly (unlike the ordered architecture of common acquired nevi) at various distances along the sides and tips of elongated rete ridges. There are variable degrees of cohesion within the nests, bridging between nests, and cytoplasmic shrinkage artifacts of the melanocytes. The junctional nests extend beyond the dermal component by at least three rete ridges ("shouldering") and the lesion may or may not be well-circumscribed (i.e. nested at both lateral edges).
- *Cytologic atypia*: Occasional melanocytes exhibit abundant cytoplasm, nuclei larger than those of adjacent keratinocytes, hyperchromasia, and prominent nucleoli; however, the consistently high-grade, extensive atypia characteristic of melanoma is not observed. DN may have a limited degree of histopathologic overlap with superficial spreading melanoma or lentigo maligna melanoma (Fig. 9.2) but the latter exhibits increased consistency and severity of atypia extensively throughout the lesion, with peripheral lentiginous proliferation (poor circumscription), and a greater degree of cytologic atypia in the junctional component. A melanocytic neoplasm exhibiting extensive features of architectural disorder and cytological atypia should indeed raise concern for melanoma arising within a DN [8]. The degrees of atypia exhibited by DN can range from a sparse presence of one or more features, to extensive manifestation of multiple atypical features, resulting in a spectrum of histopathologic phenotypes.
- *Stromal response*: The superficial dermis around DN exhibits concentric fibrosis (condensation of dense, hypocellular collagen around elongated rete ridges) and lamellar fibroplasia (delicate layered or laminated collagen in a linear array). There are increased fibroblasts in papillary dermis, fibrosis in the upper reticular dermis with widely spaced nests in the dermal component if present, and a patchy lymphocytic infiltrate, and telangiectasia.

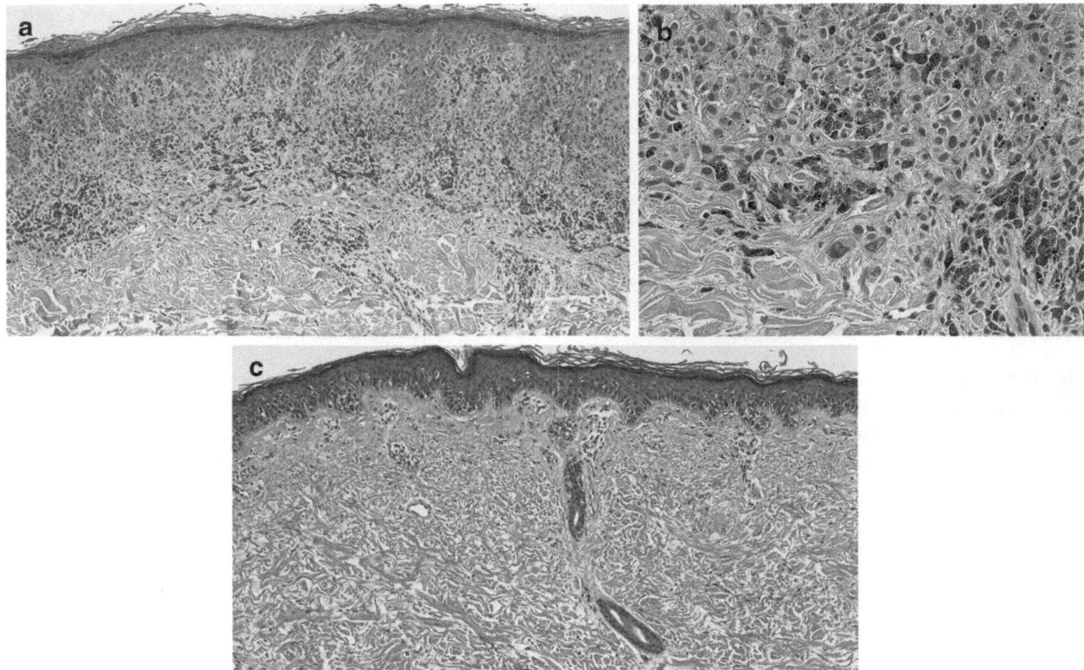

Fig. 9.2 (**a-b**) Superficial spreading melanoma histology. (**a**) ×10 magnification—Sheets of large pigmented melanocytes with very severe cytologic atypia including large pleomorphic bizarre nuclei and prominent nucleoli; severe architectural disorder with extensive pagetoid spread, and heavily pigmented melanocytes at the base. Dermal infiltrating lymphocytes and some plasma cells are noted. (**b**) ×40 magnification—sheets of atypical pigmented melanocytes; note bizarre melanocytes at base of specimen. (**c**) Lentigo maligna melanoma histology. ×10 magnification—Lentiginous proliferation of atypical melanocytes both as single cells and in poorly cohesive nests along the dermoepidermal junction and in suprabasilar regions, on a background of dermal solar elastosis. Note extension down adnexal structures (eccrine duct)

Comparison of Dysplastic Nevi with Common Acquired Nevi

Dysplastic nevi (DN) display various features that distinguish them from common acquired nevi (Table 9.1). Characteristic aspects of DN include the presence of varying levels of disordered architecture and atypical cytology, as previously discussed; a higher proliferation index; distinctive gene expression patterns including the presence of p16-INK4A gene mutation (or deletion in some cases), altered p53 expression; evidence of increased microsatellite instability; and increased presence of reactive oxygen species [7]. Expression of HMSA-2, a protein involved in melanogenesis, is present in both DN and melanoma but not in common acquired nevi [9]. There is also a lack of expression of collagen IV around the nests of common acquired nevi, but a continuous pattern of staining surrounding the junctional nests in a concentric fashion in most DN, with the remainder having a discontinuous pattern [10]. DN and common acquired nevi also share certain similarities including the presence of clonality of melanocytes; expression of apoptotic regulators and senescence marker; similar BRAF mutation rates; loss of PTEN expression; and similar rates for recurrence after biopsy [7].

Correlation of Architectural and Cytologic Dysplasia

One point of contention has been whether the diagnosis of DN must be based on cytologic or architectural features alone, or should incorporate both features. A study attempted to develop objective, reproducible criteria for grading DN and correlate architectural disorder with cytologic atypia [11]. The resulting Duke system for grading DN used a binary scoring system in which each factor was given a value of 0 or 1. The features given a value of 1 included;

- *Architectural disorder*: Junctional component not nested at both edges (poor circumscription), poor overall symmetry, less than 50 % of nests cohesive (poor cohesion), suprabasal spread prominent (in more than 2 high power field (hpf)) or present at the edge, confluence of more than 50 % of the proliferation as bridges or single cells, single-cell proliferation not focal or absent. Mild disorder (score of 0–1), moderate disorder (score of 2–3), and severe disorder (score of 4–6) were delineated.
- *Cytologic atypia* (determined in more than 50 % of cells within 2hpf of the most atypical areas): Nuclei not round/oval and euchromatic, nuclei size greater than basal keratinocyte nuclei, nucleoli prominent, and cell diameter greater than twice the size of the basal keratinocyte nuclei. Mild atypia (score 0–1), moderate atypia (score 2), and severe atypia (score 3–4) were delineated.

This study suggested that both architectural disorder and cytologic atypia were important in combination to increase the sensitivity of evaluation and diagnosis of DN (Fig. 9.3). In this study, confluence of junctional component and poor circumscription were the most frequent features of architectural disorder noted, followed by single-cell proliferation and asymmetry [11]. The data indicated that on average architectural disorder and cytological atypia tended to correlate. The authors proposed that both criteria should be considered for a complete histopathologic evaluation of DN because grading architecture may permit better clinical-pathologic correlation [7, 11, 12].

Ancillary Studies

Immunohistochemistry in Melanocytic Lesions

The histopathologic diagnosis of a significant proportion of melanocytic lesions are clear-cut on hematoxylin-eosin staining and may be confidently classified as nevi (whether dysplastic or non-dysplastic) versus melanoma (Fig. 9.3). Only a minority of lesions, such as nevi with a high degree of dysplasia and spitzoid melanocytic proliferation, necessitate use of ancillary techniques to aid in the diagnosis. Among those techniques, immunohistochemistry is the method most widely employed. Melanocyte differentiation antigens such as Mart-1/Melan-A, tyrosinase, and gp100 (HMB-45) help highlight melanocytes to better ascertain architectural behavior, such as pagetoid spread, lentiginous growth, and lack of maturation. They may be used in combination with proliferation markers (e.g., Ki-67) to determine biologic behavior. There is no single marker, or combination, that establishes an unequivocal diagnosis of melanoma or nevus. Analysis of the pattern of expression and localization can be correlative with morphologic features to facilitate getting to a diagnosis.

HMB-45

HMB-45 antibody, which recognizes the gp100 protein, originally produced by Gown and Vogel in 1980s, defines an oncofetal premelanosomal antigen, positive in fetal melanocytes and melanoma but typically negative in adult resting melanocytes [13]. This marker is valuable in determining the biologic behavior of maturation. In DN, there is a progressive morphologic change in the melanocytes with increased depth. This maturation (senescence) is captured by the antibody HMB-45, which highlights melanocytes in a top-heavy pattern, with loss of staining with increasing depth into the dermis. Overall sensitivity is approximately 85 % but this significantly decreases in spindle-cell or desmoplastic melanomas [14]. In contrast, primary cutaneous melanoma usually expresses gp100 in a patchy pattern throughout the dermal component. HMB-45 can also be used to highlight the intraepidermal component and can label confluence/lentiginous proliferation, and suprabasilar spread of melanocytes, which are features characteristic of melanoma.

Mart-1/Melan-A

Mart-1, also known as Melan-A, is a small cytoplasmic protein, not localized to premelanosomes, initially identified as a target for cytotoxic

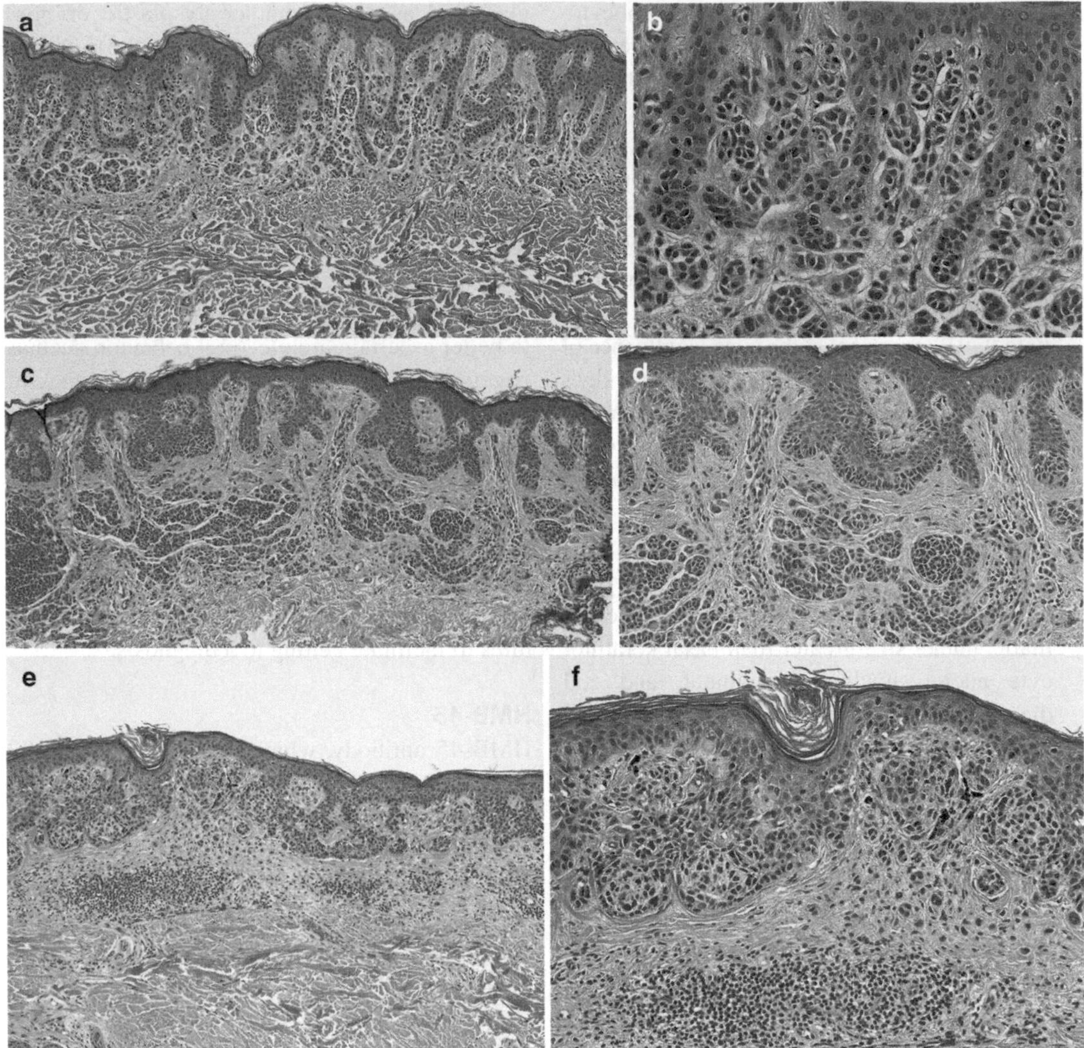

Fig. 9.3 (**a-f**) Comparision of different grade of dysplasia in DN (**a**) Compound mild DN. x10 magnification-Compound mild dysplastic nevi. ×20—Architectural disorder with elongation of rete, bridging of similar-sized cohesive nests, concentric fibrosis around rete ridges and scattered single melanocytes along dermal–epidermal junction. Presence of inflammatory infiltrate is minimal. (**b**) ×40 magnification of (**a**) —Mild pleomorphism with scattered hyperchromatic nuclei of melanocytes. (**c**) Compound moderate DN. ×10 magnification—Architectural disorder with more extensive cohesive nest of melanocytes and single cells along the DEJ extending up the rete ridges, bridging, concentric fibrosis, and an inflammatory infiltrate. (**d**) ×20 magnification of (**c**) More atypical melanocytes with hyperchromatic nuclei, as single cells and nests, extending up the rete ridges. (**e**) Compound severe DN. ×10 magnification—Architectural disorder with extensive bridging; proliferation of melanocytes in cohesive nests and as single cells along the DEJ and a few suprabasilar melanocytes. Notable dermal inflammatory infiltrate. (**f**) ×20 magnification of (**e**) Multiple melanocytes with pleomorphic hyperchromatic large nuclei and prominent nucleoli, more extensively through the lesion. (**g-i**) superficial spreading melanoma. (**g**) ×10 magnification —Sheets of large pigmented melanocytes with very severe architectural disorder with extensive pagetoid spread, and heavily pigmented melanocytes at the base. (**h**) ×20 magnification of (**g**) Dermal infiltrating lymphocytes and some plasma cells are noted. (**i**) ×40 magnification of (**g**) —Cells with severe cytologic atypia inclusing large pleomorphic bizzare-shaped nuclei with prominent nucleoli, present throught lesion including the base

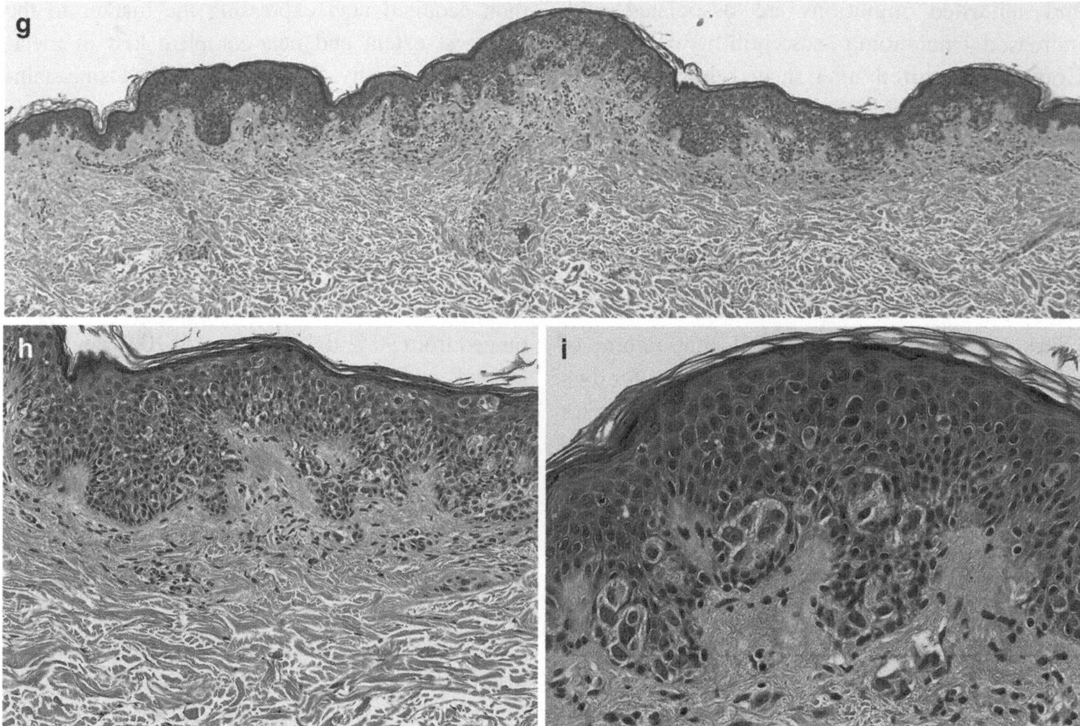

Fig. 9.3 (continued)

T-cells [15] and expressed in adult resting melanocytes as well as melanoma. Staining for this melanocyte differentiation antigen has an overall sensitivity of ~85 %, greatest in large-cell, undifferentiated malignancies [16, 17]. Anti-Mart-1 antibodies are positive not just in melanocytes but in adrenocortical adenomas/carcinomas as well as sex-cord stromal tumors of ovary, which may be a pitfall in cases of metastasis of these malignancies to the skin [18]. Anti-Mart-1 antibodies can label confluence/lentiginous proliferation, and suprabasilar spread of melanocytes, highlighting their extent, which can help distinguish DN from melanoma. Also, as a potential pitfall, there is labeling of melanophages by anti-Mart-1 antibodies, which may represent melanocytic antigens that have been phagocytized by macrophages.

MIB-1/Ki-67

MIB-1, also known as Ki-67, is a proliferation marker of cycling cells. The practice of co-labeling the nuclear Ki-67 stain with a cytoplasmic melanocytic marker such as Mart-1/Melan-A, greatly improves the identification of proliferating melanocytes. In DN, Ki-67-positive cells are few (usually <5 %) and are typically located close to the dermoepidermal junction and adnexal epithelium, or in the superficial dermis, but are absent in the deeper portion of the lesion. In contrast, melanomas have a random pattern of immunoreactivity (average ~16 % in "hot spots"), with proliferating cells present at all levels of the lesion, especially at depth, indicating a lack of maturation/senescence [19].

The p16-INK4A Protein

The p16-INK4A product of CDKN2A is a cyclin-dependent kinase inhibitor, which has critical functions at the G_1-S checkpoint of the cell cycle, This enzyme blocks the cell cycle at the G1-S checkpoint by inhibiting CDK (cyclin-dependent kinases), including CDK4, and cyclins such as cyclin D1. This suppresses the proliferation of cells with damaged DNA or with activated oncogenes and is also activated when cells are old or crowded. The p16-INK4A protein is frequently inactivated in human tumors, including melanoma, and inherited mutations are associated with increased melanoma susceptibility [20, 21]. Common acquired nevi show minimal loss of p16-INK4A, while allelic loss of this locus is common in DN and in primary and metastatic melanomas [22]. The expression pattern can be nuclear or cytoplasmic.

Microphthalmia Transcription Factor (MITF)

Clark and colleagues proposed that failure of melanocytes to differentiate is necessary for dysplasia [23]. MITF is a nuclear transcription factor that regulates development, differentiation, and survival of melanocytes [24]. MITF plays a key role in the pathway leading to melanin production. Specifically, signaling initiated by alpha-MSH binding to the MCR1 transmembrane receptor results in MITF activation and subsequent transcription of genes necessary for melanin synthesis, including the key enzyme, tyrosinase [25], as well as other melanocyte-specific genes such as MART1 and SILV (silver homolog). MITF expression can also result in cell-cycle arrest by the induction of p16-INK4A [26, 27]. MITF is amplified or mutated in ~10 % of primary cutaneous melanoma and ~20 % of metastatic melanoma [28, 29]. MITF amplification occurs in tumors with poor prognosis, being associated with resistance to therapy [28]. There is paradoxically a decrease in genes regulated by MITF, including SILV, TRPM1 (melastatin), and MART1 in certain melanoma subsets and this is thought to accompany the progression from nevus to melanoma, as well as to be a poor prognostic indicator [30, 31].

5-Hydroxymethylcytosine

5-Hydroxymethylcytosine is a recently described marker that correlates with the level of dysplasia [32]. This proves very useful in challenging lesions, including distinguishing DN from melanoma. Tumor cells in various human cancers exhibit global hypomethylation as well as selective hypermethylation at promoter regions of tumor suppressors, resulting in gene silencing and malignant transformation [33]. Progressive loss of 5-hydroxymethylcytosine was noted in one study to be associated with increasing levels of dysplasia, with the common acquired nevi expressing the marker to the strongest extent and near-complete loss in melanoma. Specifically, 5-hydroxymethylcytosine staining was highest in normal resident basal layer melanocytes, with 100 % staining darkly. Common acquired (non-dysplastic) nevi and low-grade DN (defined as those with mild or focally moderate cytologic atypia) showed 60 % of melanocytes staining darkly in this study [32]. High-grade DN (defined as those with diffusely moderate or severe atypia) ranged from 90 % lightly stained to 10 % negatively stained melanocytes. 5-Hydroxymethylcytosine exhibited near total loss in melanoma, being associated particularly with poor prognosis in superficial spreading melanoma and nodular melanoma [34]. In addition, increased nuclear size, a feature of dysplasia, had an inverse correlation with the expression of 5-hydroxymethylcytosine while being directly proportional to the degree of dysplasia [32]. Interestingly, DN showed darker staining in deep aspects of the neoplasm than the superficial aspect, likely highlighting maturation. In melanoma arising within a nevus, where delineating the extent of the melanoma for Breslow depth determination may prove challenging, there was a strong staining of 5-hydroxymethylcytosine levels in the nevus component and loss in the melanoma component [32].

SOX Proteins

SOX (Sry-HMG-box) proteins are a family of transcription factors involved in regulating a variety of biologic events including lineage restriction and terminal differentiation, through a precise pattern of expression that is cell-type specific [35]. SOX10 plays a key role in the transcriptional control of MITF, which is the master regulatory gene for melanogenesis [36]. However, SOX9, SOX18, and SOX5 have also been implicated in regulating aspects of the melanocyte life cycle. SOX9 (a nuclear stain), and SOX10 (a perinuclear and cytoplasmic stain) have been reported to be expressed in various stages of melanoma progression and in established melanoma cell lines [37–39]. Studies showed that SOX10-positive melanocytes were present in 31 % of nevi, 43 % of primary melanoma, and 50 % of metastatic melanoma [38, 39]. However, SOX9 expression was observed in a majority (~75 %) of the melanocytic neoplasms, with moderate decrease as the severity of melanoma progressed [40]. SOX9 expression has been shown to reduce proliferation of multiple melanoma cell lines [37]. The SOX protein expression in DN have not yet been fully elucidated and the combination of SOX 9 and SOX 10 expression patterns by immunohistochemistry may prove useful in better delineating the spectrum or grades of atypia that characterize DN and melanoma.

Angiogenesis Markers

Angiogenesis and microvascular density (MVD) are important characteristics in tumorigenesis, with roles in the multifactorial transition from benign to malignant states [41]. These features have been shown to affect the prognosis of malignant tumors and skin neoplasms including melanoma [42]. Benign nevi (dysplastic and non-dysplastic) have similar MVD and mean major diameters of blood vessels. However, these parameters, in addition to total vascular area, are significantly increased in melanoma [43]. Therefore melanomas, unlike DN, have a greater number of vessels over a larger area, providing evidence for correlation of malignancy with increased vascularity.

Survivin

Survivin is an antiapoptotic protein that has been detected in DN by immunohistochemistry. In one study, the majority of DN with a nuclear and cytoplasmic staining pattern for this marker had severe dysplasia [44]. A lack of nuclear staining was specifically described in benign melanocytic nevi, while 67 % of melanoma showed a positive nuclear stain, with an average index of 7 % [19].

Phosphohistone H3 (PHH3)

Phosphohistone H3 (PHH3) is a proliferative marker that highlights cells specifically in the M-phase of the cell cycle. A study by Nasr et al. showed a lack of PHH3 expression in the dermis of compound and dysplastic nevi, however an average of positivity of 25 cells/10 hpf was noted in melanomas [19]. Use of PHH3 expression can be of value in identifying the "hot spot" of greatest mitotic index within a tumor.

Confocal Microscopy in Melanocytic Neoplasms

Confocal microscopy uses point illumination via a pinhole to eliminate out-of-focus signals. The pinhole is conjugate to the focal point of the lens, allowing for optimal resolution [45]. Melanin offers the strongest contrast due to a high refractive index; therefore the cytoplasm of melanocytes is intensely white (Fig. 9.4). However, keratin has a lower refractive index and therefore less contrast, so keratinocyte cytoplasms appear darker. Nuclei appear dark and dermal collagen fibers appear very bright [46]. In vivo reflectance confocal microscopy (RCM) is a noninvasive tool that generates stacks of optical horizontal (z-axis) sections within the depth of intact living tissue. This proves to be a useful tool for studying the skin surface, and was first used in human skin in 1995 [47]. RCM enables visualization of the skin layers to a cellular level resolution (0.5–1.0 μm in the lateral dimension and 4–5 μm axially). The imaging depth is limited to 200–300 μm corresponding to depth at the dermoepidermal junction and papillary dermis, using the current commercially available RCM model [48]. An advantage of RCM is that the technology allows a section of skin to be assessed without processing (which may introduce artifact), and re-examination in order to evaluate dynamic changes over time. Characteristic architectural and cytologic features have been described, with histopathologic and dermoscopic correlates (Table 9.2).

Confocal Microscopy in Melanoma

In vivo RCM plays an important role in the characterization of the superficial aspect of melanoma, where a large number of characteristic findings are visible. However, Breslow depth determination, which has prognostic significance, is currently not possible. In the radial growth phase of melanoma, the epidermal pattern can be a disarranged honeycombed or cobblestoned pattern (i.e. an irregular epidermal pattern due to irregularly shaped keratinocytes) [49]. There can be suprabasilar/pagetoid migration of malignant melanocytes, evident as bright cells in superficial layers (Fig. 9.4). Atypical melanocytes are also noted along DEJ and in superficial layers,

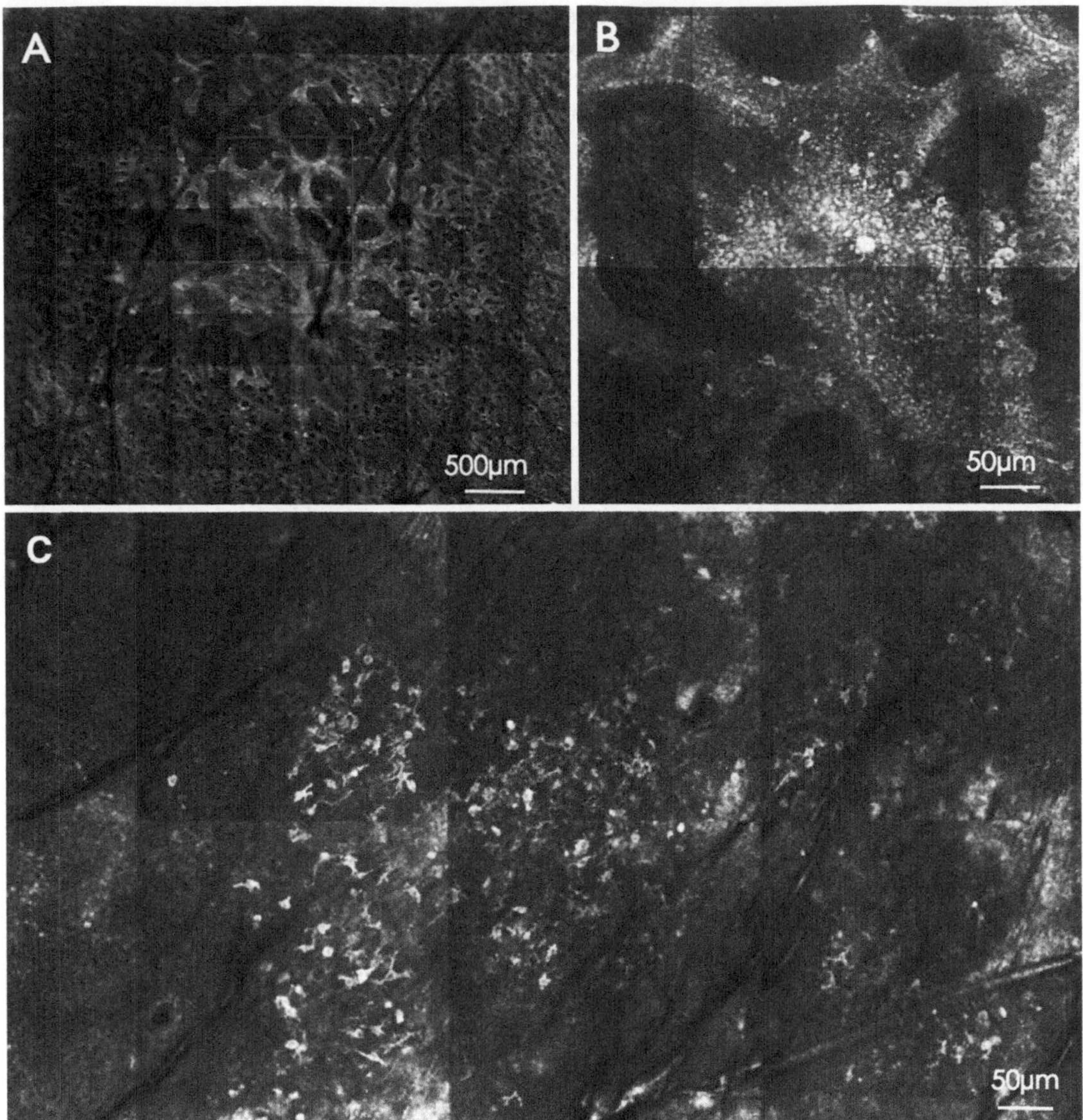

Fig. 9.4 (**a**) Confocal image of a dysplastic nevus: overview highlighting the meshwork pattern (500 μm). (**b**) Magnified view of the red box insert of (**a**): cytologic atypia (50 μm). (**c**) Confocal image of a melanoma: Florid and widespread pagetoid cells (50 μm). Courtesy Caterina Longo M.D., Ph.D. Caterina Longo, M.D., Ph.D. Skin Cancer Unit, Arcispedale Santa Maria Nuova-IRCCS, viale Risorgimento 80, 42100 Reggio Emilia, Italy

forming a nested and confluent proliferation (Fig. 9.3). In addition, atypical nucleated cells tend to infiltrate the dermal papillae and correspond histopathologically to nested melanocytic proliferation in upper dermis that invade and cause disarray of rete ridges. In almost 50 % of melanoma with microinvasion, regression is present, with an inflammatory infiltrate, and this is visualized by small bright inflammatory cells and plump bright cells (melanophages) with coarse bright collagen fibers [50]. In hypopigmented and amelanotic melanoma, confocal microscopy may still show features of melanoma due to melanin refractivity [49].

Table 9.2 Confocal terminology with dermoscopic and histopathologic correlates

Histopathologic features	Dermoscopic features	Confocal microscopic features
Elongated rete with increased melanocytes	Typical pigment network	Edged papillae and ringed pattern at DEJ
Rete ridges disarranged with atypical melanocytes. Usually in melanoma	Atypical pigment network	Non-edged papilla; irregular size and shape of dermal papillae without a clear border
Uniform nests at DEJ/papillary dermis	Regular pigment globules	Compact aggregates with sharp margins made of monomorphous polygonal cells
Combination of typical nests and compact aggregates of pleomorphic melanocytes	Irregular pigment globules	Irregular clusters with regular cytology (in benign) and atypical pleomorphic cells (in melanoma)
(A) Pagetoid spread	Pigmented dots	(A) Bright cells in superficial layers
(B) Melanophages in dermis		(B) Dermal plump bright cells
Peripheral elongated and parallel epidermal rete with nests	(A) Radial streaming	Parallel elongated lines of elongated cells projected toward the periphery
Uniform nests at peripheral	(B) Peripheral globules	Dense peripheral clusters
Well-defined nests at tips of enlarged and parallel rete	(C) Pseudopods	Globular-like bulging structures
Pigmented melanocytes in a uniform epidermal architecture	Light brown pigmentation	Regular honeycombed pattern
Keratinocyte pigmentation and transepidermal melanin loss with pagetoid spread of cells	Diffuse dark pigmentation and pigment blotches	Bright cobblestone pattern; suprabasal spread
Ortho/parakeratosis with pagetoid cells; marked basal melanocyte atypia; disarranged pattern of DEJ, malignant cells in nests, solitary in dermis with melanophages and inflammatory cells	Blue-white veil	Irregular pattern, round bright cells in superficial layers; non-edged papillae; cytologic atypia in basal layer; dishomogenous nest; nucleated and plump bright cells in papillae
Melanophages and inflammatory cells in dermis	Blue areas	Plump bright cells in dermal papillae
Thin epidermis, fibroplasia with inflammatory infiltrate with melanophages	Regression	Coarse network of ill-defined grainy fibers in dermis with intermingled bright spots and plump bright cells

Confocal Microscopy in Grading of Dysplastic Nevi

Biopsy of melanocytic lesions for histopathologic assessment is the gold standard but it interferes with the natural evolution of the lesion in vivo. Therefore histopathology-based assessments of the dynamics of the any given DN, either as a benign entity or as a precursor to melanoma, are limited. The advantage of in vivo observation in real time of tumor at the bedside is opening the clinical application of RCM for evaluation of melanocytic lesions and monitoring evolution, which is a necessary component to better understanding DN. Although limited by a small sample size, Pellacani et al. first demonstrated that histopathologic criteria i.e. architectural and cytologic features outlined by the Duke grading system had significant RCM correlates [51]. DN viewed by confocal microscopy were characterized in this study predominantly by a ringed pattern in association with a meshwork pattern, in addition to atypical junctional cells in the center of the lesion and irregular junctional nests with short interconnections (Fig. 9.3). In general, DN had cytologic atypia and atypical junctional nests, i.e. an irregular pattern with short interconnections and/or with nonhomogenous cellularity. However, pagetoid spread, widespread cytologic atypia at the junction, and non-edged papillae were suggestive of melanoma [51].

There were characteristic findings for common acquired nevi, melanoma, as well as the different grades of DN (Table 9.3). Suprabasal melanocytes most directly correlated with the level of dysplasia, i.e., 0 % in common acquired nevus and nevus with mild dysplasia 7 % in nevus with moderate dysplasia, 40 % and 100 % in nevus with severe dysplasia and melanoma, respectively [51]. Marked architectural disorder was observed in all but one melanoma (which showed severe cytologic atypia), in all severe DN, in 3 of 15 moderate DN, and in one common acquired nevus. Marked cytologic atypia was observed in some DN and melanoma but not in common acquired nevi or mildly dysplastic nevi [51].

Table 9.3 Differences among common acquired nevi, dysplastic nevi, and melanoma by in vivo RCM

Neoplasm	RCM features
Common acquired nevi	General architectural symmetry
	Ringed (rim of white small cells around dark dermal papillae) and/or clod (round large compact nests of melanocytes) patterns
	Regular epidermis at superficial layers without pagetoid spread
	Papillae at DEJ clearly visible and well outlined (edged papillae)
Dysplastic nevi	Asymmetry, ringed-meshwork pattern (greater frequency than melanoma) with a central-meshwork pattern (defined as enlarged interpapillary spaces due to nests of cells in basal layer that bulge into papilla appearing as junctional thickening) surrounded by a ringed pattern at DEJ
	Large nucleated pagetoid cells, with an increasing trend from mild to severe dysplastic nevi
	DEJ visible with an edged papilla in most cases
	Atypical roundish cells in center of lesion are characteristic
	Junctional nests are irregular in size, shape, with short interconnections (i.e. bridging on histology)
	Nonhomogenous cellularity (pleomorphism) at DEJ and coarse collagen (fibrosis), bright particles (inflammatory cells) and plump bright cells (melanophages) in the superficial dermis
Melanoma	Diffuse meshwork pattern or a diffuse nonspecific pattern frequently
	Irregular disarranged epidermal pattern with numerous pagetoid cells, and widespread pleomorphic shapes
	Marked disarray of architecture via non-edged papillae at DEJ, with occasional sheet-like structures
	Junctional and dermal nests irregular in size and shape, with numerous atypical pleomorphic cells
	More extensive pleomorphism, some cases exhibiting coarse collagen (fibrosis), and bright particles (inflammatory cells) in the superficial dermis

Molecular Genetics in Melanocytic Neoplasms

Gene expression profiles identified with molecular genetics may facilitate a better understanding and characterization of melanoma to help differentiate it from mimickers such as DN (Table 9.4), although some mutations are shared between these entities. Dr. Clark, initially characterized the DN as part of a step in the evolution of melanoma (Table 9.5). However, a consensus that DN represent formal histogenetic precursor to melanoma, as opposed to a benign entity that marks a propensity of melanoma, has not been definitely reached.

BRAF in Nevi and Melanoma

Dysplastic nevi have distinct gene expression profiles and tend to harbor BRAF mutation comparable to that of common acquired nevi. However, Ras mutations are rare in DN, unlike in melanoma. The activation of the Ras/mitogen activated protein kinase pathway (MAPK) is frequent in melanoma, with 60 % of melanoma expressing a driver

Table 9.4 Genetic mutations in nevi and melanoma

Genetic mutation	Presence in nevi	Melanoma subtype
BRAF	Acquired nevi (common and dysplastic)	Superficial spreading melanoma (rare in other types of melanoma)
NRAS	Congenital nevi	Nodular melanoma (also in other types of melanoma)
HRAS	Spitz nevi (11p gain, chromosome 7 gain, tetraploidy)	Not in melanoma
GNAQ/GNA11	Blue nevi	Uveal melanoma and blue nevus-like melanoma
BAP1	Epithelioid Spitz nevi (commonly in the setting of combined lesions)	Familial cancer syndrome with uveal melanoma; rare in cutaneous melanomas (also associated with mesothelioma)
KIT	Not in nevus	Subset of acral and mucosal melanomas and melanomas of sun-damaged skin
CDKN2A	Dysplastic nevus syndrome	Melanoma and pancreatic cancer

Table 9.5 Stepwise evolution from dysplastic nevi to melanoma

Step	Main features	Histology characteristics	Molecular events
1	Formation of the benign nevus	– Increased number of structurally normal, nested melanocytes along the basal layer	BRAF mutation
1–2	Formation of the dysplastic nevus	– Random and discontiguous architectural and cytological dysplasia	Loss of CDKN2A and PTEN tumor suppressor proteins
1–2–3	Radial growth phase melanoma	– Proliferation of malignant melanocytes throughout the epidermis and papillary dermis singly or in small nests- Failure to form colonies in soft agar	Increased cyclin D1
1–2–3–4	Vertical growth phase melanoma	– Malignant melanocytes form expansile nodules, widening the papillary dermis – Extension into the reticular dermis/fat – Capacity for growth in soft agar, and formation of tumor nodules when implanted in nude mice	Loss of E-cadherin, expression of N-cadherin, $\alpha V\beta 3$ integrin, MMP2, surviving, reduced TRPM1 (melastatin1)
1–2–3–4–5	Metastasis	– Malignant melanocytes grow in soft agar, and can form tumor nodules that may metastasize when implanted in nude mice	Absent TRPM1

Abbreviations: *PTEN* phosphatase and tensin homolog, *CDKN2A* cyclin-dependent kinase inhibitor 2A, *TRPM1* transient receptor potential cation channel, subfamily M, member 1

mutation in BRAF (especially, V600E) that may potentiate uncontrolled Ras signaling [52]. BRAF mutation is also present in nevi, including DN, with some studies showing BRAF detected in 81 % nevi including congenital nevi, common acquired nevi, and DN [53]. Specifically, BRAF mutation was detected in approximately 60 % of DN and 70 % of common acquired nevi, in one study; however, DN tended to show stronger BRAF staining than common acquired nevi, especially in the junctional component [54].

The p16-INKA Protein

The p16-INK4A enzyme inhibits transition past the G1 phase of the cell cycle to the S-phase (DNA synthesis) in the presence of DNA damage or activated oncogene by inhibiting CDKs and cyclins [55]. CDK4 and cyclin D1 (CCND1) act downstream of p16-INK4A and are mutated in some melanomas but not in DN. These targets of p16-INK4A function together as part of a complex that promotes the progression of the cell cycle by phosphorylating the retinoblastoma (Rb) protein, which is an important cell-cycle regulator. Of note, cyclin D1 may have oncogenic role in acral melanoma, in which overexpression of cyclin D1 occurs more frequently [56].

The p14-ARF Protein and p53

The p14-ARF product of CDKN2A is a tumor suppressor protein that arrests the cell cycle or promotes apoptosis when DNA damage, Rb loss, or uncontrolled activation of oncogenes, stimulates abnormal cell proliferation. The p14-ARF protein participates in the core regulatory process that controls levels of p53 by acting through MDM2 (mouse double minute 2), which triggers ubiquitination and proteosome degradation of p53. The tumor suppressor p53, which is upregulated by DNA damage, is found in more than 50 % of human cancers. Mutations in p53 are not frequently observed in common acquired nevi or DN, but may be present in melanoma [54]. The p14-ARF protein binds MDM2 and sequesters it from p53, allowing the accumulation of p53 to facilitate cell-cycle arrest at G_2-M for repair of damaged DNA, or induction of apoptosis [57]. Deficiency in p14-ARF abrogates oncogene-induced senescence and increases susceptibility for transformation [58].

Phosphatase and Tensin Homolog (PTEN)

Another genetic event involved in melanoma development is a homozygous deletion of PTEN on chromosome 10 in melanoma [59]. PTEN encodes a phosphatase that decreases a variety of growth factor-mediated signaling that are dependent on PIP3 (phosphatidylinositol phosphate) as an intracellular signal. PTEN usually keeps PIP3 levels low, however in its absence, the levels of PIP3 increase, which phosphorylates Akt in the pathway. Increased Akt activity prolongs cell survival through the inactivation of Bcl-2 antagonist of cell death (BAD) protein, and increases cell proliferation by increasing cyclin D1 expression [59]. Increased levels of the active form of Akt were found in the radial growth phase of melanomas [60].

WNT Signaling and Cadherins

Disturbances in cell adhesion contribute to tumor invasion and spread, tumor-stromal interactions, and tumor-cell signaling. E-cadherin expression in melanocytes facilitates attachment with adjacent keratinocytes [61]. The intracellular domain of cadherins is also associated with a large protein complex that includes beta catenin. The wingless-type mammary tumor virus integration site family (WNT) signaling pathway results in tyrosine phosphorylation of beta catenin, resulting in its dissociation from E-cadherin and translocation to the nucleus, where it binds to lymphoid enhancer factor-T-cell factor (LEF-TCF). Increased levels of nuclear beta catenin has been shown to increase the expression of MITF and cyclin D1 and these in turn increase survival and proliferation of melanoma cells [62–64]. Progression from radial to vertical growth phase of melanoma is marked by loss of E-cadherin and expression of N-cadherin [59]. N-cadherin is characteristic of invasive melanoma and facilitates metastatic spread by permitting the interaction of melanoma cells with other N-cadherin-expressing cells, including the dermal fibroblasts and vascular endothelium [61]. The role of E-cadherin in the biologic behavior of the varying grades of DN have not been fully elucidated.

Fluorescence In Situ Hybridization in Dysplastic Nevi Versus Melanoma

Fluorescence in situ hybridization (FISH) is a technique to visualize cytogenetic abnormalities, namely chromosomal aberrations like deletions, amplifications, and translocations. These features are frequent in cancers and many play a role in cancer development and prognosis, some serving as diagnostic markers. FISH can detect chromosomal abnormalities using targeted probes on formalin-fixed tissues section, which is conveniently the same material for routine histopathology. The probes are very sensitive, with lower cost compared to comparative genomic hybridization (CGH) and require multiple probes to achieve sufficient sensitivity. Most nevi, including DN, have not been shown to have any consistent diagnostic chromosomal aberrations [65].

One of the first reports of FISH in melanoma was published by Gerami et al. in 2009 and showed high sensitivity (87 %) and specificity (95 %) for melanoma diagnosis using four probes that target chromosomes; namely 6p25-red (RREB1), 6q23-gold (MYB), 11q13-green (CCND1), and CEP6-aqua (centromere label to identify gains and losses of chromosomes). In the study, the six histopathologically ambiguous lesions that progressed to metastatic melanoma were all positive on FISH [66]. Positive result algorithms in the above study were defined as: (1) >55 % nuclei with 6p25>CEP, (2) >29 % nuclei with >2 6p25 signals, (3) >40 % nuclei with CEP6>6q23, and (4) >38 % nuclei with >2 11q13 signals. In current practice, a melanocytic tumor that meets 1 of the 4 is considered positive for melanoma. One important utility is for measuring Breslow depth of invasion for melanoma arising from or colliding with nevi because this occurrence can be challenging and has important prognostic and clinical management implications. FISH in some studies was able to delineate the two neoplasms, being negative in the nevus area and positive in malignant foci, with sensitivity of 78 % using the four-probe system [67].

Current Controversies in Dysplastic Nevus and Melanoma

Naming the "Dysplastic Nevus"

The nosology of atypical nevi has been a point of contention in the literature, with the term "dysplasia" being poorly favored by some physicians and scientists due to its inconsistent use. No single definition or name to characterize "dysplastic nevi" has been accepted by various entities, including pathologists, dermatologists, dermatopathologists, oncologists, and epidermiologists. Some view the DN as a distinct entity with clinical significance (either as a precursor to melanoma or a risk factor for melanoma), while others dismiss the concept entirely usually in favor of the designation, "Clark nevus" in honor of W. Clark and his initial description of the entity [2, 68]. B. Ackerman argued that nevi can be characterized into four categories: (1) Unna nevus with a polypoid morphology and thickened papillary dermis; (2) Miescher nevus, with a dome-shape architecture composed on nevus cells arranged in a wedge configuration; (3) Spitz nevus, characterized by a benign silhouette of epithelioid or spindled cells having large nuclei and abundant cytoplasm; and (4) Clark nevus [68]. A major issue in naming the DN is the discordance seen in diagnosing and grading them, and the clinical significance of such endeavors.

There is a lack of convincing evidence establishing DN as true precursors to melanoma in most cases, partly due to the inconsistent terminology used by dermatologists and dermatopathologists. The NIH consensus conference defined the histopathologic basis of early melanoma and DN suggesting that the term "DN" should be abandoned and a new nomenclature adopted i.e., "nevus with architectural disorder" followed by a statement describing the presence and degree of cytologic atypia (mild, mod, or severe) [8]. However, no guideline on clinical management of these lesions have been established, which have led to debates in the field, and is one of the main critiques for use of this language to describe the DN.

Diagnostic and Grading Concordance

The concordance rate for the diagnosis of dysplastic nevi amongst multiple dermatopathologists has been reported in different studies. One study showed an overall concordance between five dermatopathologists of 77 % (kappa score: 0.55–0.84) [69]. The WHO reported a 92 % mean concordance in distinguishing common acquired nevi, dysplastic nevi, and radial growth of melanoma based on their criteria [70]. The concordance rate significantly declines with the grading of DN, and may be related to the experience of the dermatopathologist. In a study by Duncan et al., more experienced dermatopathologists had stronger congruence, ranging from 35 to 58 % (kappa 0.38–0.47), while the less experienced dermatopathologists had a wider range, from 16 to 65 % (kappa 0.05–0.24) [69]. This suggests that the main difficulty is not in the diagnosis of dysplasia but in the stratification of the variable histopathologic presentations of this entity. This discordance is complicated by the inconsistent terminologies used currently by dermatopathologists to stratify the level of dysplasia, including "low-grade/high-grade" or mild/moderate/severe, as well as the clinical significance and management of such delineation.

Dysplastic Nevi and Melanoma Risk

One complicating factor in the understanding of the DN is the inconsistent correlation of histopathologic dysplasia and clinical atypia in the literature. A study found poor correlation of clinically atypical and histopathologically dysplastic nevi (kappa 0.17), noting many nevi that were less than 5 mm in size and not clinically atypical showed evidence of histopathologic dysplasia [71]. However, it is generally accepted that the presence of multiple histopathologically DN are associated with an increased melanoma risk. A few studies have attempted to correlate the presence of DN with a risk for melanoma. In one such study of approximately 6,300 cases of nevus with architectural disorder, there was an increasing level of dysplasia correlated with an increased prevalence of a history of melanoma diagnosis. Specifically, 6 % of cases with mildly DN had melanoma history, compared to 8 % of patients with moderately DN and 20 % of patients with severely DN, suggesting that risk of melanoma increases with increasing grades of histopathologic atypia [72]. Another study attempted to estimate the risk of melanoma associated with histopathologically DN by generating a scoring system and correlating scores with clinical parameters and outcomes. In patients with nevi considered to have greater than mild dysplasia, there was an increased risk of having melanoma (odds ratio 2.60; 95 % CI 0.99–6.86). However, interobserver reliability associated with grading histopathologic dysplasia in nevi, amongst the dermatopathologists in the study was poor (weighted kappa 0.28), similar to the findings of other studies [71].

The counter-argument against dysplastic nevi being a risk factor for melanoma also exists in the literature, based on the high prevalence of histopathological DN in the population. Mildly dysplastic nevi are present in 7–32 % of population, suggesting that dysplasia is a common phenomenon and therefore not a strong predictor of melanoma [73]. In addition, Klein et al. found that in clinically benign nevi biopsied from healthy individuals, 88 % had at least one feature of dysplasia and 29 % had up to three features [74]. Some other studies have not demonstrated a direct relationship between melanoma risk and histopathologic dysplasia. Most nevi graded as mildly atypical by individual dermatopathologists are not associated with increased risk of melanoma and this is partly corroborated by a study showing an absence of DNA aneuploidy in mildly dysplastic nevi but a presence in DN graded as having at least moderate atypia [75]. The natural history of DN has been studied with transplanted histopathologically confirmed DN cells into nude (athymic) mice. In this study, there was a 90 % survival of these cells, with most developing an inflammatory response, while 30 % regressed over a 16-week period. Twenty percent of the samples developed junctional melanocytic hyperplasia in a lentiginous pattern with cytologic hypertrophy, dendritic morphology, and hypermelanization, but none progressed to melanoma [76].

Conclusion

Dysplastic nevi are a strong, consistent risk factor for melanoma but their etiology and natural history are not well characterized and may be multifactorial. No current markers exist to predict biologic behavior for DN, and histopathologic features are not always a reliable predictor of biologic behavior of these lesions. A major pitfall is that DN can mimic features of melanoma and vice versa, both histopathologically and clinically. Most DN, however, do not progress to melanoma and there is little direct evidence the individual DN progress to melanoma at a higher rate than common acquired non-dysplastic nevi. It is estimated that 10–40 % of melanomas arise from nevi, with remaining melanomas developing de novo [77, 80]. In one study, the estimated lifetime risk of any nevus transforming into melanoma by age 80 was determined to be 0.03 % for a 20-year-old male and 0.009 % for a 20-year-old female [77]. The authors estimated that the yearly transformation rate of any single nevus into melanoma ranged from 1:200,000 in patients less than 40 years of age to 1:33,000 in men older than 60 years [77, 79]. Dr Clark's early description of DN occurred in the context of evolution to melanoma but he acknowledged that most DN did not become melanoma [23].

It is well-established that DN have overlapping histopathological, molecular, and clinical features with common acquired nevi and melanoma but there is a lack of consensus or currently defined guideline for management. Novel techniques are being developed to better delineate the biology of dysplastic nevi both in vivo and ex vivo not only via assessing morphology, and cytology but also protein expression by immunohistochemistry and genetic analysis. At the current time, the DN is considered benign however in challenging cases where the similarities are more towards melanoma than common acquired nevi, these novel techniques and markers may facilitate a better prediction of malignant biological potential of subsets of this entity to better guide management decisions.

References

1. Cawley EP, Kruse WT, Pinkus HK. Genetic aspects of malignant melanoma. AMA Arch Derm Syphilol. 1952;65(4):440–50.
2. Clark Jr WH, Reimer RR, Greene M, Ainsworth AM, Mastrangelo MJ. Origin of familial malignant melanomas from heritable melanocytic lesions 'The B-K mole syndrome'. Arch Dermatol. 1978;114(5):732–8.
3. Lynch HT, Frichot 3rd BC, Lynch JF. Familial atypical multiple mole-melanoma syndrome. J Med Genet. 1978;15(5):352–6.
4. Elder DE, Goldman LI, Goldman SC, Greene MH, Clark Jr WH. Dysplastic nevus syndrome: a phenotypic association of sporadic cutaneous melanoma. Cancer. 1980;46(8):1787–94.
5. Kamb A, Shattuck-Eidens D, Eeles R, Liu Q, Gruis NA, Ding W, Hussey C, Tran T, Miki Y, Weaver-Feldhaus J, et al. Analysis of the p16 gene (CDKN2) as a candidate for the chromosome 9p melanoma susceptibility locus. Nat Genet. 1994;8(1):23–6.
6. Goldstein AM, Struewing JP, Chidambaram A, Fraser MC, Tucker MA. Genotype–phenotype relationships in U.S. melanoma-prone families with CDKN2A and CDK4 mutations. J Natl Cancer Inst. 2000;92(12):1006–10.
7. Duffy K, Grossman D. The dysplastic nevus: from historical perspective to management in the modern era: part I. Historical, histologic, and clinical aspects. J Am Acad Dermatol. 2012;67(1):1.e1–16.
8. NIH consensus conference. Diagnosis and treatment of early melanoma. JAMA. 1992;268:1314–9.
9. Jimbow K, Horikoshi T, Takahashi H, Akutsu Y, Maeda K. Fine structural and immunohistochemical properties of dysplastic melanocytic nevi: comparison with malignant melanoma. J Invest Dermatol. 1989;92(5 Suppl):304S–9S.
10. Lebe B, Pabuççuoglu U, Ozer E. Expression pattern of type IV collagen in sporadic dysplastic melanocytic nevi. Anal Quant Cytol Histol. 2008;30(5):291–6.
11. Shea CR, Vollmer RT, Prieto VG. Correlating architectural disorder and cytologic atypia in Clark (dysplastic) melanocytic nevi. Hum Pathol. 1999;30(5):500–5.
12. Duffy KL, Mann DJ, Petronic-Rosic V, Shea CR. Clinical decision making based on histopathologic grading and margin status of dysplastic nevi. Arch Dermatol. 2012;148(2):259–60.
13. Gown AM, Vogel AM, Hoak D, Gough F, McNutt MA. Monoclonal antibodies specific for melanocytic tumors distinguish subpopulations of melanocytes. Am J Pathol. 1986;123(2):195–203.
14. Yaziji H, Gown AM. Immunohistochemical markers of melanocytic tumors. Int J Surg Pathol. 2003;11(1):11–5. Review.
15. Coulie PG, Brichard V, Van Pel A, Wölfel T, Schneider J, Traversari C, Mattei S, De Plaen E, Lurquin C, Szikora JP, Renauld JC, Boon T. A new gene coding for a differentiation antigen recognized by autologous cytolytic T lymphocytes on HLA-A2 melanomas. J Exp Med. 1994;180(1):35–42.
16. Orosz Z. Melan-A/Mart-1 expression in various melanocytic lesions and in non-melanocytic soft tissue tumours. Histopathology. 1999;34(6):517–25.
17. Busam KJ, Chen YT, Old LJ, Stockert E, Iversen K, Coplan KA, Rosai J, Barnhill RL, Jungbluth AA. Expression of melan-A (MART1) in benign melanocytic nevi and primary cutaneous malignant melanoma. Am J Surg Pathol. 1998;22(8):976–82.
18. Busam KJ, Iversen K, Coplan KA, Old LJ, Stockert E, Chen YT, McGregor D, Jungbluth A. Immunoreactivity for A103, an antibody to melan-A (Mart-1), in adrenocortical and other steroid tumors. Am J Surg Pathol. 1998;22(1):57–63.
19. Nasr MR, El-Zammar O. Comparison of pHH3, Ki-67, and survivin immunoreactivity in benign and

malignant melanocytic lesions. Am J Dermatopathol. 2008;30(2):117–22.

20. Scurr LL, McKenzie HA, Becker TM, Irvine M, Lai K, Mann GJ, Scolyer RA, Kefford RF, Rizos H. Selective loss of wild-type p16(INK4a) expression in human nevi. J Invest Dermatol. 2011;131(11): 2329–32.
21. Goldstein AM, Chan M, Harland M, Gillanders EM, Hayward NK, Avril MF, Azizi E, Bianchi-Scarra G, Bishop DT, Bressac-de Paillerets B, Bruno W, Calista D, Cannon Albright LA, Demenais F, Elder DE, Ghiorzo P, Gruis NA, Hansson J, Hogg D, Holland EA, Kanetsky PA, Kefford RF, Landi MT, Lang J, Leachman SA, Mackie RM, Magnusson V, Mann GJ, Niendorf K, Newton Bishop J, Palmer JM, Puig S, Puig-Butille JA, de Snoo FA, Stark M, Tsao H, Tucker MA, Whitaker L, Yakobson E, Melanoma Genetics Consortium (GenoMEL). High-risk melanoma susceptibility genes and pancreatic cancer, neural system tumors, and uveal melanoma across GenoMEL. Cancer Res. 2006;66(20):9818–28.
22. Sini MC, Manca A, Cossu A, Budroni M, Botti G, Ascierto PA, Cremona F, Muggiano A, D'Atri S, Casula M, Baldinu P, Palomba G, Lissia A, Tanda F, Palmieri G. Molecular alterations at chromosome 9p21 in melanocytic naevi and melanoma. Br J Dermatol. 2008;158(2):243–50.
23. Clark Jr WH, Elder DE, Guerry 4th D, Epstein MN, Greene MH, Van Horn M. A study of tumor progression: the precursor lesions of superficial spreading and nodular melanoma. Hum Pathol. 1984;15(12): 1147–65.
24. Widlund HR, Fisher DE. Microphthalamia-associated transcription factor: a critical regulator of pigment cell development and survival. Oncogene. 2003; 22(20):3035–41. Review.
25. Goding CR. Mitf from neural crest to melanoma: signal transduction and transcription in the melanocyte lineage. Genes Dev. 2000;14(14):1712–28. Review.
26. Du J, Miller AJ, Widlund HR, Horstmann MA, Ramaswamy S, Fisher DE. MLANA/MART1 and SILV/PMEL17/GP100 are transcriptionally regulated by MITF in melanocytes and melanoma. Am J Pathol. 2003;163(1):333–43.
27. Loercher AE, Tank EM, Delston RB, Harbour JW. MITF links differentiation with cell cycle arrest in melanocytes by transcriptional activation of INK4A. J Cell Biol. 2005;168(1):35–40.
28. Garraway LA, Widlund HR, Rubin MA, Getz G, Berger AJ, Ramaswamy S, Beroukhim R, Milner DA, Granter SR, Du J, Lee C, Wagner SN, Li C, Golub TR, Rimm DL, Meyerson ML, Fisher DE, Sellers WR. Integrative genomic analyses identify MITF as a lineage survival oncogene amplified in malignant melanoma. Nature. 2005;436(7047):117–22.
29. Cronin JC, Wunderlich J, Loftus SK, Prickett TD, Wei X, Ridd K, Vemula S, Burrell AS, Agrawal NS, Lin JC, Banister CE, Buckhaults P, Rosenberg SA, Bastian BC, Pavan WJ, Samuels Y. Frequent mutations in the MITF pathway in melanoma. Pigment Cell Melanoma Res. 2009;22(4):435–44.
30. Salti GI, Manougian T, Farolan M, Shilkaitis A, Majumdar D, Das Gupta TK. Micropthalmia transcription factor: a new prognostic marker in intermediate-thickness cutaneous malignant melanoma. Cancer Res. 2000;60(18):5012–6.
31. Miller AJ, Du J, Rowan S, Hershey CL, Widlund HR, Fisher DE. Transcriptional regulation of the melanoma prognostic marker melastatin (TRPM1) by MITF in melanocytes and melanoma. Cancer Res. 2004;64(2):509–16.
32. Larson AR, Dresser KA, Zhan Q, Lezcano C, Woda BA, Yosufi B, Thompson JF, Scolyer RA, Mihm Jr MC, Shi YG, Murphy GF, Lian CG. Loss of 5-hydroxymethylcytosine correlates with increasing morphologic dysplasia in melanocytic tumors. Mod Pathol. 2014;27(7):936–44.
33. Jones PA, Baylin SB. The fundamental role of epigenetic events in cancer. Nat Rev Genet. 2002;3(6):415–28. Review.
34. Lian CG, Xu Y, Ceol C, Wu F, Larson A, Dresser K, Xu W, Tan L, Hu Y, Zhan Q, Lee CW, Hu D, Lian BQ, Kleffel S, Yang Y, Neiswender J, Khorasani AJ, Fang R, Lezcano C, Duncan LM, Scolyer RA, Thompson JF, Kakavand H, Houvras Y, Zon LI, Mihm Jr MC, Kaiser UB, Schatton T, Woda BA, Murphy GF, Shi YG. Loss of 5-hydroxymethylcytosine is an epigenetic hallmark of melanoma. Cell. 2012;150(6): 1135–46.
35. Wegner M. All purpose Sox: the many roles of Sox proteins in gene expression. Int J Biochem Cell Biol. 2010;42(3):381–90.
36. Elworthy S, Lister JA, Carney TJ, Raible DW, Kelsh RN. Transcriptional regulation of mitfa accounts for the sox10 requirement in zebrafish melanophore development. Development. 2003;130(12):2809–18.
37. Hoek KS, Eichhoff OM, Schlegel NC, Döbbeling U, Kobert N, Schaerer L, Hemmi S, Dummer R. In vivo switching of human melanoma cells between proliferative and invasive states. Cancer Res. 2008;68(3):650–6.
38. Bakos RM, Maier T, Besch R, Mestel DS, Ruzicka T, Sturm RA, Berking C. Nestin and SOX9 and SOX10 transcription factors are coexpressed in melanoma. Exp Dermatol. 2010;19(8):e89–94.
39. Passeron T, Valencia JC, Bertolotto C, Hoashi T, Le Pape E, Takahashi K, Ballotti R, Hearing VJ. SOX9 is a key player in ultraviolet B-induced melanocyte differentiation and pigmentation. Proc Natl Acad Sci U S A. 2007;104(35):13984–9.
40. Harris ML, Baxter LL, Loftus SK, Pavan WJ. Sox proteins in melanocyte development and melanoma. Pigment Cell Melanoma Res. 2010;23(4):496–513.
41. Barnhill RL, Fandrey K, Levy MA, Mihm Jr MC, Hyman B. Angiogenesis and tumor progression of melanoma. Quantification of vascularity in melanocytic nevi and cutaneous malignant melanoma. Lab Invest. 1992;67(3):331–7.

42. Konstantina A, Lazaris AC, Ioannidis E, Liossi A, Aroni K. Immunohistochemical expression of VEGF, HIF1-a, and PlGF in malignant melanomas and dysplastic nevi. Melanoma Res. 2011;21(5):389–94.
43. Ioannidis EN, Aroni K, Kavantzas N. Assessment of vascularity in common Blue Nevi, small/medium congenital nevocellular, common and dysplastic acquired melanocytic nevi and melanomas: a comparative study. Am J Dermatopathol. 2014;36(3):217–22.
44. Adamkov M, Lauko L, Balentova S, Pec J, Pec M, Rajcani J. Expression pattern of anti-apoptotic protein survivin in dysplastic nevi. Neoplasma. 2009;56(2):130–5.
45. Nwaneshiudu A, Kuschal C, Sakamoto FH, Anderson RR, Schwarzenberger K, Young RC. Introduction to confocal microscopy. J Invest Dermatol. 2012;132(12):e3. doi:10.1038/jid.2012.429. Review.
46. Rajadhyaksha M, González S, Zavislan JM, Anderson RR, Webb RH. In vivo confocal scanning laser microscopy of human skin II: advances in instrumentation and comparison with histology. J Invest Dermatol. 1999;113(3):293–303.
47. Rajadhyaksha M, Grossman M, Esterowitz D, Webb RH, Anderson RR. In vivo confocal scanning laser microscopy of human skin: melanin provides strong contrast. J Invest Dermatol. 1995;104(6):946–52.
48. Pellacani G, Guitera P, Longo C, Avramidis M, Seidenari S, Menzies S. The impact of in vivo reflectance confocal microscopy for the diagnostic accuracy of melanoma and equivocal melanocytic lesions. J Invest Dermatol. 2007;127(12):2759–65.
49. Carrera C, Puig S, Malvehy J. In vivo confocal reflectance microscopy in melanoma. Dermatol Ther. 2012;25(5):410–22.
50. Pellacani G, Cesinaro AM, Seidenari S. Reflectance-mode confocal microscopy of pigmented skin lesions-improvement in melanoma diagnostic specificity. J Am Acad Dermatol. 2005;53(6):979–85.
51. Pellacani G, Farnetani F, Gonzalez S, Longo C, Cesinaro AM, Casari A, Beretti F, Seidenari S, Gill M. In vivo confocal microscopy for detection and grading of dysplastic nevi: a pilot study. J Am Acad Dermatol. 2012;66(3):e109–21.
52. Davies H, Bignell GR, Cox C, Stephens P, Edkins S, Clegg S, Teague J, Woffendin H, Garnett MJ, Bottomley W, Davis N, Dicks E, Ewing R, Floyd Y, Gray K, Hall S, Hawes R, Hughes J, Kosmidou V, Menzies A, Mould C, Parker A, Stevens C, Watt S, Hooper S, Wilson R, Jayatilake H, Gusterson BA, Cooper C, Shipley J, Hargrave D, Pritchard-Jones K, Maitland N, Chenevix-Trench G, Riggins GJ, Bigner DD, Palmieri G, Cossu A, Flanagan A, Nicholson A, Ho JW, Leung SY, Yuen ST, Weber BL, Seigler HF, Darrow TL, Paterson H, Marais R, Marshall CJ, Wooster R, Stratton MR, Futreal PA. Mutations of the BRAF gene in human cancer. Nature. 2002;417(6892):949–54.
53. Wu J, Rosenbaum E, Begum S, Westra WH. Distribution of BRAF T1799A(V600E) mutations across various types of benign nevi: implications for melanocytic tumorigenesis. Am J Dermatopathol. 2007;29(6):534–7.
54. Duffy K, Grossman D. The dysplastic nevus: from historical perspective to management in the modern era: Part II. Molecular aspects and clinical management. J Am Acad Dermatol. 2012;67(1):19.e1–12. quiz 31–2.
55. Sharpless E, Chin L. The INK4a/ARF locus and melanoma. Oncogene. 2003;22(20):3092–8. Review.
56. Sauter ER, Yeo UC, von Stemm A, Zhu W, Litwin S, Tichansky DS, Pistritto G, Nesbit M, Pinkel D, Herlyn M, Bastian BC. Cyclin D1 is a candidate oncogene in cutaneous melanoma. Cancer Res. 2002;62(11):3200–6.
57. Pomerantz J, Schreiber-Agus N, Liégeois NJ, Silverman A, Alland L, Chin L, Potes J, Chen K, Orlow I, Lee HW, Cordon-Cardo C, DePinho RA. The Ink4a tumor suppressor gene product, p19Arf, interacts with MDM2 and neutralizes MDM2's inhibition of p53. Cell. 1998;92(6):713–23.
58. Sharpless NE, Ramsey MR, Balasubramanian P, Castrillon DH, DePinho RA. The differential impact of p16(INK4a) or p19(ARF) deficiency on cell growth and tumorigenesis. Oncogene. 2004;23(2):379–85.
59. Miller AJ, Mihm Jr MC. Melanoma. N Engl J Med. 2006;355(1):51–65. Review.
60. Stahl JM, Sharma A, Cheung M, Zimmerman M, Cheng JQ, Bosenberg MW, Kester M, Sandirasegarane L, Robertson GP. Deregulated Akt3 activity promotes development of malignant melanoma. Cancer Res. 2004;64(19):7002–10.
61. Hsu M, Andl T, Li G, Meinkoth JL, Herlyn M. Cadherin repertoire determines partner-specific gap junctional communication during melanoma progression. J Cell Sci. 2000;113(Pt 9):1535–42.
62. Widlund HR, Horstmann MA, Price ER, Cui J, Lessnick SL, Wu M, He X, Fisher DE. Beta-catenin-induced melanoma growth requires the downstream target Microphthalmia-associated transcription factor. J Cell Biol. 2002;158(6):1079–87.
63. Shtutman M, Zhurinsky J, Simcha I, Albanese C, D'Amico M, Pestell R, Ben-Ze'ev A. The cyclin D1 gene is a target of the beta-catenin/LEF-1 pathway. Proc Natl Acad Sci U S A. 1999;96(10):5522–7.
64. Gerami P, Busam KJ. Cytogenetic and mutational analyses of melanocytic tumors. Dermatol Clin. 2012;30(4):555–66.
65. Song J, Mooi WJ, Petronic-Rosic V, Shea CR, Stricker T, Krausz T. Nevus versus melanoma: to FISH, or not to FISH. Adv Anat Pathol. 2011;18(3):229–34.
66. Gerami P, Jewell SS, Morrison LE, Blondin B, Schulz J, Ruffalo T, Matushek 4th P, Legator M, Jacobson K, Dalton SR, Charzan S, Kolaitis NA, Guitart J, Lertsbarapa T, Boone S, LeBoit PE, Bastian BC. Fluorescence in situ hybridization (FISH) as an ancillary diagnostic tool in the diagnosis of melanoma. Am J Surg Pathol. 2009;33(8):1146–56.

67. Newman MD, Lertsburapa T, Mirzabeigi M, Mafee M, Guitart J, Gerami P. Fluorescence in situ hybridization as a tool for microstaging in malignant melanoma. Mod Pathol. 2009;22(8):989–95.
68. Ackerman AB, Magana-Garcia M. Naming acquired melanocytic nevi. Unna's, Miescher's, Spitz's Clark's. Am J Dermatopathol. 1990;12(2):193–209.
69. Duncan LM, Berwick M, Bruijn JA, Byers HR, Mihm MC, Barnhill RL. Histopathologic recognition and grading of dysplastic melanocytic nevi: an interobserver agreement study. J Invest Dermatol. 1993; 100(3):318S–21.
70. Clemente C, Cochran AJ, Elder DE, Levene A, MacKie RM, Mihm MC, Rilke F, Cascinelli N, Fitzpatrick TB, Sober AJ. Histopathologic diagnosis of dysplastic nevi: concordance among pathologists convened by the World Health Organization Melanoma Programme. Hum Pathol. 1991;22(4):313–9.
71. Annessi G, Cattaruzza MS, Abeni D, Baliva G, Laurenza M, Macchini V, Melchi F, Ruatti P, Puddu P, Faraggiana T. Correlation between clinical atypia and histologic dysplasia in acquired melanocytic nevi. J Am Acad Dermatol. 2001;45(1):77–85.
72. Arumi-Uria M, McNutt NS, Finnerty B. Grading of atypia in nevi: correlation with melanoma risk. Mod Pathol. 2003;16(8):764–71.
73. Piepkorn MW, Barnhill RL, Cannon-Albright LA, Elder DE, Goldgar DE, Lewis CM, Maize JC, Meyer LJ, Rabkin MS, Sagebiel RW, et al. A multiobserver, population-based analysis of histologic dysplasia in melanocytic nevi. J Am Acad Dermatol. 1994;30(5 Pt 1):707–14.
74. Klein LJ, Barr RJ. Histologic atypia in clinically benign nevi. A prospective study. J Am Acad Dermatol. 1990;22(2 Pt 1):275–82.
75. Schmidt B, Weinberg DS, Hollister K, Barnhill RL. Analysis of melanocytic lesions by DNA image cytometry. Cancer. 1994;73(12):2971–7.
76. Meyer LJ, Schmidt LA, Goldgar DE, Piepkorn MW. Survival and histopathologic characteristics of human melanocytic nevi transplanted to athymic (nude) mice. Am J Dermatopathol. 1995;17(4): 368–73.
77. Tsao H, Bevona C, Goggins W, Quinn T. The transformation rate of moles (melanocytic nevi) into cutaneous melanoma: a population-based estimate. Arch Dermatol. 2003;139(3):282–8.
78. Shors AR, Kim S, White E, Argenyi Z, Barnhill RL, Duray P, Erickson L, Guitart J, Horenstein MG, Lowe L, Messina J, Rabkin MS, Schmidt B, Shea CR, Trotter MJ, Piepkorn MW. Dysplastic naevi with moderate to severe histological dysplasia: a risk factor for melanoma. Br J Dermatol. 2006;155(5): 988–93.
79. Goldstein AM, Tucker MA. Dysplastic nevi and melanoma. Cancer Epidemiol Biomarkers Prev. 2013; 22(4):528–32.
80. Rhodes AR. Acquired dysplastic melanocytic nevi and cutaneous melanoma: precursors and prevention Ann Intern Med. 1985 Apr;102(4):546–8.

Blue Nevus Versus Pigmented Epithelioid Melanocytoma

10

Jon A. Reed, Victor G. Prieto, and Christopher R. Shea

Melanocytic lesions containing abundant melanin pigment pose a unique diagnostic challenge. Some benign nevi and malignant melanomas are heavily pigmented. The amount of melanin may be so great in some lesions that it confounds accurate diagnosis. Differentiating heavily pigmented nevi from melanomas obviously has significant clinical implications. Heavily pigmented melanocytic lesions also must be distinguished from other inflammatory and neoplastic conditions with pigmentary alterations caused by melanin incontinence and from lesions containing other pigments (exogenous and endogenous) that resemble melanin. One of the more clinically important differential diagnoses is between blue nevus (dermal melanocytoma), its variants, and the so-called "pigmented epithelioid melanocytoma" (PEM). This chapter will focus on that challenge, but will include a discussion of the differential diagnosis of other pigmented lesions (melanocytic and non-melanocytic) that clinically and microscopically resemble blue nevi. Common to each of these lesions is the presence of abundant cytoplasmic pigmented material. In some cases, cytoplasmic pigment obscures nuclear detail necessitating histochemical, immunohistochemical, or other techniques to improve diagnostic accuracy.

J.A. Reed, M.S., M.D. (✉)
Baylor College of Medicine,
1 Baylor Plaza, Houston, TX 77030, USA

CellNetix Pathology & Laboratories,
1124 Columbia St., Suite 200, Seattle,
WA 98117, USA
e-mail: jreed@bcm.edu; jreed@cellnetix.com

V.G. Prieto, M.D., Ph.D.
MD Anderson Cancer Center, University of Houston,
1515 Holcombe Blvd., Unit 85, Houston,
TX 77030, USA

C.R. Shea, M.D.
University of Chicago Medicine,
5841 S. Maryland Ave., MC 5067, L502,
Chicago, IL 60637, USA

Blue Nevus (Dermal Melanocytoma)

Clinical Features

Blue nevi derive their name from their clinical appearance. They present as poorly circumscribed blue or blue-gray macules and patches, although hypopigmented and multi-pigmented forms also exist [1]. More heavily pigmented lesions are blue-gray, dark blue, brown, or even black. Most blue nevi are acquired lesions, but their appearance may mimic other bluish lesions of congenital onset, including sacral dermal melanocytosis, and the nevus of Ota and the nevus of Ito with which they share similar microscopic features [2, 3]. Blue nevi occur at any location (including visceral sites), but scalp, buttocks, and the dorsal surfaces of the hands and feet are most common [1, 4]. Lesions may enlarge slowly over time and the pigmentation may become more intense or may vary in

C.R. Shea et al. (eds.), *Pathology of Challenging Melanocytic Neoplasms: Diagnosis and Management*,
DOI 10.1007/978-1-4939-1444-9_10, © Springer Science+Business Media New York 2015

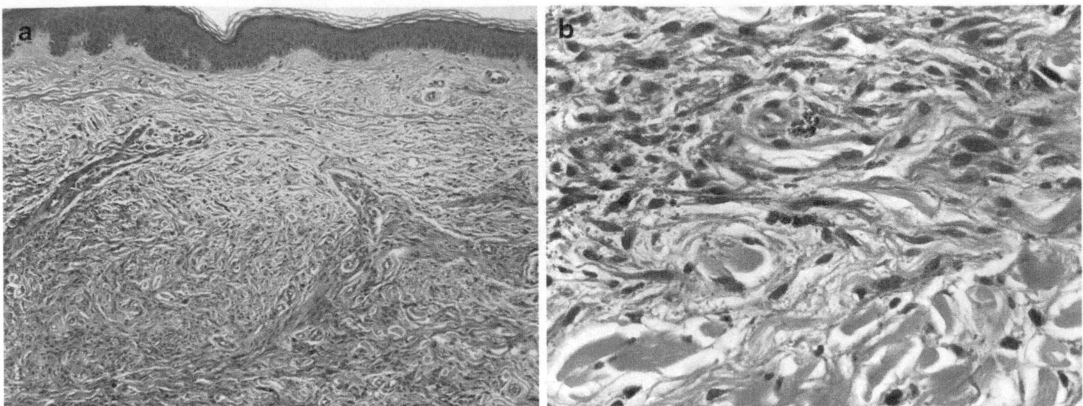

Fig. 10.1 Blue nevus. (**a**) Pigmented fusiform and dendritic cells between thickened collagen fibers (×10). (**b**) Note the delicate branched dendritic processes (×40)

color. Cellular lesions may be raised and often are more circumscribed. The deep penetrating nevus (plexiform spindle cell nevus) has an appearance similar to that of the cellular blue nevus, but occurs predominantly in younger patients on the head, neck, and proximal extremities [5–7].

Microscopic Features

Blue nevi that are believed to arise from a population of melanocytes is the dermis. As such, blue nevi usually do not have an intraepidermal component. A lesion with an intraepidermal component should be considered a combined melanocytic nevus with a blue nevus component [8, 9]. Blue nevi are characterized by a proliferation of fusiform and dendritic cells singly or in small clusters between dermal collagen fibers (Fig. 10.1). Collagen fibers may be considerably thickened in the sclerotic variant of blue nevus. Most of the fusiform and dendritic melanocytes in blue nevi contain abundant cytoplasmic melanin. Dendritic melanocytes have elongated, delicate branched cellular processes. Nuclei are small and uniform in appearance. Mitotic figures are infrequent. Smaller epithelioid melanocytes usually are present as well, but the presence of nested epithelioid cells favors a diagnosis of combined intradermal nevus with a blue nevus component.

Cellular Blue Nevus

The cellular variant of blue nevus contains aggregates of melanocytes with either a fusiform or small epithelioid morphology arranged into elongated nests or fascicles [1, 10]. The nests may concentrate in the adventitial dermis surrounding adnexal structures or in a perivascular or perineural distribution. These fascicular collections of melanocytes may protrude into the underlying subcutis producing a plexiform or "dumbbell" shaped lesion (Fig. 10.2). The nests are surrounded by more heavily pigmented melanophages. Pigmented fusiform and dendritic cells typical of ordinary blue nevus are present in variable numbers, often more peripherally distributed in the lesion. Most lesions lack significant cytologic atypia and have few mitotic figures. Atypia, when present, may present a diagnostic challenge [11]. Cytogenetic aberrations have been documented in lesions with significant cytologic atypia and with high mitotic rates [12]. So-called "ancient changes" also have been reported in cellular blue nevi, but these features do not affect the benign clinical behavior [13].

Deep Penetrating Nevus

The deep penetrating nevus has microscopic features that overlap ordinary blue nevus, cellular

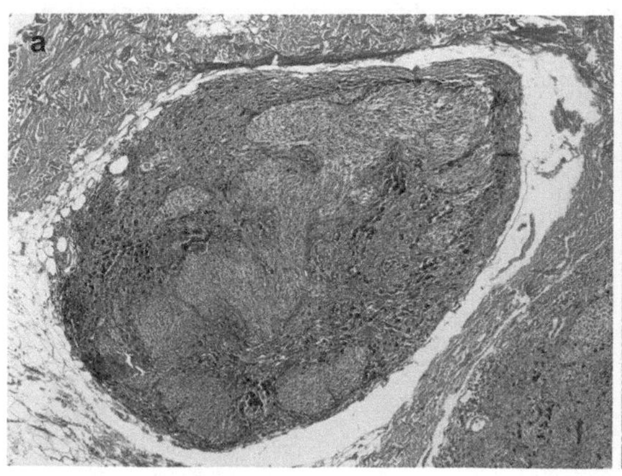

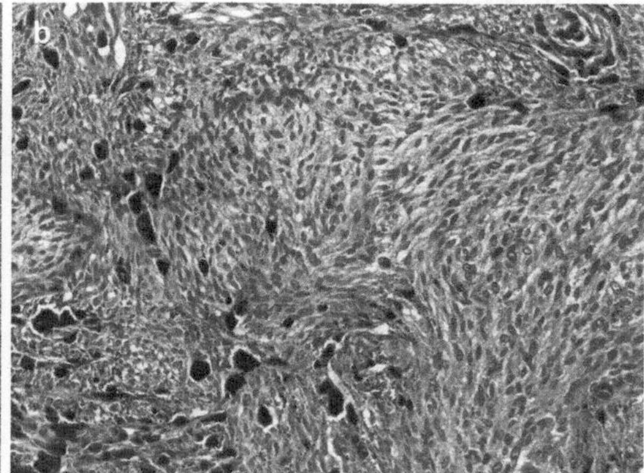

Fig. 10.2 Cellular blue nevus. (**a**) Elongated nests of fusiform and epithelioid cells in a plexiform pattern extending into the subcutaneous adipose tissue (×4). (**b**) Most of the cells have a fusiform or small epithelioid appearance and contain finely granular cytoplasmic melanin. Note the more heavily pigmented melanophages toward the periphery of the nests (×20)

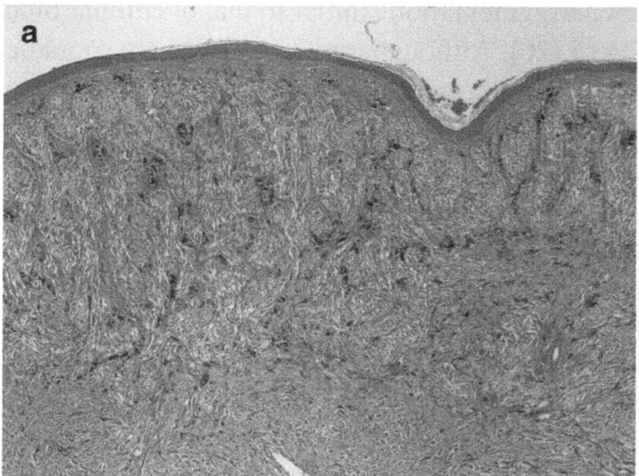

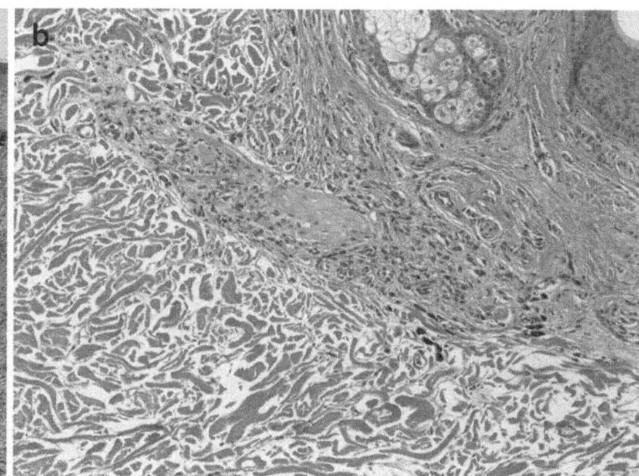

Fig. 10.3 Deep penetrating nevus. (**a**) Superficial portion of the lesion with elongated nests of fusiform cells surrounded by more heavily pigmented melanophages (×4). (**b**) Deeper portion of the lesion with melanocytes following adnexal structures and nerves (×10)

blue nevus, and spindle and epithelioid cell (Spitz) nevus [5–7]. Similar to cellular blue nevus, the less-pigmented spindle and epithelioid cells toward the base of the lesion may concentrate around blood vessels and nerves producing a plexiform pattern of growth reminiscent of a neurofibroma (Fig. 10.3). Deep penetrating nevus also has been described as a component of a combined nevus [5, 8, 9].

Immunohistochemical Features

The Immunohistochemical features are similar for each of the variants of blue nevus. As would be expected for cells having abundant cytoplasmic melanin, labeling for melanosomal glycoproteins such as gp100 (using HMB-45) is present (Fig. 10.4) [10, 14, 15]. Interpretation of Immunohistochemical markers of melanosomal

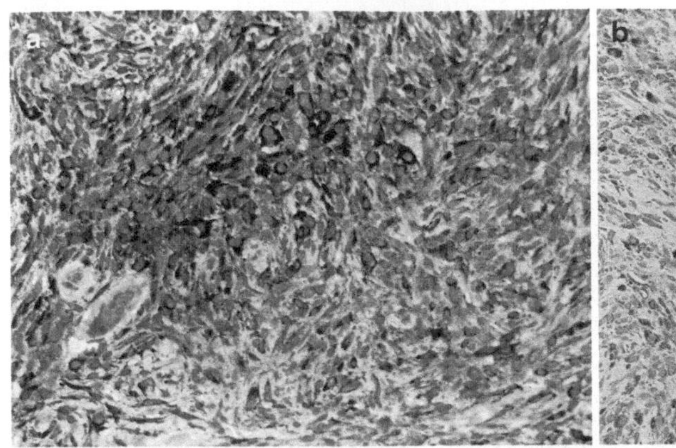

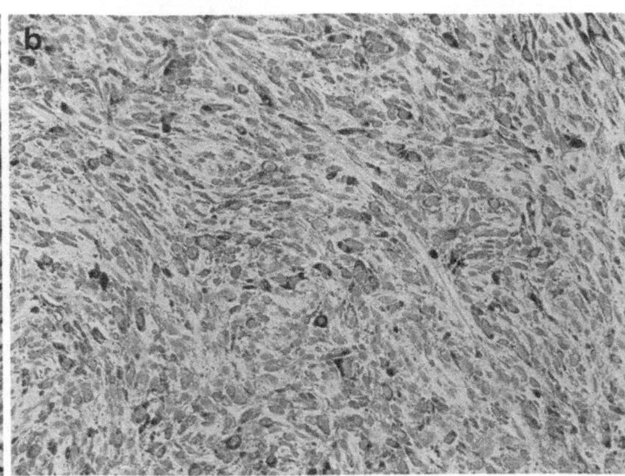

Fig. 10.4 Immunohistochemistry of cellular blue nevus. (**a**) Prominent labeling for gp100 (using HMB45) by most of the fusiform and small epithelioid melanocytes (×20). (**b**) Very few of the melanocytes display nuclear labeling for Ki-67 (using MIB-1) (×20)

proteins is facilitated by use of a red chromogenic substrate to avoid interference with brown cytoplasmic melanin. Labeling typically is uniform throughout the nevus including the melanocytes toward the base. The pattern of maturation typical of an ordinary acquired compound or intradermal nevus having diminished expression with progressive dermal descent (see Chap. 4) is not observed. Labeling for Ki-67 antigen (MIB-1) is not increased (Fig. 10.4) [15].

Pigmented Epithelioid Melanocytoma

Clinical Features

The appellation pigmented epithelioid melanocytoma (PEM) was recently proposed for a lesion that has large epithelioid melanocytes with abundant cytoplasmic melanin [16]. Initially, PEM was proposed to include epithelioid blue nevi associated with Carney Complex (a syndrome characterized by lentigines, myxomas, schwannomas, and endocrine abnormalities) and possibly the pigment synthesizing "animal-type" melanoma, an often less biologically aggressive pigmented melanoma resembling lesions described in horses [17–19]. PEM occur as solitary, usually well-circumscribed nodular lesions with pigmentation similar to that of cellular blue nevi [20]. Although rare, most PEM are sporadic and are not associated with an underlying syndrome. Clinical follow-up suggests that most of these lesions have a benign clinical course, although local recurrence, regional lymph node metastasis, and rare cases of distant metastasis were reported [16, 21]. Recently, it was shown that the large epithelioid melanocytes in most PEM lack expression of one cAMP-dependent protein kinase A regulatory subunit isoform (PKA R1alpha) similar to that observed in the epithelioid blue nevi associated with the Carney Complex [22]. Loss of expression correlated with loss of heterozygosity (LOH) of the PKA R1alpha gene locus at 17q22–24, the same gene mutated in Carney Complex. Loss of expression of PKA R1alpha was not observed in several pigment synthesizing (animal-type) melanomas. This difference and the low rate of distant metastasis, suggest that PEM is a unique neoplasm of lower malignant potential.

Microscopic Features

PEM is characterized by intradermal collections of large epithelioid cells containing abundant cytoplasmic melanin (Fig. 10.5). The lesion may be hypercellular and contain areas in which the

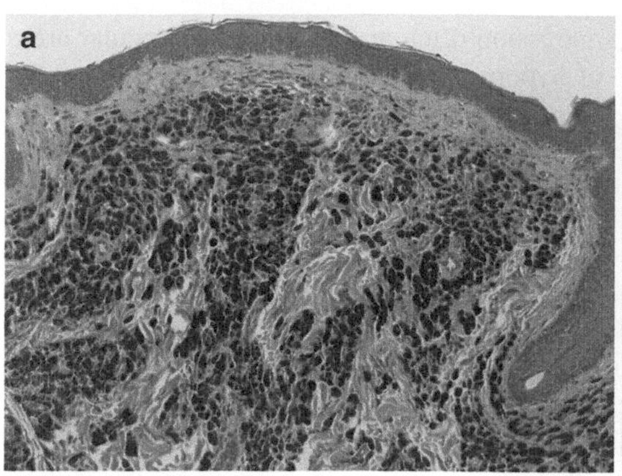

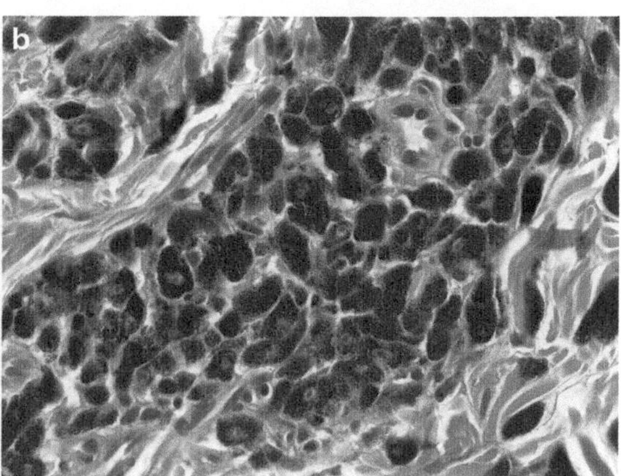

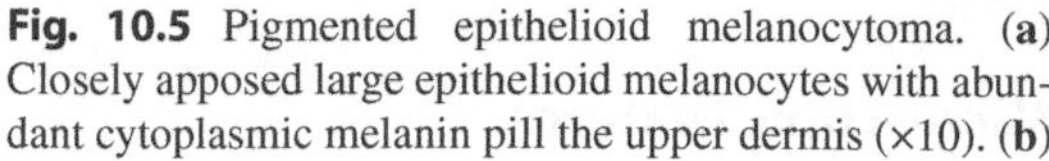

Fig. 10.5 Pigmented epithelioid melanocytoma. (**a**) Closely apposed large epithelioid melanocytes with abundant cytoplasmic melanin pill the upper dermis (×10). (**b**) Most of the cells have an enlarged nucleus containing one or two prominent eosinophilic nucleolus/nucleoli (×40)

epithelioid cells are closely apposed, but not forming cohesive nests. Numerous melanophages are present within the lesion as well. The melanophages typically are smaller than the epithelioid melanocytes. Larger nodules may be ulcerated and some lesions have a small junctional component. Most of the epithelioid melanocytes have an enlarged nucleus with a single prominent nucleolus. Mitotic figures are rare, but if present, should raise suspicion for a more aggressive clinical course. In some PEM, cytoplasmic melanin may obscure the nucleus and obviate assessment of mitotic rate necessitating histochemical bleaching procedures. It is important to remember that subsequent immunohistochemical studies may be unreliable on sections previously bleached of melanin.

Immunohistochemical Features

Similar to blue nevi, markers of melanosomal glycoproteins such as gp100, and Melan A/MART-1 are expressed in cells of PEM. Labeling for Ki-67 antigen may be useful to identify "hot spots" of proliferative activity not observed in cellular blue nevi. Loss of expression of PKA R1alpha can be documented by immunohistochemistry and LOH of 17q22–24 confirmed by molecular genetic analysis [22].

Differential Diagnosis: Post-Inflammatory Pigmentary Alteration (PIPA)

Clinical Features

Melanocytic lesions containing heavily pigmented dermal melanocytes must be distinguished from other neoplasms and inflammatory dermatoses rich in melanophages. Dermal aggregates of melanophages may elicit a clinical appearance similar to that of blue nevi. Any neoplasm or inflammatory dermatosis resulting in cytolysis of melanin-containing cells may lead to melanin incontinence and a subsequent infiltrate of melanophages [23, 24]. Epidermal keratinocytes provide the source of melanin incontinence for many of the inflammatory dermatoses associated with PIPA. Lichenoid interface dermatoses such as lichen planus or lupus erythematosus often result in areas of PIPA as does physical trauma such as chronic rubbing/excoriation or thermal injury.

Microscopic Features

The common finding in PIPA regardless of etiology is the presence of melanophages in the

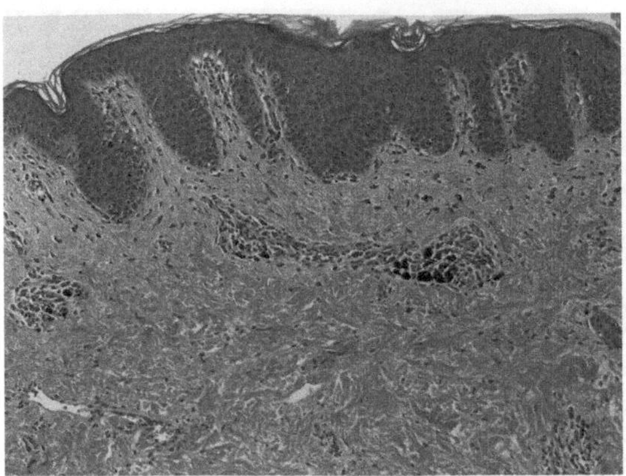

Fig. 10.6 Postinflammatory pigmentary alteration. Example of a partially resolved fixed drug eruption with clusters of melanophages in a perivascular distribution in the upper dermis (×10). The melanophages are small and lack dendritic processes or nuclear atypia

dermis (Fig. 10.6). Resolved inflammatory dermatoses may have few other inflammatory cells suggestive of an active process. Epidermal rete ridges may be attenuated in resolved lichenoid interface dermatitis and the basement membrane zone may be thickened in long-standing lesions of discoid lupus erythematosus. Individual melanophages have a small epithelioid appearance. Most contain coarse granular melanin and a small nucleus with inconspicuous nucleoli. Some melanophages may be elongated, but delicate branched dendritic processes are not present. This feature is critical for distinguishing PIPA from blue nevus. Similarly, melanophages are much smaller and lack the nuclear changes typical of the epithelioid cells in PEM.

Differential Diagnosis: Regressed Malignant Melanoma

Clinical Features

Clinical history of a changing melanocytic lesion with asymmetry, irregular borders, and variation in color should raise suspicion of an atypical melanocytic nevus or malignant melanoma. Some melanomas and atypical nevi undergo spontaneous regression mediated by the host immune system. Clinical features of regression often are manifest by irregular areas of hypopigmentation/depigmentation, hyperpigmentation or erythema within a preexisting pigmented lesion. A melanocytic lesion undergoing spontaneous regression may exhibit multiple shades of blue, brown, black, and red or may have zones devoid of melanin. Long-standing regression may produce a depigmented/hypopigmented patch resembling a lesion of vitiligo or an old scar. Clinical knowledge of a prior pigmented lesion at the site may thus be necessary for accurate diagnosis.

Microscopic Features

Many of the histologic features described for PIPA above also are present in regressed melanomas (Fig. 10.7) [25–27]. In fact, regression involves an immunoregulatory response that results in melanoma cell death and melanin incontinence with subsequent melanophage activity of variable degree. Other features suggestive of regression include alterations of dermal collagen fibers, vascular proliferation, and attenuation of overlying epidermal rete ridges, features also present in scars and recurrent nevi [28, 29]. Partially regressed lesions also contain residual melanoma cells in the epidermis and/or in the dermis in addition to the infiltrate of melanophages. Immunohistochemistry may be helpful to identify a small residual focus of melanoma partially obscured by the inflammation associated with regression. Histologic features suggestive of regression in the absence of a melanocytic lesion require adequate clinical correlation to determine if the biopsy is a representative sample of the lesion.

Differential Diagnosis: Foreign Body Reaction to Tattoo

Clinical Features

Clinical history of prior trauma may be the best clue for the diagnosis of a foreign body tattoo. Pigmented material commonly found in traumatic

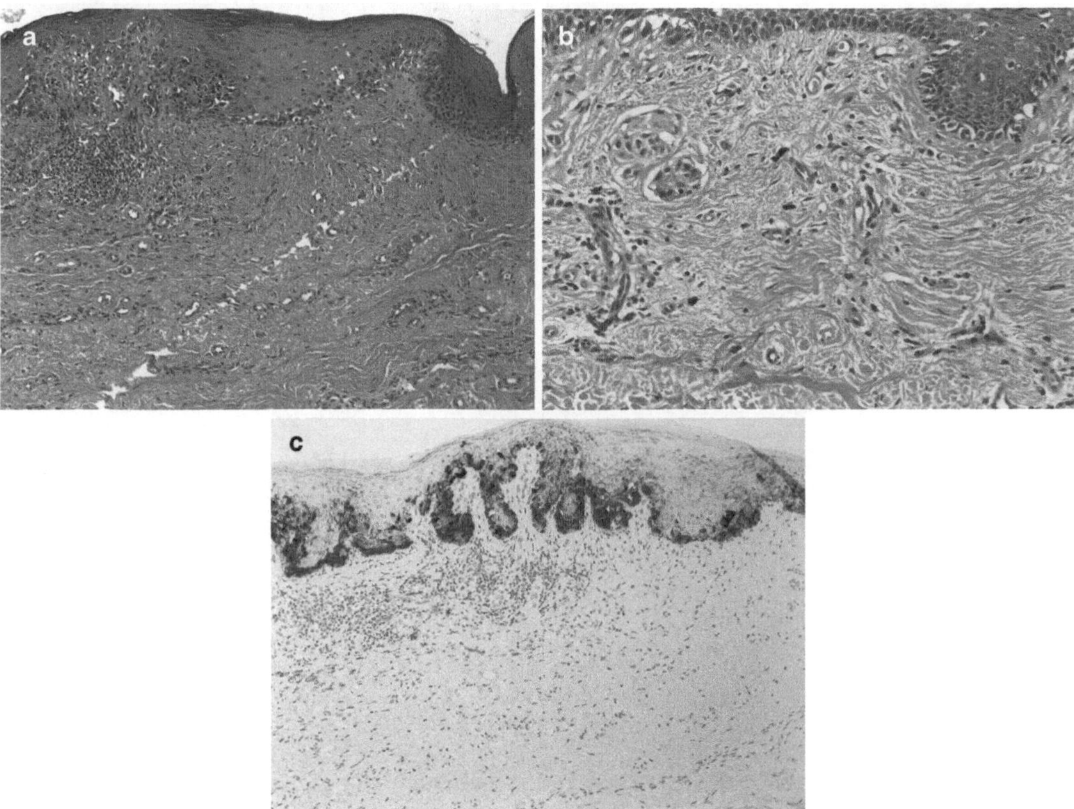

Fig. 10.7 Malignant melanoma with partial regression. (**a**) Melanoma in situ with features of regression in the subjacent dermis (×20). (**b**) Clusters of small epithelioid melanophages are scattered within an area of dermis having lamellar fibroplasia and vascular proliferation (×20). Note the nests of larger epithelioid invasive melanoma cells toward the left edge. (**c**) Anti-Melan A/MART-1 highlights the intraepidermal melanoma cells, but does not reveal a residual invasive dermal component (×20). Numerous small melanophages within the area of regression are not immunolabeled

tattoos include graphite, metals such as aluminum, and components of soil. Intentional (ornamental) tattoos also may be seen as an incidental finding in biopsies of an adjacent neoplastic or inflammatory process.

Microscopic Features

Traumatic tattoos have a dermal scar containing scattered pigmented macrophages (Fig. 10.8). Pigmented material also may be present in the extracellular space. The color of pigmented material will depend on its source. Graphite and many tattoo inks appear black in histologic sections; red tattoo ink may be more obvious. Traumatic tattoos may contain additional non-pigmented foreign material such as cotton fibers or silicates/glass. Larger particles of foreign material may induce histological sectioning artifact drawing attention to its presence. Observation with polarized light also may reveal smaller particles of non-pigmented material thereby implicating prior trauma as a source for the associated pigmented material as well. Associated features of an allergic hypersensitivity reaction can be seen with certain ornamental tattoo dyes [30, 31].

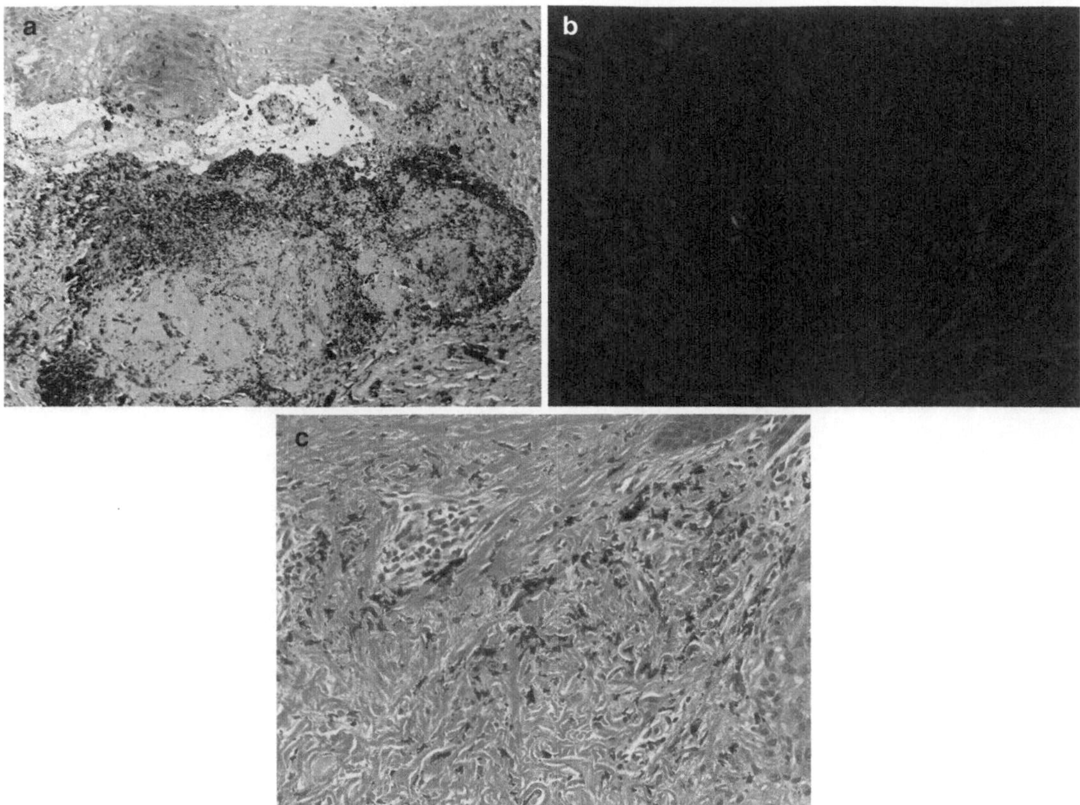

Fig. 10.8 Traumatic tattoo. (**a**) Black graphite pigment from a pencil-stick injury (×10). Note histological artifact caused by the foreign material in the section. (**b**) Observation with polarized light reveals refractile foreign body within the tattoo (×20). (**c**) Intentional/ornamental tattoo with red pigment (×20)

Differential Diagnosis: Ferrugination of Biopsy Site (Monsel Tattoo)

Clinical Features

Clinical history of a prior biopsy (most often a shave biopsy) is helpful to recognize this iatrogenic foreign body reaction. Monsel solution (20 % ferric subsulfate solution) is an agent used for hemostasis following a superficial biopsy [32–34]. Over time, oxidation of the ferruginous crystals may lead to brown pigmentation within the prior biopsy scar. This may be concerning for recurrence of a melanocytic lesion at the site of prior removal.

Microscopic Features

Features of scar should be present in the dermis. Collections of macrophages with brown or yellow–brown granular cytoplasmic pigment are scattered throughout the scar (Fig. 10.9). Importantly, similar pigmented material often is present on collagen fibers giving the entire scar a brownish hue on low magnification of hematoxylin- and eosin-stained sections. The ferruginous material also can be seen in the subcutaneous tissues including skeletal muscle [32]. Observation with polarized light may reveal suture material associated with a prior biopsy/surgical site, but the pigmented material itself is not birefringent. A histochemical stain for iron often is helpful to distinguish the pigmented macrophages in a

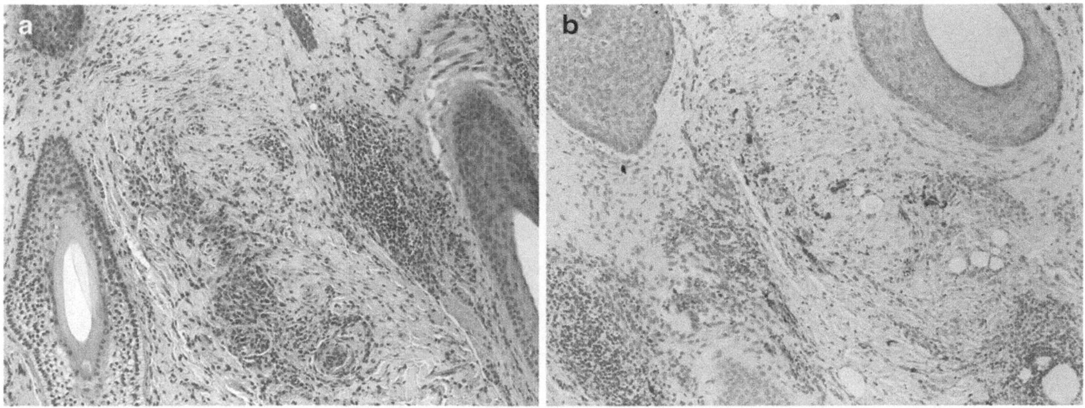

Fig. 10.9 Ferrugination of Biopsy Site (Monsel Tattoo). (**a**) Clusters of epithelioid macrophages containing cytoplasmic brown granular pigment within a biopsy scar (×10). (**b**) Stain for iron highlights the macrophages (×10)

Monsel tattoo from carbonaceous material in traumatic tattoo or from melanophages in PIPA or in a regressed melanocytic lesion.

Differential Diagnosis: Minocycline Hyperpigmentation

Clinical Features

Another form of iatrogenic hyperpigmentation may be seen in patients on long-standing therapy with minocycline. Several distinct clinical presentations of minocycline hyperpigmentation have been reported, one of which appears to be limited to preexisting scars [35–37]. Individual hyperpigmented scars may resemble melanocytic lesions.

Microscopic Features

The histologic features are very similar to those of PIPA, a regressed melanocytic lesion, and of Monsel tattoo, although extracellular pigmented material is not obvious. The dermis often contains a scar and has scattered epithelioid and fusiform cells containing brown–black finely granular cytoplasmic pigment (Fig. 10.10). Pigment also may coat elastic fibers and be present in eccrine myoepithelial cells and in the subcutis [35, 38]. The precise mechanism for hyperpigmentation is unclear, but several known metabolites of minocycline have been shown to chelate iron and/or form a complex with melanin [39–41]. Not unexpectedly, histochemical stains for iron and for melanin often are positive. Both of these stains would thus be needed to rule out PIPA and Monsel tattoo.

Conclusions

The initial diagnostic approach toward a cutaneous lesion with abundant pigmentation should include careful consideration of the clinical history and review of any prior biopsy from the same anatomic site. Observation with polarized light may help to rule out foreign bodies, and histochemical stains for iron and/or for melanin may be necessary in select cases to determine the composition of the pigmented material. Cellular size and nuclear features are an important determinant in the differential diagnosis of melanocytic lesions. Immunohistochemistry also may help to distinguish blue nevi with atypia from PEM. Rare cases may require molecular cytogenetic studies if the amount of pigmentation confounds interpretation of immunohistochemistry.

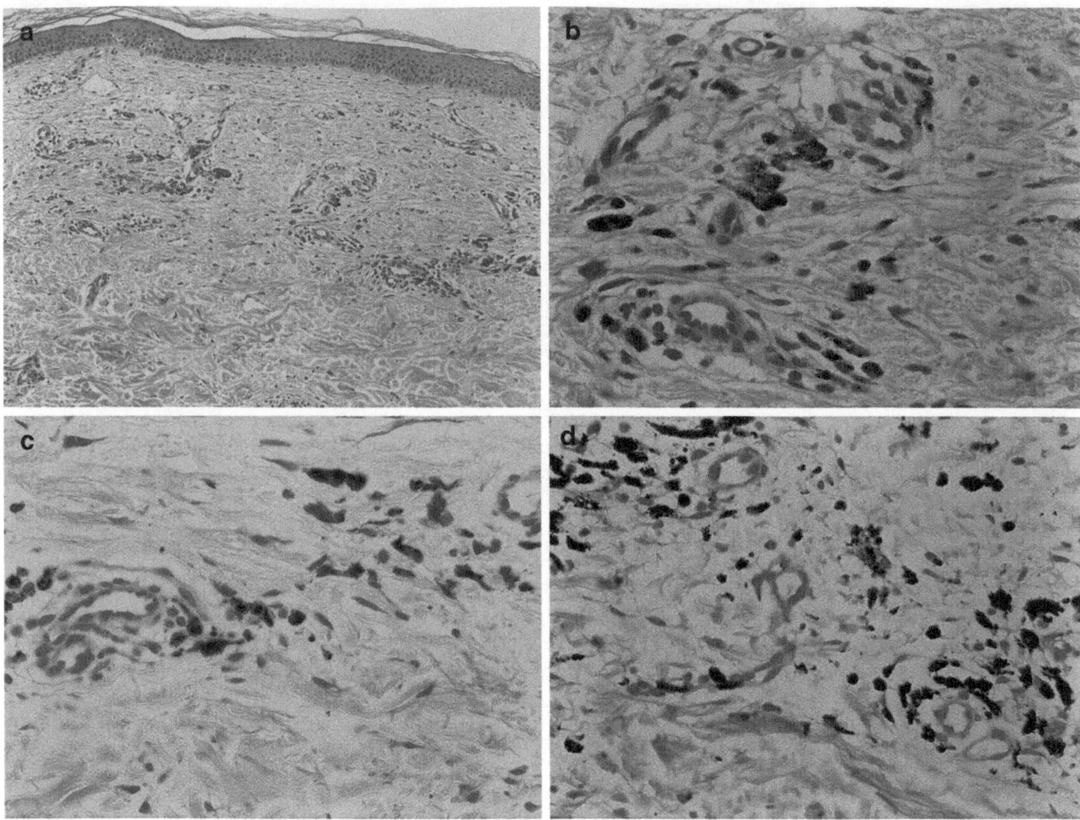

Fig. 10.10 Minocycline hyperpigmentation. (**a**) Perivascular collections of pigmented epithelioid and fusiform cells (×10). (**b**) Most of the cells contain dark brown-to-black granular material in their cytoplasm (×40). (**c**) Stain for iron highlights the cells with granular pigment (×40). (**d**) Fontana stain for melanin also highlights the pigmented cells (×40)

References

1. Ferrara G, Soyer HP, Malvehy J, et al. The many faces of blue nevus: a clinicopathologic study. J Cutan Pathol. 2007;34:543–51.
2. Harrison-Balestra C, Gugic D, Vincek V. Clinically distinct form of acquired dermal melanocytosis with review of published work. J Dermatol. 2007;34: 178–82.
3. Lee JY, Lee JS, Kim YC. Histopathological features of acquired dermal melanocytosis. Eur J Dermatol. 2010;20:345–8.
4. Gonzalez-Campora R, Galera-Davidson H, Vazquez-Ramirez FJ, Diaz-Cano S. Blue nevus: classical types and new related entities. A differential diagnostic review. Pathol Res Pract. 1994;190:627–35.
5. Cooper PH. Deep penetrating (plexiform spindle cell) nevus. A frequent participant in combined nevus. J Cutan Pathol. 1992;19:172–80.
6. Mehregan DA, Mehregan AH. Deep penetrating nevus. Arch Dermatol. 1993;129:328–31.
7. Seab JAJ, Graham JH, Helwig EB. Deep penetrating nevus. Am J Surg Pathol. 1989;13:39–44.
8. Baran JL, Duncan LM. Combined melanocytic nevi: histologic variants and melanoma mimics. Am J Surg Pathol. 2011;35:1540–8.
9. Scolyer RA, Zhuang L, Palmer AA, Thompson JF, McCarthy SW. Combined naevus: a benign lesion frequently misdiagnosed both clinically and pathologically as melanoma. Pathology. 2004;36:419–27.
10. Murali R, McCarthy SW, Scolyer RA. Blue nevi and related lesions: a review highlighting atypical and newly described variants, distinguishing features and diagnostic pitfalls. Adv Anat Pathol. 2009;16: 365–82.
11. Barnhill RL, Argenyi Z, Berwick M, et al. Atypical cellular blue nevi (cellular blue nevi with atypical features): lack of consensus for diagnosis and distinction from cellular blue nevi and malignant melanoma ("malignant blue nevus"). Am J Surg Pathol. 2008; 32:36–44.
12. Maize JCJ, McCalmont TH, Carlson JA, Busam KJ, Kutzner H, Bastian BC. Genomic analysis of blue

nevi and related dermal melanocytic proliferations. Am J Surg Pathol. 2005;29:1214–20.
13. Cerroni L, Borroni RG, Massone C, Kerl H. "Ancient" blue nevi (cellular blue nevi with degenerative stromal changes). Am J Dermatopathol. 2008;30:1–5.
14. Skelton HG, Smith KJ, Barrett TL, Lupton GP, Graham JH. HMB-45 staining in benign and malignant melanocytic lesions. A reflection of cellular activation. Am J Dermatopathol. 1991;13:543–50.
15. Wang Q, Prieto V, Esmaeli B, et al. Cellular blue nevi of the eyelid: a possible diagnostic pitfall. J Am Acad Dermatol. 2008;58:257–60.
16. Zembowicz A, Carney JA, Mihm MC. Pigmented epithelioid melanocytoma: a low-grade melanocytic tumor with metastatic potential indistinguishable from animal-type melanoma and epithelioid blue nevus. Am J Surg Pathol. 2004;28:31–40.
17. Antony FC, Sanclemente G, Shaikh H, Trelles AS, Calonje E. Pigment synthesizing melanoma (so-called animal type melanoma): a clinicopathological study of 14 cases of a poorly known distinctive variant of melanoma. Histopathology. 2006;48:754–62.
18. Crowson AN, Magro CM, Mihm MCJ. Malignant melanoma with prominent pigment synthesis: "animal type" melanoma—a clinical and histological study of six cases with a consideration of other melanocytic neoplasms with prominent pigment synthesis. Hum Pathol. 1999;30:543–50.
19. Groben PA, Harvell JD, White WL. Epithelioid blue nevus: neoplasm Sui generis or variation on a theme? Am J Dermatopathol. 2000;22:473–88.
20. Howard B, Ragsdale B, Lundquist K. Pigmented epithelioid melanocytoma: two case reports. Dermatol Online J. 2005;11:1.
21. Mandal RV, Murali R, Lundquist KF, et al. Pigmented epithelioid melanocytoma: favorable outcome after 5-year follow-up. Am J Surg Pathol. 2009;33:1778–82.
22. Zembowicz A, Knoepp SM, Bei T, et al. Loss of expression of protein kinase a regulatory subunit 1alpha in pigmented epithelioid melanocytoma but not in melanoma or other melanocytic lesions. Am J Surg Pathol. 2007;31:1764–75.
23. Chance EW. Treatment of unwanted pigment. Facial Plast Surg. 2014;30:16–25.
24. Ruiz-Maldonado R, Orozco-Covarrubias ML. Postinflammatory hypopigmentation and hyperpigmentation. Semin Cutan Med Surg. 1997;16:36–43.
25. Emanuel PO, Mannion M, Phelps RG. Complete regression of primary malignant melanoma. Am J Dermatopathol. 2008;30:178–81.
26. Fontaine D, Parkhill W, Greer W, Walsh N. Partial regression of primary cutaneous melanoma: is there an association with sub-clinical sentinel lymph node metastasis? Am J Dermatopathol. 2003;25:371–6.
27. High WA, Stewart D, Wilbers CR, Cockerell CJ, Hoang MP, Fitzpatrick JE. Completely regressed primary cutaneous malignant melanoma with nodal and/or visceral metastases: a report of 5 cases and assessment of the literature and diagnostic criteria. J Am Acad Dermatol. 2005;53:89–100.
28. Duray PH, Livolsi VA. Recurrent dysplastic nevus following shave excision. J Dermatol Surg Oncol. 1984;10:811–5.
29. King R, Hayzen BA, Page RN, Googe PB, Zeagler D, Mihm MCJ. Recurrent nevus phenomenon: a clinicopathologic study of 357 cases and histologic comparison with melanoma with regression. Mod Pathol. 2009;22:611–7.
30. Mortimer NJ, Chave TA, Johnston GA. Red tattoo reactions. Clin Exp Dermatol. 2003;28:508–10.
31. Steinbrecher I, Hemmer W, Jarisch R. Adverse reaction to the azo dye Pigment Red 170 in a tattoo. J Dtsch Dermatol Ges. 2004;2:1007–8.
32. Amazon K, Robinson MJ, Rywlin AM. Ferrugination caused by Monsel's solution. Clinical observations and experimentations. Am J Dermatopathol. 1980;2:197–205.
33. Olmstead PM, Lund HZ, Leonard DD. Monsel's solution: a histologic nuisance. J Am Acad Dermatol. 1980;3:492–8.
34. Wood C, Severin GL. Unusual histiocytic reaction to Monsel's solution. Am J Dermatopathol. 1980;2:261–4.
35. Argenyi ZB, Finelli L, Bergfeld WF, et al. Minocycline-related cutaneous hyperpigmentation as demonstrated by light microscopy, electron microscopy and X-ray energy spectroscopy. J Cutan Pathol. 1987;14:176–80.
36. Patterson JW, Wilson B, Wick MR, Heath C. Hyperpigmented scar due to minocycline therapy. Cutis. 2004;74:293–8.
37. Simons JJ, Morales A. Minocycline and generalized cutaneous pigmentation. J Am Acad Dermatol. 1980;3:244–7.
38. Bowen AR, McCalmont TH. The histopathology of subcutaneous minocycline pigmentation. J Am Acad Dermatol. 2007;57:836–9.
39. Fenske NA, Millns JL, Greer KE. Minocycline-induced pigmentation at sites of cutaneous inflammation. JAMA. 1980;244:1103–6.
40. Ridgway HA, Sonnex TS, Kennedy CT, Millard PR, Henderson WJ, Gold SC. Hyperpigmentation associated with oral minocycline. Br J Dermatol. 1982;107:95–102.
41. Sato S, Murphy GF, Bernhard JD, Mihm MCJ, Fitzpatrick TB. Ultrastructural and X-ray microanalytical observations of minocycline-related hyperpigmentation of the skin. J Invest Dermatol. 1981;77:264–71.

Recurrent Melanocytic Nevus Versus Melanoma

11

Alexander D. Means, Victor G. Prieto, Jon A. Reed, and Christopher R. Shea

Introduction

Recurrent melanocytic nevi (RMN) present a diagnostic dilemma for both clinician and pathologist. The term refers to the development of another melanocytic lesion at the site of a previously incompletely excised or injured melanocytic neoplasm. The word "pseudomelanoma," occasionally used to reference recurrent nevi but additionally variously ascribed over the last century to lesions clinically resembling melanoma (including pigmented basal cell carcinomas, sclerosing hemangiomas, blue nevi, seborrheic keratoses, congenital nevi, Spitz nevi, onychomycosis, and acquired benign or atypical nevi) [1–7], continues to be used in the ophthalmologic literature to refer to lesions clinically mimicking melanoma of the eye [8]; however we recommend that this term be avoided in dermatologic communications in favor of the far less ambiguous term, recurrent nevus. While the exact mechanisms of recurrence are still an active area of research, the underlying cause is invariably due to subsequent proliferation and migration of melanocytes within and around the residual dermal scar, which manifest as irregular and variably pigmented macules or papules with a characteristic appearance on histopathology.

A.D. Means • C.R. Shea, M.D. (✉)
University of Chicago Medicine, 5841 S. Maryland Ave., MC 5067, L502, Chicago, IL 60637, USA
e-mail: cshea@medicine.bsd.uchicago.edu

V.G. Prieto
MD Anderson Cancer Center, University of Houston, 1515 Holcombe Blvd., Unit 85, Houston, TX 77030, USA

J.A. Reed
CellNEtix Pathology & Laboratories, 1124 Columbia St., Suite 200, Seattle, WA 98117, USA

Mechanisms of Recurrence of Nevi

There have been no studies to date that convincingly demonstrate the physiology of nevi recurrence. Several mechanisms, from seeding of existing melanocytes during excision [9] and trauma-induced reversion to a more primitive proliferative stage of nevogenesis, to growth factor signaling by surviving melanocytes, have been proposed but without experimental data to support their claim [9–12]. Immunofluorescence studies have lent substantiation to contributions of dendritic eccrine- and follicular-derived melanocytes in repopulating junctional and dermal nests along appendageal structures [13]; this may be mediated through adnexal melanocytic stem cells as demonstrated in vivo using a murine model [14]. The notion that junctional melanocytes in RMN must originate from existing epithelial melanocytic populations including those in adnexae has also been suggested given the absence of gp100 (HMB-45) immunostaining that

C.R. Shea et al. (eds.), *Pathology of Challenging Melanocytic Neoplasms: Diagnosis and Management*, DOI 10.1007/978-1-4939-1444-9_11,

would be expected for dermally derived progenitors [15]. Residual dermal melanocytes resembling fibroblasts have however been detected within scars of re-excised recurrent nevi as staining S100 (+) [positive], factor VIII/XIIIa (–) [negative] [16], suggesting a possible perivascular migration from the deep dermis to the dermal–epidermal junction. Further research is clearly needed into this topic, and it is likely that still other mechanisms are at play.

Epidemiology

The diagnosis of RMN is suggested by a history of prior biopsy, but nonsurgical trauma can also alter the architecture of a melanocytic neoplasm and initiate the same wound-healing response that leads to an RMN phenotype on histology. Injury to the site may not be recalled by the patient presenting for dermatologic evaluation, or may be of a chronic irritant nature as from clothing, further complicating matters [9]. RMN have also occurred following the use of CO_2, erbium:yttrium aluminum garnet, alexandrite, and Q-switched ruby lasers for destruction of melanocytic nevi, likely second to incomplete destruction of deeper dermal components [3, 17–19]. Given these concerns, the use of any laser for cosmetic removal of clinically benign melanocytic nevi is not recommended, though there may be situations (such as large congenital nevi) where elective surgical removal may not be feasible. Similar reports have also been published of RMN resulting from treatment with radiotherapy for lung cancer [20], Solcoderm (a proprietary mixture of organic and inorganic acids and copper ions) application for destruction of benign pigmented lesions [21, 22], intralesional triamcinolone injection intended to prevent keloid formation [23], electrodesiccation [24], dermabrasion [25], and following shave biopsy with Monsel solution [26]. Recurrent nevi have been described on oral mucosa [27] as well as cutaneous genital [28], glabrous, and hair-bearing skin, with a predilection for the back more than the face and extremities [29–31]. There is a 4:1 female predominance, with mean age at diagnosis of around 30 years old [32]. Both common and atypical melanocytic nevi have been shown in large, separate studies to recur more frequently than other types of pigmented lesions, and conclusions cannot be drawn regarding which has a higher rate of recurrence at this time [29, 33].

Clinical Features

Clinically, RMN present within a few weeks to up to 6 months after trauma as irregular, variably pigmented macules or papules with stippled, streaked, halo, or diffuse pigmented networks. A history of prior biopsy or nonsurgical trauma is usually elicited. Pigment is often most intense initially, and fades with time. Reactive pigmented lesions may develop in the scars of both melanocytic and non-melanocytic tumors, and are suggested by the presence of a regular pigment network and/or streaks on dermoscopy [34]. Benign RMN on dermoscopy tend to display radial lines, symmetry, and a centrifugal growth pattern [35]; a starburst pattern has also been described [36]. With few exceptions (see below), they grow within the margins of the scar, as opposed to malignant melanomas, which often invade into surrounding healthy skin [37] (Table 11.1, Fig. 11.1).

Histopathologic Features

When entertaining the diagnosis of RMN, it is preferable, if not essential, to have for comparison slides of the patient's initial biopsy for comparison. Any unusual features such as atypia initially present in the nevus would be expected

Table 11.1 Clinical features of recurrent nevi

Women 20–40 years old
Back > face, extremities
History of biopsy or excision, with or without free margins
Appear within weeks–months after excision
Pigment usually within margins of scar
Pigment fades with time
Benign or atypical nevi most commonly recur

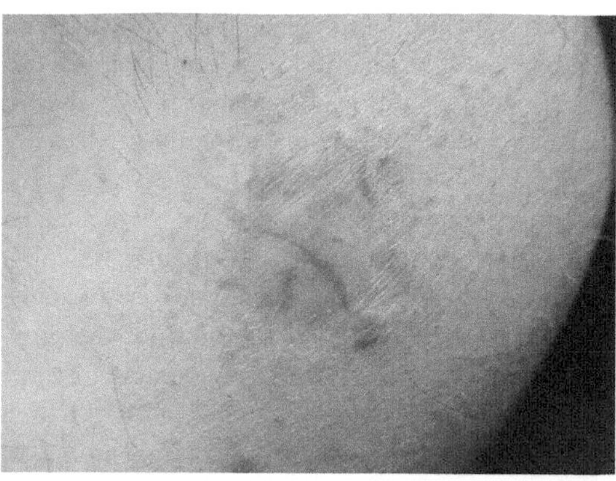

Fig. 11.1 Recurrent melanocytic nevus. Multiple irregularly shaped pigmented streaks are present within the margins of an atrophic scar. The patient had a history of shave excision of a junctional melanocytic nevus 17 years prior

Table 11.2 Histopathologic features of recurrent nevi

Junctional confluence
Orderly central fibrosis
Dermal nests with normal maturation
Cytologic atypia usually contained in junctional component or superficial scar
Single-cell proliferation contained in the junctional component
Compound or intradermal nevi most common
Epithelioid melanocytes predominate
Focal hyperplasia, rare mitoses, or pagetoid spread may be seen in isolation

to similarly manifest in a recurrence. Larger case series have shown up to 60 % of recurrent nevi are compound, followed by intradermal and then junctional nevi [29–31]. A distinguishing feature of recurrent nevi is the presence of a central dermal scar, interposed between a confluent junctional melanocytic component and deeper nests of residual melanocytes and melanophages—the so-called "trizonal"pattern [9]. Epithelioid melanocytes with bland and evenly staining nuclei are usually seen, though atypical histopathologic features such as confluence of melanocytic nests, cytologic atypia of melanocytes, suprabasal spread, and dermal mitotic figures are not uncommon in the junctional component, hence the historical pathologic correlate for the term "pseudomelanoma" [30, 38].

In one of the largest studies to date, 112 out of 357 recurrent nevi (26 %) demonstrated single-cell proliferation [29]. Extension and suprabasal spread of melanocytes down the adnexal structures was present in 6 % of cases. A confluent lentiginous growth pattern was observed in 2 % of the cases. 26 % of cases showed cytologic atypia, defined as hyperchromasia and nuclear enlargement. Usually, the irregular architectural and cytologic patterns seen in recurrent nevi are restricted to the epidermis and dermis immediately above the scar [39], and most RMN display a normal maturation pattern. However, focal lentiginous hyperplasia, moderate nuclear atypia, rare mitotic figures, and pagetoid spread (not beyond the granular layer) have been reported in decreasing order from 35 to 3 %, usually in isolation [30]. Furthermore, the appropriate diagnosis of RMN may be obscured by features consistent with intermediate/late stage regression of melanoma and dermal scar extending to the margin of the biopsy specimen [29]. Clinical-pathologic correlation is of particular importance in such cases as distinction from melanoma can be difficult without a pertinent history.

Reflectance confocal microscopy is an emerging in vivo adjunct for the characterization of pigmented lesions [40]. One case series of three patients with recurrent nevi showed some atypical but cytologically monomorphous junctional melanocytes consistent with histopathologic analysis, without any pagetoid or lateral spread of melanocytes or atypical nests [41] (Table 11.2, Fig. 11.2).

Immunohistochemistry

Like their original nevi counterparts, RMN usually display a normal maturation gradient, with decreased expression of tyrosinase and gp100 deeper into the dermis and persistently low mitotic activity (<5 %) by Ki67 [15, 39]. Melanomas typically immunolabel strongly for all three stains, though exceptions have been described [42, 43]. Unfortunately, MART-1 (Melan-A) and S100 proteins have not been shown to be of use in distinguishing between these two entities [39]. Future utility of soluble

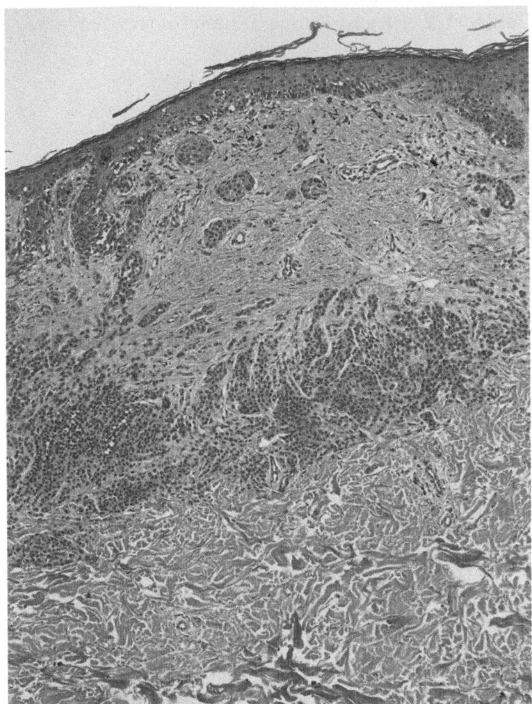

Fig. 11.2 Characteristic trizonal pattern of fibrosis in a recurrent nevus. Note the (1) confluent junctional component with epidermal pigmentation overlying an area of (2) central fibrosis and finally (3) nests of smaller nevus cells

adenylyl cyclase has been suggested in one small newer study, in which histopathologically benign recurrent nevi displayed an immunostaining pattern similar to the original lesion when compared to melanomas [44].

Special Types of Recurrent Nevi

Recurrent Atypical (Dysplastic) Nevus

Atypical nevi, first recognized in families with an increased risk of melanoma as nevi with unusual clinicopathologic features [45, 46] and autosomal dominant inheritance [47], present a challenge for many pathologists given their subjective and evolving controversial diagnostic criteria and association with melanoma [48]. They tend to show lentiginous and nesting proliferations, varying degrees of cytologic atypia with accompanying host inflammatory response, elongation and bridging of rete ridges, fibroplasia around rete pegs with proliferation of dermal capillaries, and horizontally arranged, usually spindle-shaped melanocytes [49]. In one study of mild-moderately atypical nevi followed for at least 2 years compared to benign nevi, fewer than 4 % of nevi in either group were found to recur clinically. Recurrence was associated with the use of shave biopsy technique for sampling but not the presence of positive margins or congenital features [50]. Other retrospective studies with up to 5 years follow-up have not shown melanoma to occur from excised atypical nevi, irrespective of margin involvement [51, 52].

Recurrent Spitz Nevi

Recurrent Spitz (spindled and epithelioid cell) nevi often demonstrate unusual features when compared to typical recurrent melanocytic nevi, not least of which is that their clinical presentation tends to be nodular rather than macular and can extend beyond the margins of the scar [53, 54]. Despite the presence of positive margins in many Spitz nevi, they infrequently recur. In a larger case series of 16 patients, the average time to recurrence was around 13 months, with predominately intradermal nests of spindled or epithelioid cells that extended into the deep reticular dermis and subcutis within an almost keloidal stroma [55]. These lesions histopathologically resembled desmoplastic Spitz nevus rather than the primary Spitz nevus. Other case series have shown less of a histopathological discordance between primary and recurrent Spitz nevi [56–58], and supported the observations of a desmoplastic stroma, a nodular growth pattern with low mitotic indices, maturation as assessed by immunostaining, and junctional nesting with intraepidermal spread above a dermal scar, such that many recurrent nevi can simulate melanoma. Recurrent Spitz nevi have reportedly resulted in metastasis and death [59], but in such extraordinary cases the diagnosis of Spitz nevus rather than melanoma must be questioned. The use of fluorescent in situ hybridization (FISH) or comparative genomic hybridization (CGH) can be used in conjunction with histopathologic and immunostains for further help in distinguishing between melanoma and recurrent Spitz nevi [57].

Recurrent Blue Nevi

There are even fewer reports of recurrent blue nevi than recurrent Spitz or atypical nevi, but they have been described as recurring from cutaneous (including 1 report of recurrence from a plaque-type blue nevus with malignant transformation and mortality [60]) and mucocutaneous surfaces as well as lymph nodes [61–63], the latter of which can further complicate the already difficult distinction between metastatic melanoma and benign nodal blue nevi [64]. Recurrences have been reported in all subsets and histotypes, and occur an average of 2.7 years after initial biopsy. Extension beyond the margins of the original scar has been described. In the largest case series reported to date, seven of nine recurrences resembled the original biopsy, occasionally with a more cellular deep component. The other two recurrences demonstrated a higher degree of cytologic atypia when compared to prior, although follow-up (mean 3.7 years) did not support malignant tumor progression [61].

Sclerosing Nevus with Features of Recurrent Nevi

Sclerosing nevi with pseudomelanomatous features, first described in 2008 [65] and similarly detailed in a larger case series as nevi with regression-like fibrosis in 2009 [66, 67], are relatively new entities to the recurrent nevi family characterized on the basis of their unique clinical and pathologic features including an absence of preceding trauma or biopsy. All of the 19 reported sclerosing nevi with pseudomelanomatous features had clinical features suggestive of regression in conjunction with architecturally disordered junctional and dermal melanocytic nests with pagetoid spread but few to no mitotic figures and no high-grade cytologic atypia or pleomorphism, flanking a central band of fibrous scar-like tissue. They were primarily from the truncal sites in young to middle-aged patients, as were the 90 reported nevi with regression-like fibrosis cases, and did not recur or metastasize at 2–9 year follow-up. Etiology is thought to be related to chronic, asymptomatic trauma over years, leading to atypical regenerative hyperplasia and fibrosis.

Epidermolysis Bullosa Nevi

Acquired nevi arising within scarred areas of former blistering in patients with hereditary epidermolysis bullosa have been shown to have clinical and histopathologic features similar to recurrent nevi, and these so-called "EB nevi" should be considered in the differential diagnosis of recurrent nevi when supported by history and clinical exam [68].

Differential Diagnosis

In addition to the special types mentioned above, the most important diagnoses to consider in the differential of a recurrent benign melanocytic nevus include melanoma arising from a dermal nevus, and a nevus with changes of regression.

The junctional confluence and atypia in melanomas tend to be more severe than in recurrent nevi, and should raise suspicion when seen in combination with prominent pagetoid spread and/or mitoses, features which individually can be seen in recurrent nevi but not altogether. While fibrosis can be seen in melanoma, it will not usually be in an orderly, trizonal pattern. A prominent lymphocytic infiltrate will also be seen [69]. Additional stains such as Ki-67, Melan-A, and HMB-45 (anti-gp100) should be employed if there is even the slightest doubt about whether or not a melanoma is present [29, 70].

RMN can have the same architecture as a regressed melanoma, and is more common in atypical nevi. Fibrosis is again present, but will be irregular and in association with prominent melanophages.

Table 11.3 Recurrent nevus vs melanoma

	Recurrent nevus	Melanoma arising with a nevus	Nevus with regression[a]
Pagetoid spread	Can be present in isolation	Often present with other concerning features	Absent
Single-cell proliferation	Can be present in isolation	Often present with other concerning features	Absent
Confluence	Present in junctional component	Present throughout	Absent
Cytologic atypia	Present in junctional component	Present throughout	Absent
Fibrosis	Central, trizonal	Haphazard	Usually non-fibrotic response
Architectural disorder	Superficial	Throughout	Same as melanoma with regression
Cell populations	Uniform	Two populations of large atypical melanoma cells and small nevus cells	Uniform
Nesting	Confluent above scar, orderly below	Expansile	Orderly
Patient demographics	Usually history of biopsy or trauma	Longstanding nevus that is evolving or suddenly symptomatic	Asymptomatic, younger patients
Melanophages	Absent	Can be present or absent	Present
Neovascularity	Absent	Present	Present
Epidermal atrophy	Absent	Can be present or absent	Present
Immunostaining	Normal	Abnormal	Normal

[a]Excluding melanomas with regression, which would have features more similar to melanoma arising within a nevus

The halo phenomenon can confound examination, but generally does not produce a fibrotic response. A melanoma with regression will have epidermal atrophy and neovascularity in addition to melanophages and irregular dermal fibrosis (Table 11.3, Figs. 11.3, 11.4, 11.5).

Treatment

Complete re-excision of all recurrent nevi should be considered, both for ease of future surveillance as well as to limit the number of additional invasive procedures to the patient. If a nevus with regression is suspected, clear surgical margins are recommended as what has already regressed is unknown and a component of regressed malignant melanoma cannot be excluded. When excising congenital nevi, it has been recommended to biopsy for histopathologic subtype beforehand, as over one-third of lesions in one study showed a depth of invasion into the deep dermis and subcutis that predicted a higher likelihood of recurrence [71].

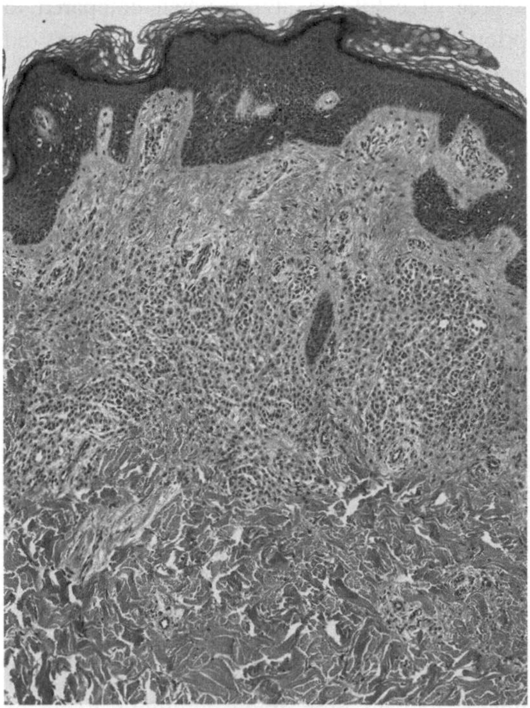

Fig. 11.3 Recurrent atypical nevus. A trizonal pattern of fibrosis is observed, with cellular atypia and pleomorphism of both junctional and dermal nests

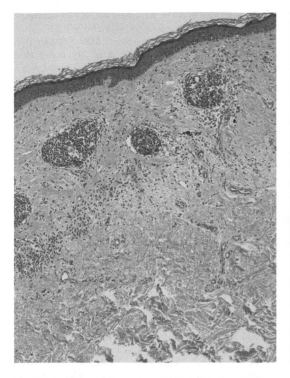

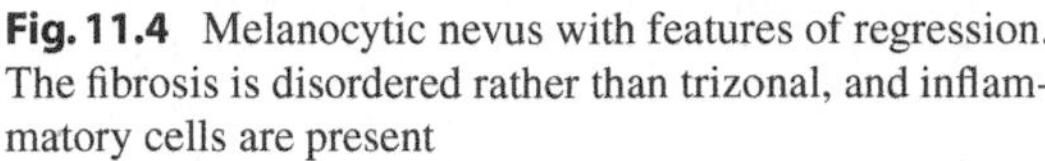

Fig. 11.4 Melanocytic nevus with features of regression. The fibrosis is disordered rather than trizonal, and inflammatory cells are present

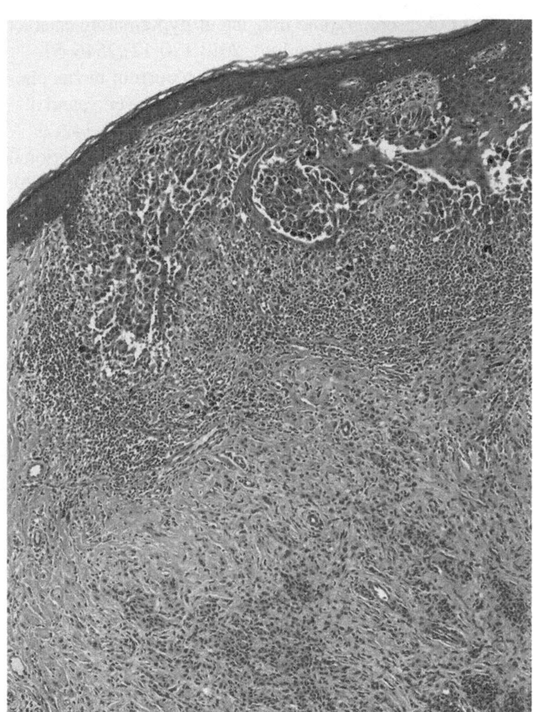

Fig. 11.5 Melanoma arising within a nevus. A dense lymphocytic infiltrate and erratic fibrosis are present alongside poorly cohesive melanocytic cells that display bizarre architectural and cellular disorder

Summary

Recurrent nevi can pose an intimidating histopathologic evaluation that is difficult to distinguish from malignant melanoma or a melanocytic neoplasm (including melanoma) with regression. Fortunately, there are some distinguishing features that should aid the prepared dermatopathologist in making its diagnosis, and avoiding patient morbidity associated with overdiagnosing melanoma. A clinical history of prior biopsy or excision should first raise suspicion for the presence of a recurrent nevus, and a time course of regrowth within a matter of weeks to months after initial sampling should further highlight the need to place this entity on the differential. Salient histopathologic findings include an orderly trizonal pattern of fibrosis; while atypia may be present it tends to be less severe than what would be, expected in an invasive melanoma or melanoma in situ. Finally, and perhaps most importantly, any and all previous biopsy specimens from the lesion in question should be obtained for review.

References

1. Kerl H, Smolle J, Hodl S, Soyer HP. Congenital pseudomelanoma. Z Hautkr. 1989;64(7):564, 7–8.
2. Reed BW. Pseudomelanoma. Arch Dermatol. 1976;112(11):1611–2.
3. Trau H, Orenstein A, Schewach-Miller M, Tsur H. Pseudomelanoma following laser therapy for congenital nevus. J Dermatol Surg Oncol. 1986;12(9): 984–6.
4. Nagy R, Vasily DB. Pseudomelanoma in nevus sebaceus of Jadassohn. Arch Dermatol. 1979;115(8):1004–5.
5. Grupper C, Tubiana R. Spitz' juvenile melanoma or pseudomelanoma. Bull Soc Fr Dermatol Syphiligr. 1955;3:300–2.
6. Brehm G. On the subject of "pseudomelanoma": onychomycosis nigricans. Med Welt. 1967;48:2923–4.
7. Hiss Y, Shafir R. "Pseudomelanoma" in a keloid. J Dermatol Surg Oncol. 1978;4(12):938–9.
8. Shields CL, Pellegrini M, Kligman BE, Bianciotto C, Shields JA. Ciliary body and choroidal pseudomelanoma

from ultrasonographic imaging of hypermature cataract in 20 cases. Ophthalmology. 2013;120(12):2546–51.
9. Fox JC, Reed JA, Shea CR. The recurrent nevus phenomenon: a history of challenge, controversy, and discovery. Arch Pathol Lab Med. 2011;135(7):842–6.
10. Cox AJ, Walton RG. The induction of junctional changes in pigmented nevi. Arch Pathol. 1965;79: 428–34.
11. Lund HZ, Stobbe GD. The natural history of the pigmented nevus; factors of age and anatomic location. Am J Pathol. 1949;25(6):1117–55. incl 4 pl.
12. Schoenfeld RJ, Pinkus H. The recurrence of nevi after incomplete removal. AMA Arch Dermatol. 1958;78(1): 30–5.
13. Imagawa I, Endo M, Morishima T. Mechanism of recurrence of pigmented nevi following dermabrasion. Acta Derm Venereol. 1976;56(5):353–9.
14. Nishimura EK, Jordan SA, Oshima H, Yoshida H, Osawa M, Moriyama M, et al. Dominant role of the niche in melanocyte stem-cell fate determination. Nature. 2002;416(6883):854–60.
15. Sexton M, Sexton CW. Recurrent pigmented melanocytic nevus. A benign lesion, not to be mistaken for malignant melanoma. Arch Pathol Lab Med. 1991; 115(2):122–6.
16. Arrese Estrada J, Pierard-Franchimont C, Pierard GE. Histogenesis of recurrent nevus. Am J Dermatopathol. 1990;12(4):370–2.
17. Hwang K, Lee WJ, Lee SI. Pseudomelanoma after laser therapy. Ann Plast Surg. 2002;48(5):562–4.
18. Lee HW, Ahn SJ, Lee MW, Choi JH, Moon KC, Koh JK. Pseudomelanoma following laser therapy. J Eur Acad Dermatol Venereol. 2006;20(3):342–4.
19. Sohn S, Kim S, Kang WH. Recurrent pigmented macules after q-switched alexandrite laser treatment of congenital melanocytic nevus. Dermatol Surg. 2004; 30(6):898–907 [discussion].
20. Arpaia N, Cassano N, Vena GA. Melanocytic nevus with atypical dermoscopic features at the site of radiodermatitis. Dermatol Surg. 2006;32(1):100–2.
21. Grunwald MH, Gat A, Amichai B. Pseudomelanoma after Solcoderm treatment. Melanoma Res. 2006; 16(5):459–60.
22. Goldenhersh MA, Scheflan M, Zeligovsky A. Recurrent melanocytic nevi after Solcoderm therapy: a new cause of pseudomelanoma. J Am Acad Dermatol. 1992;27(6 Pt 1):1012–3.
23. Ronnen M, Sokol MS, Huszar M, Kahana M, Schewach-Millet M. Pseudomelanoma following treatment with surgical excision and intralesional triamcinolone acetonide to prevent keloid formation. Int J Dermatol. 1986;25(8):533–4.
24. Walton RG, Sage RD, Farber EM. Electrodesiccation of pigmented nevi; biopsy studies: a preliminary report. AMA Arch Dermatol. 1957;76(2):193–9.
25. Dwyer CM, Kerr RE, Knight SL, Walker E. Pseudomelanoma after dermabrasion. J Am Acad Dermatol. 1993;28(2 Pt 1):263–4.
26. Duray PH, Livolsi VA. Recurrent dysplastic nevus following shave excision. J Dermatol Surg Oncol. 1984;10(10):811–5.
27. Dyer PV, Eveson JW. Recurrent compound naevus of gingiva. J Periodontol. 1993;64(8):739–41.
28. Gleason BC, Hirsch MS, Nucci MR, Schmidt BA, Zembowicz A, Mihm Jr MC, et al. Atypical genital nevi. A clinicopathologic analysis of 56 cases. Am J Surg Pathol. 2008;32(1):51–7.
29. King R, Hayzen BA, Page RN, Googe PB, Zeagler D, Mihm Jr MC. Recurrent nevus phenomenon: a clinicopathologic study of 357 cases and histologic comparison with melanoma with regression. Mod Pathol. 2009;22(5):611–7.
30. Park HK, Leonard DD, Arrington 3rd JH, Lund HZ. Recurrent melanocytic nevi: clinical and histologic review of 175 cases. J Am Acad Dermatol. 1987;17(2 Pt 1):285–92.
31. Walton RG, Cox AJ. Electrodesiccation of pigmented nevi. Arch Dermatol. 1963;87:342–9.
32. Brenn T. Pitfalls in the evaluation of melanocytic lesions. Histopathology. 2012;60(5):690–705.
33. Sommer LL, Barcia SM, Clarke LE, Helm KF. Persistent melanocytic nevi: a review and analysis of 205 cases. J Cutan Pathol. 2011;38(6):503–7.
34. Botella-Estrada R, Nagore E, Sopena J, Cremades A, Alfaro A, Sanmartin O, et al. Clinical, dermoscopy and histological correlation study of melanotic pigmentations in excision scars of melanocytic tumours. Br J Dermatol. 2006;154(3):478–84.
35. Blum A, Hofmann-Wellenhof R, Marghoob AA, Argenziano G, Cabo H, Carrera C, et al. Recurrent melanocytic nevi and melanomas in dermoscopy: results of a multicenter study of the international dermoscopy society. JAMA Dermatol. 2014;150(2): 138–45.
36. Yoshida Y, Yamada N, Adachi K, Tanaka M, Yamamoto O. Traumatized recurrent melanocytic naevus with typical starburst pattern on dermoscopy. Acta Derm Venereol. 2008;88(4):408–9.
37. Kelly JW, Shen S, Pan Y, Dowling J, McLean CA. Post-excisional melanocytic regrowth extending beyond the initial scar: a novel clinical sign of melanoma. Br J Dermatol. 2014;170(4):961–4.
38. Kornberg R, Ackerman AB. Pseudomelanoma: recurrent melanocytic nevus following partial surgical removal. Arch Dermatol. 1975;111(12):1588–90.
39. Hoang MP, Prieto VG, Burchette JL, Shea CR. Recurrent melanocytic nevus: a histologic and immunohistochemical evaluation. J Cutan Pathol. 2001;28(8):400–6.
40. Larre Borges A, Zalaudek I, Longo C, Dufrechou L, Argenziano G, Lallas A, et al. Melanocytic nevi with special features: clinical-dermoscopic and reflectance confocal microscopic-findings. J Eur Acad Dermatol Venereol. 2014;28(7):833–45.
41. Longo C, Moscarella E, Pepe P, Cesinaro AM, Casari A, Manfredini M, et al. Confocal microscopy of recurrent naevi and recurrent melanomas: a retrospective morphological study. Br J Dermatol. 2011;165(1):61–8.
42. Ruhoy SM, Kolker SE, Murry TC. Mitotic activity within dermal melanocytes of benign melanocytic nevi: a study of 100 cases with clinical follow-up. Am J Dermatopathol. 2011;33(2):167–72.

43. Ruhoy SM, Prieto VG, Eliason SL, Grichnik JM, Burchette Jr JL, Shea CR. Malignant melanoma with paradoxical maturation. Am J Surg Pathol. 2000; 24(12):1600–14.
44. Magro CM, Crowson AN, Desman G, Zippin JH. Soluble adenylyl cyclase antibody profile as a diagnostic adjunct in the assessment of pigmented lesions. Arch Dermatol. 2012;148(3):335–44.
45. Clark Jr WH, Reimer RR, Greene M, Ainsworth AM, Mastrangelo MJ. Origin of familial malignant melanomas from heritable melanocytic lesions 'The B-K mole syndrome'. Arch Dermatol. 1978;114(5): 732–8.
46. Elder DE, Goldman LI, Goldman SC, Greene MH, Clark Jr WH. Dysplastic nevus syndrome: a phenotypic association of sporadic cutaneous melanoma. Cancer. 1980;46(8):1787–94.
47. Lynch HT, Frichot 3rd BC, Lynch JF. Familial atypical multiple mole-melanoma syndrome. J Med Genet. 1978;15(5):352–6.
48. Rhodes AR, Harrist TJ, Day CL, Mihm Jr MC, Fitzpatrick TB, Sober AJ. Dysplastic melanocytic nevi in histologic association with 234 primary cutaneous melanomas. J Am Acad Dermatol. 1983;9(4): 563–74.
49. Blessing K. Benign atypical naevi: diagnostic difficulties and continued controversy. Histopathology. 1999;34(3):189–98.
50. Goodson AG, Florell SR, Boucher KM, Grossman D. Low rates of clinical recurrence after biopsy of benign to moderately dysplastic melanocytic nevi. J Am Acad Dermatol. 2010;62(4):591–6.
51. Kmetz EC, Sanders H, Fisher G, Lang PG, Maize Sr JC. The role of observation in the management of atypical nevi. South Med J. 2009;102(1):45–8.
52. Abello-Poblete MV, Correa-Selm LM, Giambrone D, Victor F, Rao BK. Histologic outcomes of excised moderate and severe dysplastic nevi. Dermatol Surg. 2014;40(1):40–5.
53. Omura EF, Kheir SM. Recurrent Spitz's nevus. Am J Dermatopathol. 1984;6(Suppl):207–12.
54. Tanaka K, Mihara M, Shimao S, Taniguchi K. The local recurrence of pigmented Spitz nevus after removal. J Dermatol. 1990;17(9):575–80.
55. Stern JB. Recurrent Spitz's nevi. A clinicopathologic investigation. Am J Dermatopathol. 1985;7(Suppl): 49–50.
56. Gambini C, Rongioletti F. Recurrent Spitz nevus. Case report and review of the literature. Am J Dermatopathol. 1994;16(4):409–13.
57. Harvell JD, Bastian BC, LeBoit PE. Persistent (recurrent) Spitz nevi: a histopathologic, immunohistochemical, and molecular pathologic study of 22 cases. Am J Surg Pathol. 2002;26(5):654–61.
58. Kaye VN, Dehner LP. Spindle and epithelioid cell nevus (Spitz nevus). Natural history following biopsy. Arch Dermatol. 1990;126(12):1581–3.
59. Barnhill RL. The Spitzoid lesion: rethinking Spitz tumors, atypical variants, 'Spitzoid melanoma' and risk assessment. Mod Pathol. 2006;19 Suppl 2:S21–33.
60. Held L, Metzler G, Eigentler TK, Leiter U, Messina J, Gogel J, et al. Recurrent nodules in a periauricular plaque-type blue nevus with fatal outcome. J Cutan Pathol. 2012;39(12):1088–93.
61. Harvell JD, White WL. Persistent and recurrent blue nevi. Am J Dermatopathol. 1999;21(6):506–17.
62. Jakobiec FA, Nguyen J, Bhat P, Fay A. Recurrent blue nevus of the corneoscleral limbus. Cornea. 2010; 29(8):947–51.
63. Shih L, Hawkins DB. Recurrent postauricular blue nevus with lymph node involvement. Otolaryngol Head Neck Surg. 1987;97(5):491–4.
64. Lambert WC, Brodkin RH. Nodal and subcutaneous cellular blue nevi. A pseudometastasizing pseudomelanoma. Arch Dermatol. 1984;120(3):367–70.
65. Fabrizi G, Pennacchia I, Pagliarello C, Massi G. Sclerosing nevus with pseudomelanomatous features. J Cutan Pathol. 2008;35(11):995–1002.
66. Ferrara G, Amantea A, Argenziano G, Broganelli P, Cesinaro AM, Donati P, et al. Sclerosing nevus with pseudomelanomatous features and regressing melanoma with nevoid features. J Cutan Pathol. 2009;36(8):913–5. author reply 6.
67. Ferrara G, Giorgio CM, Zalaudek I, Broganelli P, Pellacani G, Tomasini C, et al. Sclerosing nevus with pseudomelanomatous features (nevus with regression-like fibrosis): clinical and dermoscopic features of a recently characterized histopathologic entity. Dermatology (Basel, Switzerland). 2009;219(3):202–8.
68. Bauer JW, Schaeppi H, Kaserer C, Hantich B, Hintner H. Large melanocytic nevi in hereditary epidermolysis bullosa. J Am Acad Dermatol. 2001;44(4):577–84.
69. Strungs I. Common and uncommon variants of melanocytic naevi. Pathology. 2004;36(5):396–403.
70. Tschandl P. Recurrent nevi: report of three cases with dermatoscopic-dermatopathologic correlation. Dermatol Pract Concept. 2013;3(1):29–32.
71. Stenn KS, Arons M, Hurwitz S. Patterns of congenital nevocellular nevi. A histologic study of thirty-eight cases. J Am Acad Dermatol. 1983;9(3):388–93.

12 Neurothekeoma Versus Melanoma

Kristen M. Paral, Jon A. Reed, Victor G. Prieto, and Christopher R. Shea

Introduction

Although many current textbooks place neurothekeoma under the heading of nerve sheath tumors [1–5], others, such as the most recent WHO Classification of Tumours of Soft Tissue and Bone [6], omit neurothekeoma altogether. This phenomenon likely has roots in the contentious nosological history of neurothekeoma. Introduced into the literature in 1980, the tumor's name reflected its purported nerve sheath origin [7]. Early observers noted some histomorphologic resemblance to dermal nerve sheath myxoma (DNSM), most notably in neurothekeomas with a pronounced myxoid matrix [8]. Consequently, the two lesions were placed on a morphologic continuum, with DNSM often being regarded as a myxoid variant of neurothekeoma[1] (so-called "myxoid neurothekeoma") [9].

However, subsequent studies provided convincing morphologic, ultrastructural, and immunophenotypic evidence that DNSM and "myxoid neurothekeoma" are distinct entities, with demonstrable nerve sheath differentiation in DNSM but not in neurothekeoma [10–13]. Nevertheless, DNSM and "myxoid neurothekeoma" had become intertwined and entrenched in the literature and in textbooks. The term "cellular neurothekeoma"[2] is preferred by some authors [14–17] to emphasize the distinction from the confused and contaminated myxoid end of the spectrum. The ensuing text employs "neurothekeoma" to encompass all morphologic patterns thought to be true neurothekeomas, whether cellular or with myxoid matrix, based on the present understanding of this tumor. Regardless of the adjective placed before it, the appellation "neurothekeoma" has been acknowledged as inappropriate [9, 14] but will likely remain in place until the tumor origin or differentiation is elucidated.

K.M. Paral • C.R. Shea, M.D. (✉)
University of Chicago Medicine,
5841 S. Maryland Ave., MC 5067, L502,
Chicago, IL 60637, USA
e-mail: cshea@medicine.bsd.uchicago.edu

J.A. Reed
CellNEtix Pathology & Laboratories,
1124 Columbia St., Suite 200, Seattle,
WA 98117, USA

V.G. Prieto
MD Anderson Cancer Center, University of Houston,
1515 Holcombe Blvd., Unit 85, Houston,
TX 77030, USA

[1] Other terms that may have been lumped together with "myxoid neurothekeoma" include myxoid tumor of nerve sheath, perineurial myxoma, Pacinian neurofibroma, and bizarre cutaneous neurofibroma [8, 15].

[2] The term "cellular neurothekeoma" was introduced by Barnhill and Mihm [15] as a distinctive subtype of neurothekeoma, but currently, it is best understood as a morphologic pattern on a spectrum of cellular ↔ myxoid rather than as an actual subtype.

C.R. Shea et al. (eds.), *Pathology of Challenging Melanocytic Neoplasms: Diagnosis and Management*,
DOI 10.1007/978-1-4939-1444-9_12, © Springer Science+Business Media New York 2015

Features of Neurothekeoma

Clinical Presentation

Neurothekeoma preferentially affects a young patient population, with greater than 85 % of patients being younger than 40 years (Fig. 12.1). Women are affected nearly twice as often as men. The most commonly involved body sites are the head and neck (especially the face) followed by the shoulder region and upper arms [9, 14]. No consistent association with other disease conditions has been established. The lesion is most often solitary, but multifocal cases have been reported [18, 19]. The tumor most often presents as a dome-shaped, pink-tan to red-brown papule or nodule (Fig. 12.2), usually measuring about 1 cm (range 0.3–6 cm). The vast majority are asymptomatic but, rarely, patients report pain or itching. Most are slow-growing, with some patients reporting a 10-year history at presentation. The clinical differential diagnosis usually consists of benign entities such as a cyst, dermatofibroma, or nevus; skin adnexal tumors or basal cell carcinoma may also be considered [9, 14].

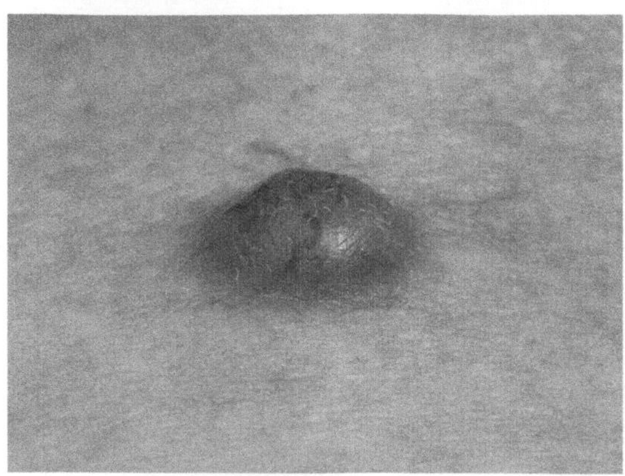

Fig. 12.2 Neurothekeoma, shown here as a well-defined, red-pink nodule. The unusually prominent, arborizing vasculature seen beneath the surface in this case led to a clinical impression of basal cell carcinoma. Original figure from Aydingoz IE, Mansur AT, Dikicioglu-Cetin E. Arborizing vessels under dermoscopy: a case of cellular neurothekeoma instead of basal cell carcinoma. Dermatol Online J. 2013;19(3):5. Retrieved from: http://escholarship.org/uc/item/1nx5r21x. ©2013 Dermatology Online Journal. Reproduced with permission

Prognosis or Course

No reported case of neurothekeoma has metastasized, and there is only a small risk of recurrence or regrowth associated with incomplete excision (15 % at most) [9, 14]. Therefore, complete excision is the cornerstone of therapy. Location in the head and neck is also correlated with higher recurrence risk, likely reflecting more conservative excisions. There are no established histopathologic features that predict recurrence (see below) [9, 14].

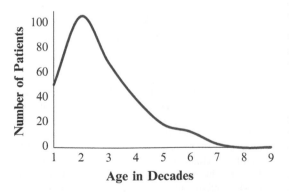

Fig. 12.1 Age distribution for 302 patients with neurothekeoma (compiled from [9, 14])

Etiology/Pathogenesis

Neurothekeoma is a tumor of uncertain origin and unclear differentiation. Based on light microscopy, immunohistochemistry, and ultrastructural examination, various lines of differentiation have been proposed, including (myo)fibroblastic (fibro)histiocytic, and neuroectodermal [9, 20–23]. Microarray data comparing DNSM with neurothekeoma revealed that not only do the two tumors demonstrate divergent expression profiles, but DNSM clustered with schwannoma, while neurothekeoma clustered with cellular fibrous histiocytoma [24]. However, this study utilized a limited number and range of cases, so further investigation is necessary.

Histopathology

Microscopic examination discloses a multinodular, variably circumscribed mass in the dermis and/or subcutis (Fig. 12.3a). The epidermis is not directly involved by tumor but may be atrophic, and a Grenz zone is often seen (Fig. 12.3b) [14, 15, 25]. The mass is composed of whorled nests and bundles of cells (Fig. 12.3c). The whorled, concentric arrangements of cells have been deemed *neuroid* characteristics and likened to *endoneurial-like structures* [15]. The constituent cells range from epithelioid to spindled, with abundant, faintly eosinophilic cytoplasm and indistinct cell borders (Fig. 12.3d). Fetsch et al. [9] noted a somewhat granular quality to the cytoplasm. Nuclei are usually ovoid with fine chromatin and indistinct nucleoli. Dense collagen bands often separate the cellular nests and bundles (Fig. 12.3e). For cases exhibiting florid stromal sclerosis, the term "*desmoplastic cellular neurothekeoma*" has been endorsed by some authors [18, 25, 26]. Myxoid matrix is variably present in neurothekeoma (Fig. 12.3f), accounting for much of its morphologic variability, which is delineated in Table 12.1. Osteoclast-like giant cells are present in 15–39 % of cases, and rarely, Touton giant cells are seen [9, 14]. Mitotic activity varies from none to 41 per 10 high-power fields, with an average of 2–3 per 10 high-power fields [9, 14].

Overall, most neurothekeomas have a banal appearance, but atypical features are well documented [9, 14, 21, 27]. A minority of cases (12–25 %) exhibit focal or scattered atypical cells with enlarged nuclei, coarse chromatin, and prominent nucleoli [9, 14], including tumor giant cells in 5 % of cases [14]. Other atypical features, such as tumor size >2 cm, high mitotic rate, atypical mitotic figures, and infiltration of fat or skeletal muscle, are seemingly insignificant with respect to biologic behavior [9, 14, 25, 27]. Vascular and perineural invasion have been described [21, 27, 28]. Necrosis is exceptional [14]. Other unusual features in neurothekeoma include collagen trapping, hemorrhage, lymphocytic cuffing, chondroid stroma, and cellular vacuolization. In rare cases exhibiting sheet-like growth, there is at least focal nesting of epithelioid and spindled cells characteristic of neurothekeoma [21]. Extensive calcification and even ossification have been reported [29, 30].

Immunophenotype

The immunophenotype of neurothekeoma is nonspecific but fairly consistent (Fig. 12.4) and thus can be supportive of the microscopic impression. S100 protein and GFAP are almost always negative [9, 10, 14], with few reports of focal S100 positivity [16], supporting the argument that it is distinct from DNSM and is not a nerve sheath tumor. Care must be taken to distinguish lesional from non-lesional cells, as S100-positive dendritic cells may be peppered throughout the tumor (Fig. 12.5) [9]. Other markers that are consistently negative in neurothekeoma include Melan-A, tyrosinase, neurofilament, CD34, desmin, and cytokeratins. gp100 (HMB-45) is usually negative, but rare cases demonstrate minimal expression [9].

Notwithstanding the consistent S100 negativity in lesional cells, the frequent expression of MITF, NK1/C3, PGP9.5, and NSE has led several authors to propose a neuroectodermal origin for neurothekeoma [19, 23, 27, 31, 32]. However, this suggestion has been heavily criticized on the basis of the restricted specificities and sensitivities of these markers. For example, MITF expression was observed in over 80 % of neurothekeomas in two large series [9, 14], but a smaller subsequent study reported focal or no expression in most of their cases [33]. MITF also suffers from questionable specificity, with expression reported in many reactive and neoplastic cells of non-neuroectodermal origin [34–36]. Similarly, NK1/C3 expression has been reported in a wide array of neoplasms of many lineages aside from melanocytic, including (fibro)histiocytic tumors [37]. PGP9.5 was originally reported as a marker for neurothekeoma based on a study of 12 cases [32], but its promiscuity was later exposed in a report of strong expression in the vast majority of

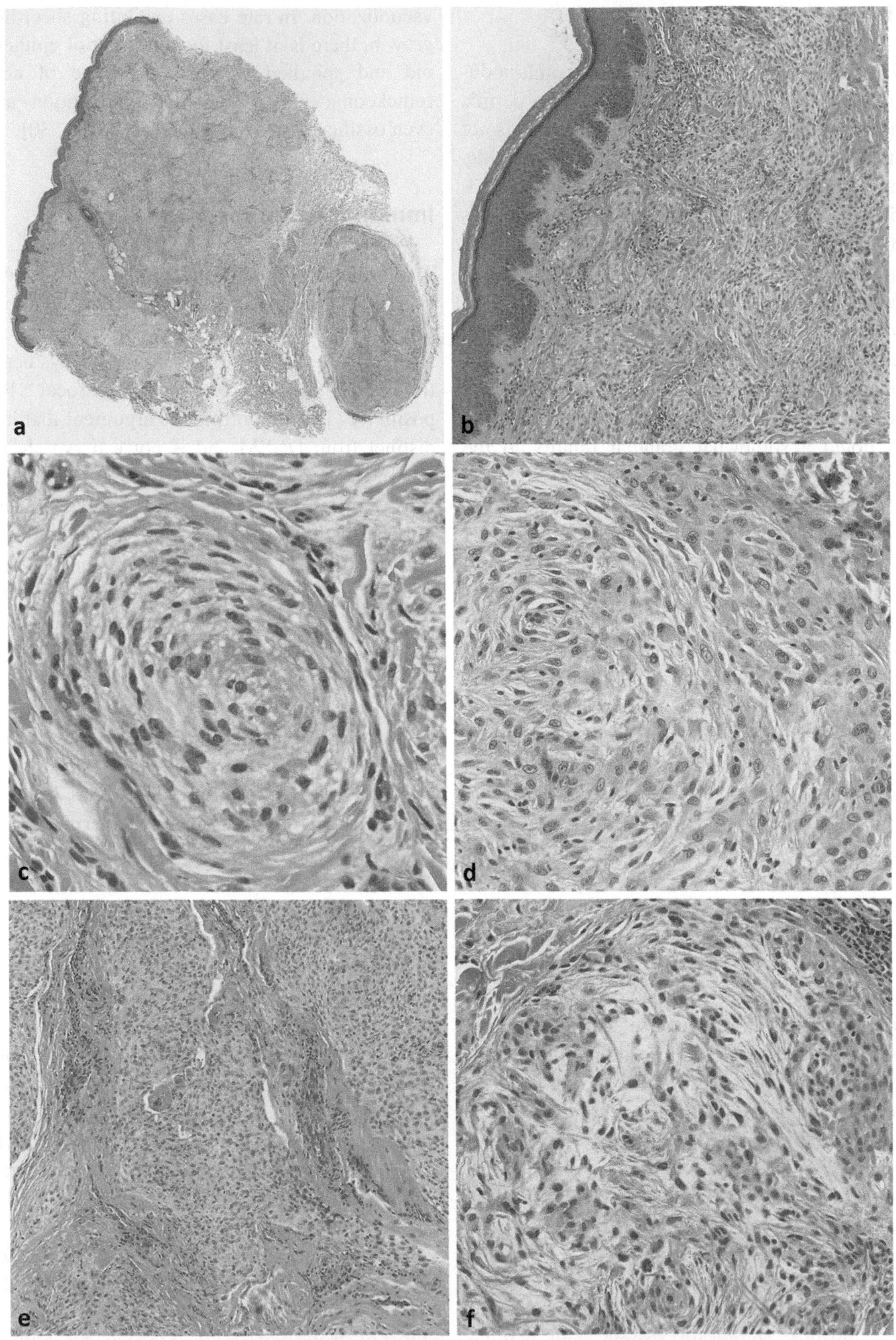

Fig. 12.3 Neurothekeoma. (**a**) Low-power view shows a multinodular, variably circumscribed mass in the dermis and subcutis (H&E, ×1). (**b**) The epidermis is spared (H&E, ×10). (**c**) A whorled nest of cells is depicted (H&E, ×40). (**d**) Cells range from epithelioid to spindled, with abundant, faintly eosinophilic cytoplasm (H&E, ×20). (**e**) Dense collagen bands may separate the nests of cells (H&E, ×10). (**f**) Myxoid matrix is apparent in this view (H&E, ×20)

Table 12.1 Morphologic spectrum of neurothekeoma [9, 14]

	Morphologic patterns[a]			
	Cellular	Mixed	Myxoid	Desmoplastic
Myxoid matrix	≤10 %	>10 % and ≤50 %	>50 %	Focal or absent
Architectural features	Multinodular configuration of whorled nests and bundles, sometimes fascicles Dense collagen among the nests and bundles		Larger nests Cell growth pattern is more random and less whorled/fascicular Dense collagen not as evident	Multinodular, haphazardly arranged fascicles Prominent sclerotic, fibrotic background
Cytologic features	Shape spindled to epithelioid (most have both) Cytoplasm abundant and faintly eosinophilic Cell borders indistinct			
Nuclear features[b]	Shape ovoid Chromatin usually fine Nucleoli usually inconspicuous or pinpoint			
Mitotic figures	Number variable (average 2–3 per 10 HPF, range 0–41 per 10 HPF) Atypical forms rarely seen (2 % of cases)			
Non-lesional cells	Osteoclast-like giant cells in 15–39 % of cases Occasional dendritic cells, mast cells 5 % of cases have Touton or tumor giant cells			
Melanocytic lesions in the differential diagnosis	Spitz nevus (amelanotic intradermal) Melanoma (metastatic or primary intradermal) Nevus (amelanotic intradermal)		Myxoid melanoma	Desmoplastic melanoma or nevi

[a]There is no established clinical significance to subdividing neurothekeomas; rather, the significance lies in illustrating patterns and their corresponding differential diagnoses

[b]Most cases demonstrate minimal nuclear atypia, with a minority (12–25 %) showing focal or scattered atypical cells with enlarged nuclei, coarse chromatin, and prominent nucleoli

non-neuroectodermal and neuroectodermal neoplasms [38]. Two studies endorse S100A6[3] as a more sensitive alternative to PGP9.5 but report a similar poor specificity [16, 31]. Finally, SOX-10, a marker of neuroectodermal differentiation, has been reported as negative in all of 25 neurothekeomas in one series [33]. Therefore, the notion of a neuroectodermal origin for neurothekeoma seems tenuous at best.

Genetic and Molecular Findings

As mentioned previously, microarray analysis revealed disparate expression profiles for neurothekeoma and DNSM, with the former resembling cellular fibrous histiocytoma and the latter resembling dermal schwannoma [24]. No recurring chromosomal abnormalities have been described for neurothekeoma.

[3] S100A6 must not be confused with S100 protein, with which it is in the same family [16].

Differential Diagnosis: Non-melanocytic Lesions

The most common alternative diagnoses rendered by pathologists for neurothekeoma cases include melanocytic lesions, neural tumors, fibrohistiocytic proliferations, and DNSM (Fig. 12.6) [9, 14], each of which can present as an amelanotic dermal proliferation of epithelioid or spindled cells [15]. The salient discriminatory features for neurothekeoma versus non-melanocytic lesions are reviewed in Table 12.2. Of special note is that neurothekeoma and plexiform fibrohistiocytic tumor are best distinguished on morphologic grounds, as no immunohistochemical marker can

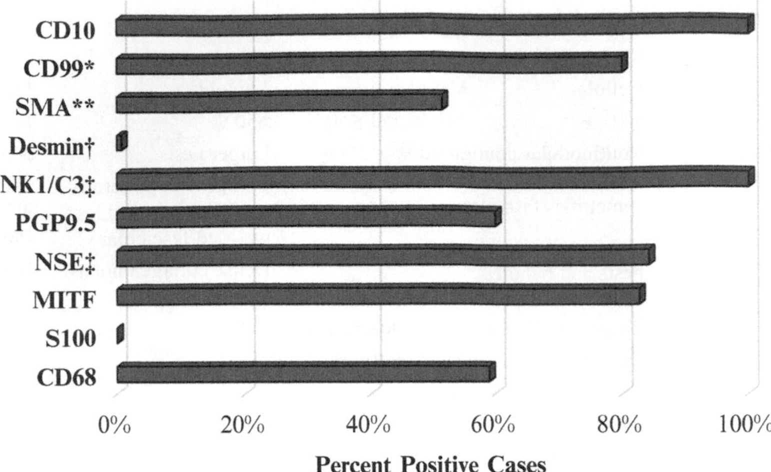

Fig. 12.4 Immunophenotype of neurothekeoma, compiled from the two largest series to date [9, 14]. *Based on only 10 cases. **Focally or diffusely positive. †A single case demonstrated focal desmin positivity. ‡Mostly diffuse positivity

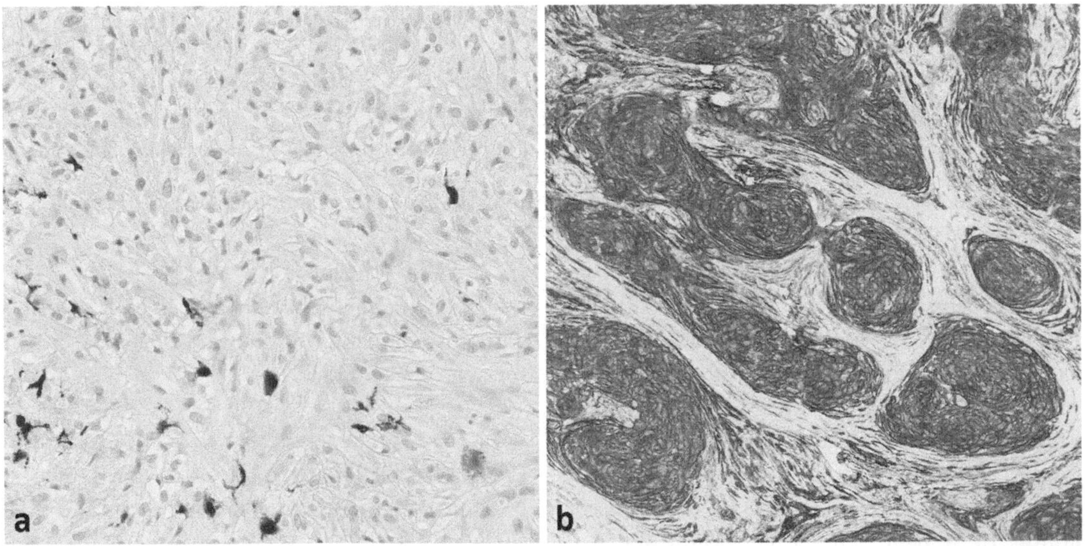

Fig. 12.5 (**a**) The lesional cells are negative for S100, but scattered S100-positive dendritic cells are noted (×20). (**b**) Strong CD10 expression, although not specific, is consistently seen (×10)

distinguish the two with certainty [14, 16, 39]. The distinction is important, as plexiform fibrohistiocytic tumor has some metastatic potential [6]. Other non-melanocytic lesions entering into the differential for neurothekeoma include reticulohistiocytoma and variants of fibrous histiocytoma [9]. Architectural features, such as a lack of whorled growth in reticulohistocytoma or the presence of storiform growth in fibrous histiocytoma, can lead to the correct diagnosis without a need for ancillary studies. Another diagnosis that may be considered is a pilar leiomyoma [40] in cases expressing smooth-muscle actin (SMA). Although neurothekeomas contain spindle cells with eosinophilic cytoplasm, they lack the characteristic cigar-shaped or corkscrew nuclei of

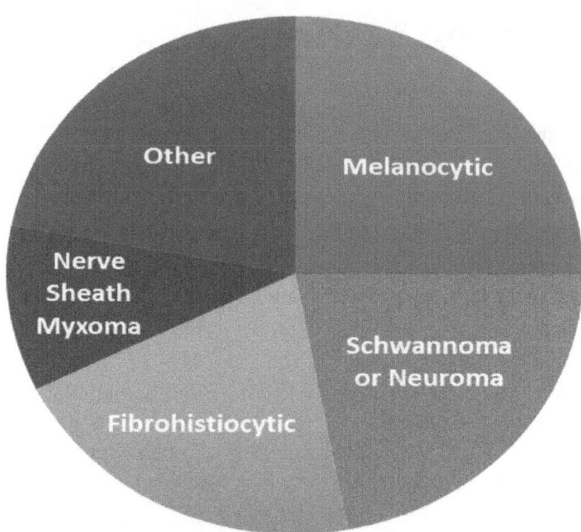

Fig. 12.6 Frequencies of alternative diagnoses for cases of neurothekeoma offered by contributing pathologists in the largest series to date [9]. A malignant diagnosis was considered in 21 % of cases. Diagnoses within the "Other" category include granulomatous processes, skin adnexal tumors, smooth-muscle tumors, granular cell tumors, and various sarcomas

smooth-muscle tumors. Desmin expression can exclude neurothekeoma. Likewise, S100 positivity can exclude neurothekeoma, which resolves the neuronal and Schwannian differentials.

Differential Diagnosis: Melanocytic Lesions

The broad morphologic spectrum of neurothekeoma notoriously overlaps with that of various melanocytic lesions. Although most neurothekeomas have a banal microscopic appearance, a wide range of mitotic activity and cytologic atypia can be seen, permitting consideration of benign and malignant melanocytic lesions alike. As reviewed in Table 12.1, each morphological pattern of neurothekeoma corresponds to its own group of melanocytic entities. Neurothekeomas with the more cellular patterns, owing to their nests or "theques" of spindled to epithelioid cells, overlap with intradermal nevi, Spitz tumors, and melanomas. The so-called *desmoplastic cellular* pattern of neurothekeoma can be confused with desmoplastic melanoma [18, 25, 26]. In cases of neurothekeoma with prominent myxoid matrix, myxoid melanoma may be considered [41–47]. The distinguishing clinicopathologic features of each are discussed below. In any case, the most invaluable distinguishing tool for neurothekeoma versus any melanocytic lesion (aside from careful microscopic scrutiny) is S100 immunohistochemistry. A lack of S100 expression is a hallmark of neurothekeoma, whereas nearly all melanocytic lesions express S100 [41]. Distinguishing neurothekeoma from any malignant melanocytic lesion is of paramount importance, as the clinical ramifications can be drastic.

Neurothekeoma vs. Intradermal Spitz Nevus

In the largest neurothekeoma series to date [9], Spitz nevus was the most commonly considered melanocytic entity in the differential. Neurothekeoma—namely, the cellular pattern—overlaps significantly with amelanotic, intradermal Spitz nevi, both clinically and morphologically. Both affect predominantly young patients (Fig. 12.7) with a female preponderance. The amelanotic Spitz nevus also exhibits a proclivity for the head and neck, where it typically presents as a dome-shaped, red-to-pink papule or nodule [48]. Intradermal Spitz accounts for up to 20 % of Spitz lesions [49]. Histologically, the epidermal changes associated with Spitz nevi tend to be hyperplastic [50–52], which is not a usual feature of neurothekeoma [9, 14, 15]. The overall multinodular shape of neurothekeoma contrasts with the classic wedge shape of Spitz nevi [50]. Although both lesions contain spindled to epithelioid cells in a collagenous stroma, only Spitz nevi show maturation. Additionally, the cellular whorling that is characteristic of neurothekeoma is not a feature of Spitz nevi [15]. Myxoid matrix, if present, steers toward the interpretation of neurothekeoma, as it is very rare in Spitz nevi [53, 54]. Although both lesions can have giant cells, those of neurothekeoma are described as osteoclastic, which are not described in Spitz nevi [49, 51, 52]. The lesions are compared in Table 12.3 and Fig. 12.8.

Table 12.2 The non-melanocytic differential diagnosis of neurothekeoma [6, 9, 10, 14]

	Neurothekeoma	Dermal nerve sheath myxoma (DNSM)	Plexiform fibrohistiocytic tumor	Superficial angiomyxoma (cutaneous myxoma)
Clinical features	Young women>men	Young to middle-aged adults	Children and young adults	Sporadic or associated with Carney's
	Head and neck, especially the face	Distal extremities	Upper extremities, especially the forearm	Trunk, legs, head and neck (eyelids in Carney's)
	Benign; low recurrence rate (<15 %) when incompletely excised	Benign; high local recurrence rate (up to 50 %) when incompletely excised	Metastatic potential; 13–38 % local recurrence rate	Benign, but local recurrence is common (up to 40 %)
Cellular architecture	Poorly marginated, multinodular mass of whorled nests and bundles, sometimes fascicles	Multilobulated mass of sharply demarcated lobules with highly myxoid matrix Prominent peripheral fibrous border	Multinodular mass composed of nodules of histiocyte-like cells and fascicles of spindle cells in varying proportions (fascicles usually longer and better defined compared to neurothekeoma)	Multinodular, myxoid, paucicellular mass with variable dermarcation Cleft-like spaces at the interface of the nodule and surrounding tissue
	Variable myxoid matrix (architecture is more random with more myxoid matrix) Dense collagen among the nests and bundles		Myxoid stromal change can be seen but is not prominent	Wispy collagen fibers throughout the stroma Delicate vasculature
Cellular morphology	Shape is spindled to epithelioid Cytoplasm is abundant and faintly eosinophilic Cell borders are indistinct	Shape is spindled, stellate, ring-shaped (resembling adipocytes), or epithelioid (often forming cords and syncytial aggregates)	The spindled cells are (myo) fibroblastic in appearance The histiocyte-like cells may appear epithelioid Less nuclear variability than that seen in neurothekeoma	Shape is spindled or stellate Mononuclear or multinucleated Nuclear chromatin often "smudgy" Cytoplasmic-nuclear invaginations common
Osteoclast-like giant cells	Frequent	None	Frequent	None
Immunohistochemical differences	:S100 –, GFAP –, CD34 –	S100 +, GFAP +	No clear distinguishing markers	S100 –, CD34 –

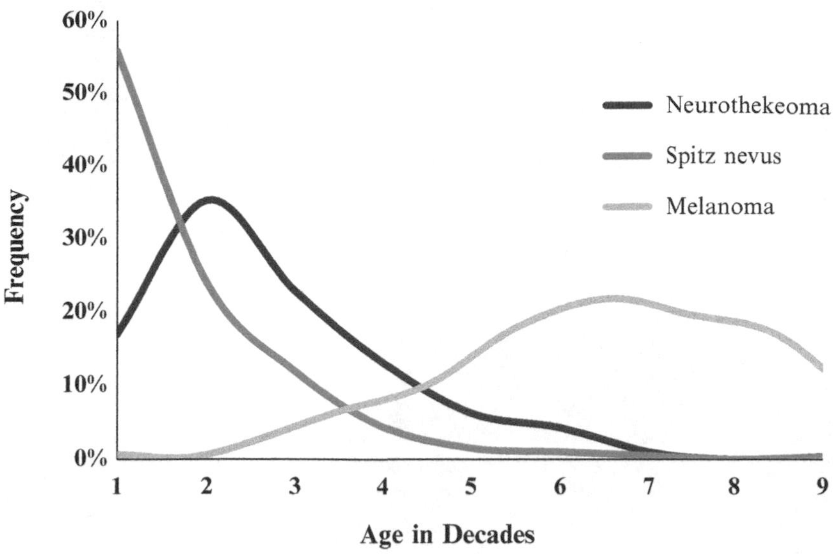

Fig. 12.7 Frequency distribution of age for neurothekeoma [9, 14] versus Spitz nevus [65] and melanoma [66]. Note: melanoma curve approximately reflects the following percentages for age groups: <20 (0.6 %), 20–34 (6.5 %), 35–44 (10 %), 45–54 (17.8 %), 55–64 (21.8 %), 65–74 (19.6 %), 75–84 (16.8 %), and >84 (7 %)

Table 12.3 Neurothekeoma versus intradermal Spitz nevus [9, 14, 15, 50–52]

	Neurothekeoma (cellular pattern)	Intradermal Spitz nevus
Epidermal changes	Effacement of rete pattern, usually with a Grenz zone ± Epidermal atrophy	Epidermis tends to show hyperplastic changes
Shape & location	Multinodular dermal or subcutaneous mass	Often symmetrical, wedge-shaped dermal mass
Architecture	Whorled nests and bundles Margins often infiltrative Dense collagen bands	Small nests, fascicles, and single cells ± Clefting/retraction around nests Collagenous stroma
Cytology	Cells are spindled to epithelioid Cytoplasm is palely eosinophilic, maybe granular No maturation	Cells are spindled to epithelioid Cytoplasm is eosinophilic, amphophilic, or even basophilic, sometimes glassy Maturation
Atypical features	Rarely, marked pleomorphism is present but focal Mitotic activity is variable and not worrisome if present	Limited mitotic activity and nuclear pleomorphism (worrisome if present)
Other features	± Osteoclastic giant cells ± Myxoid matrix ± Ectatic vessels, patchy perivascular lymphoid infiltrates	± Multinucleated cells (not osteoclastic) No myxoid matrix (with rare exceptions) ± Ectatic vessels, patchy perivascular lymphoid infiltrates
Immunohistochemistry	S100 –, Melan-A –	S100 +, Melan-A +

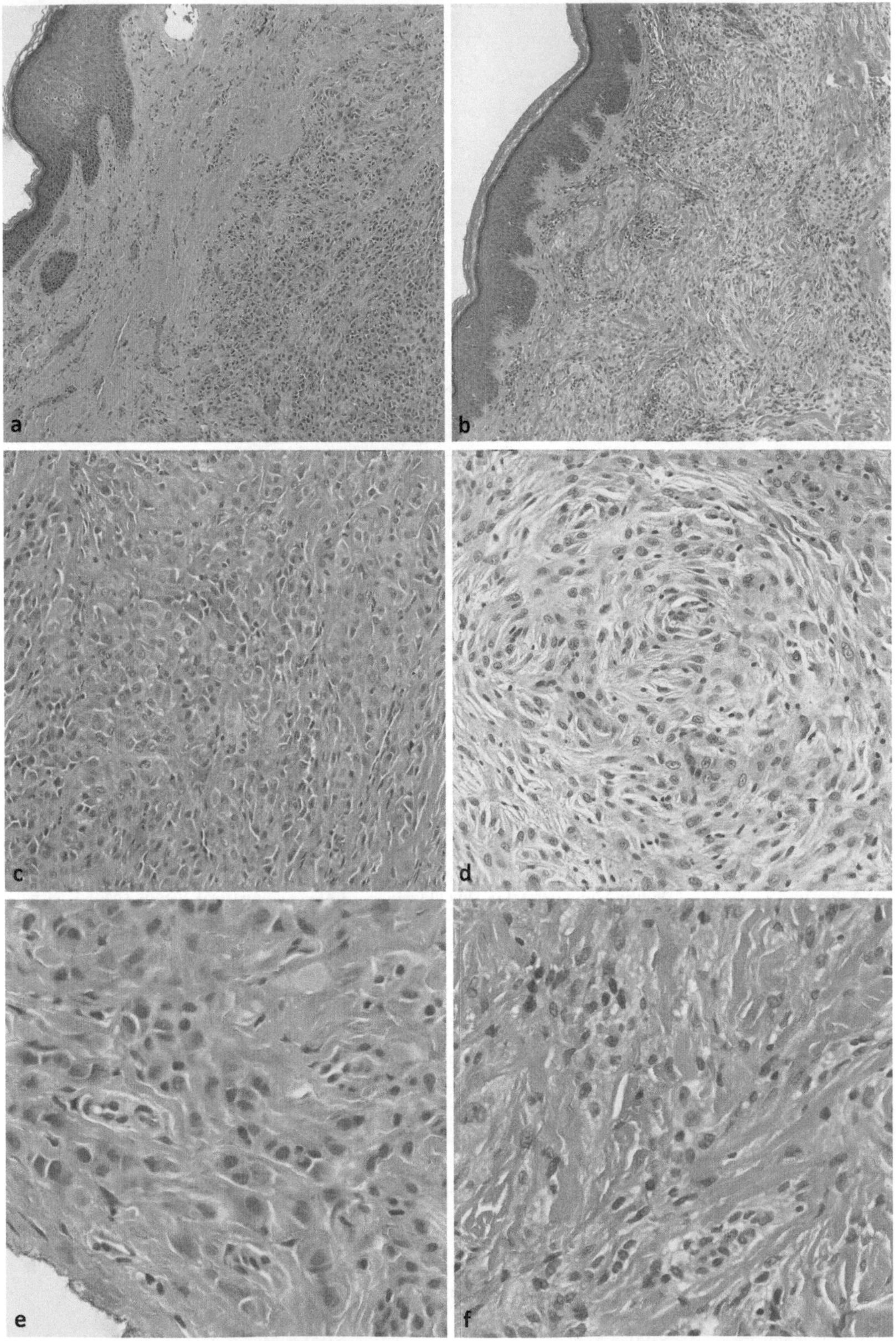

Fig. 12.8 Intradermal Spitz nevus versus neurothekeoma. The panel illustrates Spitz nevus on the left and neurothekeoma on the right. (**a**, **b**) Note that the epidermis is hyperplastic in the Spitz nevus but not in the neurothekeoma (H&E, ×10). (**c**, **d**) Both lesions exhibit spindled and epithelioid cells, but the nests in the Spitz nevus tend to be small and do not form whorls (H&E, ×20). (**e**, **f**) The Spitz nevus exhibits maturation at its base. The cells of neurothekeoma may also disperse and appear smaller at the periphery. However, the cytoplasm is glassy and the cell borders are better defined in the Spitz nevus compared to the neurothekeoma (H&E, ×40)

A very rare variant of Spitz nevus that can masquerade as neurothekeoma is the so-called *plexiform Spitz nevus* [53]. Two cases have been described as symmetrical, plexiform arrangements of fascicles and whorled bundles, circumscribed by a rim of fibrous tissue. Both cases had myxoid stroma and scattered multinucleated giant cells. The cells were eosinophilic, without evidence of maturation or melanin pigment. The lesions were strongly positive for S100 protein, which allowed for definitive separation from neurothekeoma.

Neurothekeoma vs. Intradermal Melanoma

Neurothekeoma can masquerade as metastatic melanoma, and vice versa. The usual patient with metastatic melanoma is older (Fig. 12.7) and has a history of melanoma, but clinical history is not always clear in practice. Moreover, the clinical appearance of both lesions can overlap, with metastatic melanoma often presenting as a variably pigmented nodule. Microscopic examination discloses a nodular proliferation in the dermis or subcutis. Metastatic melanoma does not display the whorled nests of cells typical for neurothekeoma. In addition, dense collagen coursing among cellular nests is not a feature of metastatic melanoma [55]. While the cells of neurothekeoma range from spindled to epithelioid, the cells of metastatic melanoma are often monomorphic and atypical [55]. Most neurothekeomas have a bland appearance; if marked pleomorphism is present, it is focal. Necrosis is exceptional in neurothekeoma but not uncommon in the center of a metastatic melanoma nodule [55]. Osteoclastic giant cells and myxoid matrix favor neurothekeoma, although both have been reported in melanoma [41]. Table 12.4 and Fig. 12.9 compare neurothekeoma to metastatic melanoma.

Table 12.4 Neurothekeoma versus metastatic melanoma [9, 14, 41, 55]

	Neurothekeoma	Metastatic melanoma
Epidermis	Not involved by tumor	Usually no epidermal component ± Epidermal collarette in superficial nodules
Shape & location	Multinodular dermal or subcutaneous mass	Single or multiple dermal or subcutaneous nodules
Architecture	Whorled nests and bundles	Clusters and strands in early metastases; sheet-like growth in developed metastases
	Dense collagen bands	Little or no fibrosis
Cytology	Cells are spindled to epithelioid	Cells are spindled, epithelioid, or small nevoid
Atypical features	Atypia is minimal; marked atypia is focal Average mitotic count: 2–3 per 10 HPF, range 0–41 per 10 HPF	Cells are atypical and variably pleomorphic Mitotic activity usually > 6/mm^2 Intranuclear cytoplasmic pseudoinclusions are common
Other features	± Osteoclastic giant cells Necrosis is almost never seen ± Myxoid matrix ± Ectatic vessels, patchy perivascular lymphoid infiltrates	Frequent vascular invasion Necrosis is not uncommon Inflammation is sparse or absent ± Pigment Any variant of melanoma can have myxoid change
Immunohistochemistry	S100 –, Melan-A –, HMB-45 – (almost always)	S100 +, Melan-A + HMB-45 +

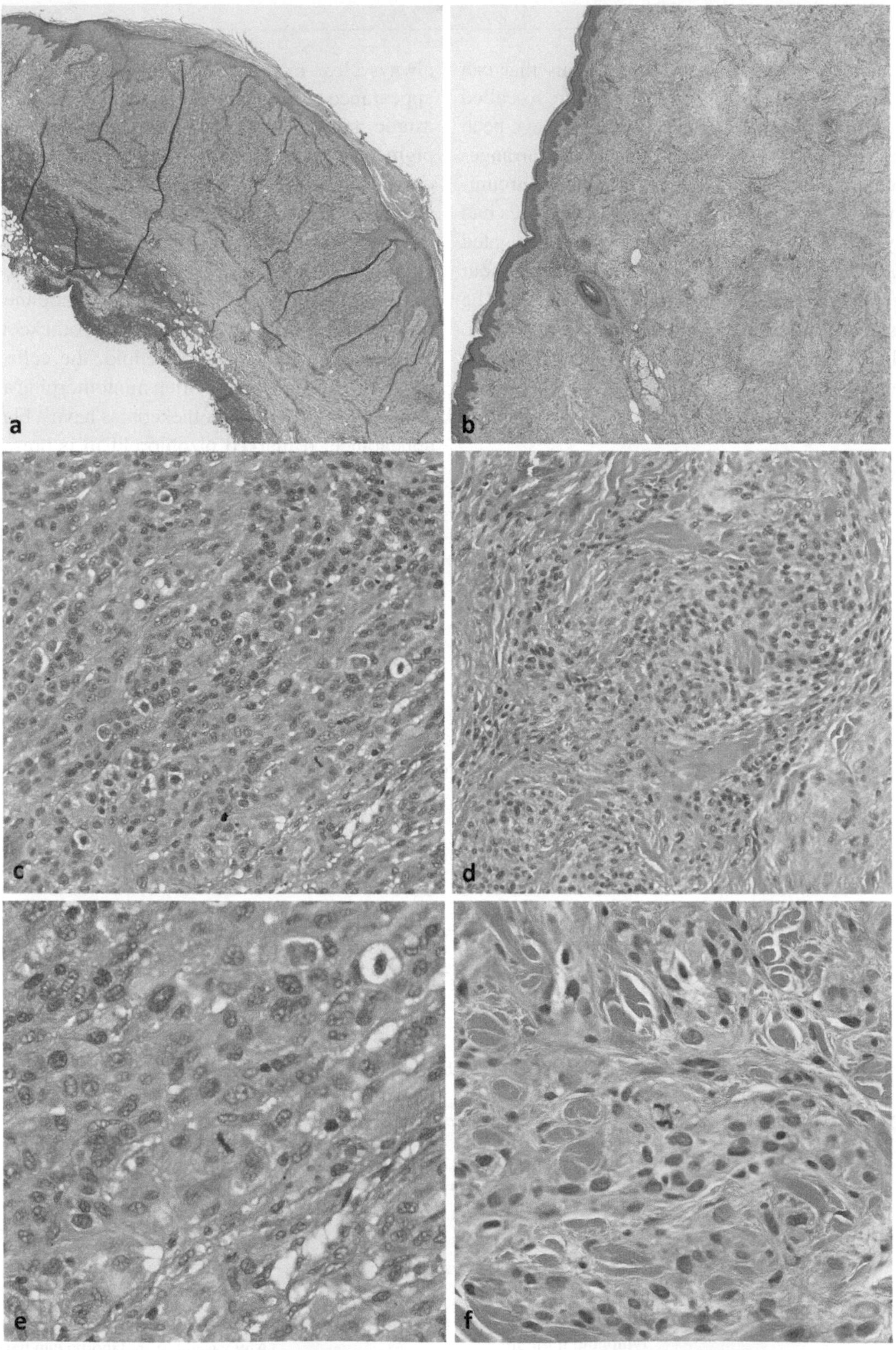

Fig. 12.9 Metastatic melanoma versus neurothekeoma. The panel illustrates melanoma on the left and neurothekeoma on the right. (**a**, **b**) Note that the epidermis forms a collarette around the metastatic melanoma, but no such collarette is present in neurothekeoma (H&E, ×2). (**c**, **d**) The growth pattern in the metastatic melanoma is more diffuse here, not nested or whorled (H&E, ×20). (**e**, **f**) The cells of metastatic melanoma are significantly more atypical than those of neurothekeoma. Both lesions demonstrate mitotic figures in the centers of the images (H&E, ×40)

An entity deemed *primary dermal melanoma* has been proposed as a distinct variant of melanoma that simulates a metastasis but lacks evidence of a primary lesion and has a better prognosis than metastatic melanoma [56]. Clinically, these cases commonly involve the head and neck as well as extremities, where they present as a subcutaneous nodule. Microscopically, they are deep dermal or subcutaneous proliferations of epithelioid or spindled cells (sometimes rhabdoid) with malignant cytologic features and frequent mitotic figures. Some cases demonstrate necrosis and hemorrhage. These tumors express melanocytic markers.

Neurothekeoma vs. Desmoplastic Melanoma

Neurothekeomas with floridly sclerotic stroma, referred to by some as *desmoplastic cellular neurothekeoma*, may evoke a differential that includes desmoplastic melanoma [18, 25, 26]. Like neurothekeoma, desmoplastic melanoma most commonly involves the head and neck, but the typical patient is much older (average 71) [57]. Some desmoplastic melanomas present as a small papule or nodule, and most lack pigmentation [41], which overlaps with neurothekeoma. Both lesions are characterized by a haphazard arrangement of spindle cells, occasionally in bundles, set within a densely collagenous matrix. Neurotropism and Meissner-like corpuscles in desmoplastic melanoma [41] can resemble the *neuroid* features of neurothekeoma. The cytologic features of desmoplastic melanoma can be deceptively bland or clearly malignant. Mitotic activity is variable but usually low [57], like neurothekeoma. Osteoclastic giant cells are more likely in neurothekeoma. The presence of solar elastosis and a lymphoplasmacytic infiltrate within and around the lesion [57] may favor desmoplastic melanoma, although these findings are not specific. As with the other melanocytic tumors, S100 can distinguish the lesions, but with the caveat of very focal expression in some cases [58], warranting careful scrutiny at high power. Additionally, desmoplastic melanoma usually does not express HMB-45 or Melan-A [58, 59]. Notably, SMA can be positive in both[4] [58]. Table 12.5 compares desmoplastic neurothekeoma and melanoma.

Neurothekeoma vs. Myxoid Melanoma

Myxoid change in primary cutaneous and metastatic melanoma has been known to generate confusion with many tumor types [41–47], neurothekeoma among them. Clinically, these melanomas usually present on the limbs and are otherwise similar to primary and metastatic melanomas in general [42]. Microscopic inspection at scanning magnification often reveals a lobulated lesion with fibrovascular septa demarcating the lobules, which resembles the myxoid pattern of neurothekeoma. The myxoid component may be focal or diffuse [41, 43]. Certain features of myxoid melanoma overlap with DNSM more so than neurothekeoma (e.g., the arrangement of cells in cords or strands within mucin pools, scattered pseudolipoblast cells) [41]. Cells within mucin pools may appear smaller than those elsewhere in the lesion [43]. In the nonmyxoid regions, cell shape ranges from stellate to spindled to epithelioid. There may be cellular condensations around vessels or around the septa [41, 43]. Mitotic rate is variable [41, 43]. Some cases show confluent necrosis [43, 44], a feature that favors melanoma. Another feature favoring melanoma is any in-situ component. Osteoclastic giant cells favor neurothekeoma. Although melanin pigment is often sparse in myxoid melanomas [41], the tumor's identity is ultimately revealed by S100 immunohistochemistry [41, 42, 47]. Notably, HMB-45 can be focal or negative, especially within myxoid zones [42, 60]. Overall, myxoid melanoma is only rarely encountered, but it carries great potential for diagnostic blunder.

[4] SMA-positive cells in desmoplastic melanoma are likely non-lesional cells (reactive stromal myofibroblasts) [58].

Table 12.5 Desmoplastic cellular neurothekeoma versus desmoplastic melanoma [41, 57, 58, 60]

	Desmoplastic cellular neurothekeoma	Desmoplastic melanoma
Epidermis	No epidermal component Underlying Grenz zone	Overlying epidermis is atrophic or acanthotic ± Atypical intraepidermal melanocytes
Architecture	Multinodular, haphazardly arranged fascicles	Haphazard and scattered cells but sometimes bundled or storiform Can have markedly elongated fascicles of cells Variable cellularity
	Prominent sclerotic, fibrotic background	Mild to marked stromal fibrosis
Cytology	Cells are spindled to epithelioid with pale, eosinophilic cytoplasm	Cells are spindled and may resemble fibroblasts
Atypical features	Usually bland; focal, marked pleomorphism and high mitotic activity in a minority of cases	Variable pleomorphism and mitotic activity Usually some elongated, hyperchromatic nuclei
Other features	± Osteoclastic giant cells ± Myxoid matrix ± Ectatic vessels, patchy perivascular lymphoid infiltrates	± Lymphoplasmacytic infiltrates at tumor front, ± solar elastosis Myxoid matrix is rarely seen
Immunohistochemistry	S100 –, HMB-45 – (almost always)	S100 + (sometimes focal) HMB-45 – (rare, focal expression) Melan-A – (usually)
Pitfalls	Both tumors can have neuroid features SMA expression can be seen in both tumors S100 expression can be focal in desmoplastic melanoma	

Neurothekeoma vs. Intradermal Nevus

Neurothekeoma can exhibit overlapping clinical and histopathologic features with a variety of benign intradermal nevi. For instance, hypopigmented cellular blue nevus occurs in a young population and can involve any body site [61]. Microscopic examination demonstrates a multinodular dermal tumor composed of bundles of spindle cells. Myxoid change can even be seen [62]. Ultimately, its usual dumbbell shape, dendritic or epithelioid melanocytes, and S100 expression reveal its true identity [61]. Deep penetrating nevus may be considered for reasons similar to cellular blue nevus, but pigmentation is a constant feature of this lesion [63]. Desmoplastic (sclerotic) nevus [64] can overlap with the desmoplastic pattern of neurothekeoma. If ever there is uncertainty, S100 expression readily unearths the melanocytic lesions.

Key Points

- Neurothekeoma is a misnamed tumor of uncertain origin and differentiation that has been previously confused with DNSM (a tumor with nerve sheath differentiation).
- It is a benign neoplasm with a proclivity for the head and neck of young women.
- Its histomorphologic plasticity—i.e., its cellular, myxoid, mixed, and desmoplastic patterns—results in overlap with various benign and malignant melanocytic neoplasms.
- Even in the face of marked cellular atypia, there is no evidence of any malignant potential.
- Neurothekeoma lacks a specific immunoprofile:
  - The literature does not suggest a particular panel for supporting the diagnosis, so the choice is ad hoc.
  - Its lack of S100 expression distinguishes it from numerous entities in the differential.

- Consider neurothekeoma when confronted with any unusual dermal tumor that recapitulates, to a variable degree, features of melanocytic, (fibro)histiocytic, and/or neural proliferations, but that does not express S100.

References

1. Weedon D. Weedon's Skin Pathology. 3rd ed. London: Churchill Livingstone Elsevier; 2010.
2. Gnepp D, editor. Diagnostic Surgical Pathology of the Head and Neck, 2nd ed. Philadelphia: Saunders Co. (Elsevier); 2009.
3. Fisher C, Montgomery E, Thway K. In: Epstein J, editor. Biopsy Interpretation of Soft Tissue Tumors. Philadelphia: Wolters Kluwer/Lippincott Williams & Wilkins; 2011.
4. Busam K. Dermatopathology. Volume in the series: Foundations in Diagnostic Pathology. Elsevier Health Sciences; 2010 [cited 2014 Feb 15]. Available from: Expert Consult
5. Weiss SW, Goldblum JR. Benign tumors of peripheral nerves. Enzinger and Weiss's Soft Tissue Tumors. 5th ed. St. Louis: Mosby; 2007.
6. Fletcher CDM, Bridge JA, Hogendoorn PCW, Mertens F, editors. WHO Classification of Tumours of Soft Tissue and Bone. Lyon: IARC Press; 2013.
7. Gallager RL, Helwig EB. Neurothekeoma—a benign cutaneous tumor of neural origin. Am J Clin Pathol. 1980;74(6):759–64.
8. Pulitzer DR, Reed RJ. Nerve-sheath myxoma (perineurial myxoma). Am J Dermatopathol. 1985;7(5): 409–21.
9. Fetsch JF, Laskin WB, Hallman JR, Lupton GP, Miettinen M. Neurothekeoma: an analysis of 178 tumors with detailed immunohistochemical data and long-term patient follow-up information. Am J Surg Pathol. 2007;31(7):1103–14.
10. Fetsch JF, Laskin WB, Miettinen M. Nerve sheath myxoma: a clinicopathologic and immunohistochemical analysis of 57 morphologically distinctive, S-100 protein- and GFAP-positive, myxoid peripheral nerve sheath tumors with a predilection for the extremities and a high local recurrence rate. Am J Surg Pathol. 2005;29(12):1615–24.
11. Zelger BG, Zelger B. Cellular "neurothekeoma": an epithelioid variant of dermatofibroma? Verh Dtsch Ges Pathol. 1998;82:239–45.
12. Laskin WB, Fetsch JF, Miettinen M. The "neurothekeoma": immunohistochemical analysis distinguishes the true nerve sheath myxoma from its mimics. Hum Pathol. 2000;31(10):1230–41.
13. Argenyi ZB, LeBoit PE, Santa Cruz D, Swanson PE, Kutzner H. Nerve sheath myxoma (neurothekeoma) of the skin: light microscopic and immunohistochemical reappraisal of the cellular variant. J Cutan Pathol. 1993;20(4):294–303.
14. Hornick JL, Fletcher CD. Cellular neurothekeoma: detailed characterization in a series of 133 cases. Am J Surg Pathol. 2007;31(3):329–40.
15. Barnhill RL, Mihm MC. Cellular neurothekeoma. A distinctive variant of neurothekeoma mimicking nevomelanocytic tumors. Am J Surg Pathol. 1990; 14(2):113–20.
16. Plaza JA, Torres-Cabala C, Evans H, Diwan AH, Prieto VG. Immunohistochemical expression of S100A6 in cellular neurothekeoma: clinicopathologic and immunohistochemical analysis of 31 cases. Am J Dermatopathol. 2009;31(5):419–22.
17. de Giorgi V, Alfaioli B, Franchi A, Gori A, Sestini S, Papi F, et al. Cellular neurothekeoma in a girl: could oestrogens favour the development and growth of this rare tumour? J Eur Acad Dermatol Venereol. 2008;22(9):1149–50.
18. García-Gutiérrez M, Toussaint-Caire S, González-Sánchez P, Ortiz-Hidalgo C. Multiple desmoplastic cellular neurothekeomas localized to the face of a 16-year-old boy. Am J Dermatopathol. 2010;32(8): 841–5.
19. Mahalingam M, Alter JN, Bhawan J. Multiple cellular neurothekeomas—a case report and review on the role of immunohistochemistry as a histologic adjunct. J Cutan Pathol. 2006;33(1):51–6.
20. Misago N, Satoh T, Narisawa Y. Cellular neurothekeoma with histiocytic differentiation. J Cutan Pathol. 2004;31(8):568–72.
21. Stratton J, Billings SD. Cellular neurothekeoma: analysis of 37 cases emphasizing atypical histologic features. Mod Pathol. 2014;27(5):701–10.
22. Chang SE, Lee TJ, Ro JY, Choi JH, Sung KJ, Moon KC, et al. Cellular neurothekeoma with possible neuroendocrine differentiation. J Dermatol. 1999;26(6): 363–7.
23. Page RN, King R, Mihm MC, Googe PB. Microphthalmia transcription factor and NKI/C3 expression in cellular neurothekeoma. Mod Pathol. 2004;17(2):230–4.
24. Sheth S, Li X, Binder S, Dry SM. Differential gene expression profiles of neurothekeomas and nerve sheath myxomas by microarray analysis. Mod Pathol. 2011;24(3):343–54.
25. Zedek DC, White WL, McCalmont TH. Desmoplastic cellular neurothekeoma: clinicopathological analysis of twelve cases. J Cutan Pathol. 2009;36(11):1185–90.
26. D'Antonio A, Cuomo R, Angrisani B, Memoli D, Angrisani P. Desmoplastic cellular neurothekeoma mimicking a desmoplastic melanocytic tumor. J Am Acad Dermatol. 2011;65(2):e57–8.
27. Busam KJ, Mentzel T, Colpaert C, Barnhill RL, Fletcher CD. Atypical or worrisome features in cellular neurothekeoma: a study of 10 cases. Am J Surg Pathol. 1998;22(9):1067–72.
28. Cardoso J, Calonje E. Cellular neurothekeoma with perineural extension: a potential diagnostic pitfall. J Cutan Pathol. 2012;39(6):662–4.
29. Goette DK. Calcifying neurothekeoma. J Dermatol Surg Oncol. 1986;12(9):958–60.

30. Rooney MT, Nascimento AG, Tung RL. Ossifying plexiform tumor. Report of a cutaneous ossifying lesion with histologic features of neurothekeoma. Am J Dermatopathol. 1994;16(2):189–92.
31. Fullen DR, Lowe L, Su LD. Antibody to S100a6 protein is a sensitive immunohistochemical marker for neurothekeoma. J Cutan Pathol. 2003;30(2):118–22.
32. Wang AR, May D, Bourne P, Scott G. PGP9.5: a marker for cellular neurothekeoma. Am J Surg Pathol. 1999;23(11):1401–7.
33. Fried I, Sitthinamsuwan P, Muangsomboon S, Kaddu S, Cerroni L, McCalmont TH. SOX-10 and MiTF expression in cellular and 'mixed' neurothekeoma. J Cutan Pathol. 2014.
34. Busam KJ, Iversen K, Coplan KC, Jungbluth AA. Analysis of microphthalmia transcription factor expression in normal tissues and tumors, and comparison of its expression with S-100 protein, gp100, and tyrosinase in desmoplastic malignant melanoma. Am J Surg Pathol. 2001;25(2):197–204.
35. Granter SR, Weilbaecher KN, Quigley C, Fletcher CD, Fisher DE. Microphthalmia transcription factor: not a sensitive or specific marker for the diagnosis of desmoplastic melanoma and spindle cell (non-desmoplastic) melanoma. Am J Dermatopathol. 2001; 23(3):185–9.
36. Folpe AL, Cooper K. Best practices in diagnostic immunohistochemistry: pleomorphic cutaneous spindle cell tumors. Arch Pathol Lab Med. 2007;131(10): 1517–24.
37. Sachdev R, Sundram UN. Frequent positive staining with NKI/C3 in normal and neoplastic tissues limits its usefulness in the diagnosis of cellular neurothekeoma. Am J Clin Pathol. 2006;126(4):554–63.
38. Campbell LK, Thomas JR, Lamps LW, Smoller BR, Folpe AL. Protein gene product 9.5 (PGP 9.5) is not a specific marker of neural and nerve sheath tumors: an immunohistochemical study of 95 mesenchymal neoplasms. Mod Pathol. 2003;16(10):963–9.
39. Wartchow EP, Goin L, Schreiber J, Mierau GW, Terella A, Allen GC. Plexiform fibrohistiocytic tumor: ultrastructural studies may aid in discrimination from cellular neurothekeoma. Ultrastruct Pathol. 2009;33(6):286–92.
40. Calonje E, Wilson-Jones E, Smith NP, Fletcher CD. Cellular 'neurothekeoma': an epithelioid variant of pilar leiomyoma? Morphological and immunohistochemical analysis of a series. Histopathology. 1992;20(5):397–404.
41. Banerjee SS, Harris M. Morphological and immunophenotypic variations in malignant melanoma. Histopathology. 2000;36(5):387–402.
42. Patel P, Levin K, Waltz K, Helm KF. Myxoid melanoma: immunohistochemical studies and a review of the literature. J Am Acad Dermatol. 2002;46(2): 264–70.
43. Hitchcock MG, McCalmont TH, White WL. Cutaneous melanoma with myxoid features: twelve cases with differential diagnosis. Am J Surg Pathol. 1999;23(12):1506–13.
44. Hitchcock MG, White WL. Malicious masquerade: myxoid melanoma. Semin Diagn Pathol. 1998;15(3): 195–202.
45. Ulamec M, Soldo-Belić A, Vucić M, Buljan M, Kruslin B, Tomas D. Melanoma with second myxoid stromal changes after personally applied prolonged phototherapy. Am J Dermatopathol. 2008;30(2): 185–7.
46. Zelger BG, Steiner H, Wambacher B, Zelger B. Malignant melanomas simulating various types of soft tissue tumors. Dermatol Surg. 1997;23(11): 1047–54.
47. Collina G, Losi L, Taccagni GL, Maiorana A. Myxoid metastases of melanoma: report of three cases and review of the literature. Am J Dermatopathol. 1997; 19(1):52–7.
48. Dal Pozzo V, Benelli C, Restano L, Gianotti R, Cesana BM. Clinical review of 247 case records of Spitz nevus (epithelioid cell and/or spindle cell nevus). Dermatology. 1997;194(1):20–5.
49. Weedon D. The Spitz Naevus. Clin Oncol. 1984; 3(3):493–507.
50. Piepkorn M. On the nature of histologic observations: the case of the Spitz nevus. J Am Acad Dermatol. 1995;32(2 Pt 1):248–54.
51. Mérot Y, Frenk E. Spitz nevus (large spindle cell and/ or epithelioid cell nevus). Age-related involvement of the suprabasal epidermis. Virchows Arch A Pathol Anat Histopathol. 1989;415(2):97–101.
52. Binder SW, Asnong C, Paul E, Cochran AJ. The histology and differential diagnosis of Spitz nevus. Semin Diagn Pathol. 1993;10(1):36–46.
53. Spatz A, Peterse S, Fletcher CD, Barnhill RL. Plexiform spitz nevus: an intradermal spitz nevus with plexiform growth pattern. Am J Dermatopathol. 1999;21(6):542–6.
54. Hoang MP. Myxoid Spitz nevus. J Cutan Pathol. 2003;30(9):566–8.
55. Heenan P, Maize J, Cook M, LeBoit P. Persistent melanoma and local metastasis of melanoma. In: LeBoit P, Burg G, Weedon D, Sarasin A, editors. Pathology and genetics of skin tumours. IARC WHO Classification of Tumours. Lyon: IARC Press; 2005. p. 90–2.
56. Cassarino DS, Cabral ES, Kartha RV, Swetter SM. Primary dermal melanoma: distinct immunohistochemical findings and clinical outcome compared with nodular and metastatic melanoma. Arch Dermatol. 2008;144(1):49–56.
57. de Almeida LS, Requena L, Rütten A, Kutzner H, Garbe C, Pestana D, et al. Desmoplastic malignant melanoma: a clinicopathologic analysis of 113 cases. Am J Dermatopathol. 2008;30(3):207–15.
58. Longacre TA, Egbert BM, Rouse RV. Desmoplastic and spindle-cell malignant melanoma. An immunohistochemical study. Am J Surg Pathol. 1996; 20(12):1489–500.

59. Prieto VG, Shea CR. Immunohistochemistry of melanocytic proliferations. Arch Pathol Lab Med. 2011;135(7):853–9.
60. Prieto VG, Kanik A, Salob S, McNutt NS. Primary cutaneous myxoid melanoma: immunohistologic clues to a difficult diagnosis. J Am Acad Dermatol. 1994;30(2 Pt 2):335–9.
61. Calonje E, Blessing K, Glusac E, Strutton G. Blue naevi. In: LeBoit P, Burg G, Weedon D, Sarasin A, editors. Pathology and genetics of skin tumours. IARC WHO classification of tumours. Lyon: IARC Press; 2005. p. 95–9.
62. Rongioletti F, Innocenzi D. Sclerosing 'mucinous' blue naevus. Br J Dermatol. 2003;148(6):1250–2.
63. Luzar B, Calonje E. Deep penetrating nevus: a review. Arch Pathol Lab Med. 2011;135(3):321–6.
64. Harris GR, Shea CR, Horenstein MG, Reed JA, Burchette JL, Prieto VG. Desmoplastic (sclerotic) nevus: an underrecognized entity that resembles dermatofibroma and desmoplastic melanoma. Am J Surg Pathol. 1999;23(7):786–94.
65. Vollmer RT. Use of Bayes rule and MIB-1 proliferation index to discriminate Spitz nevus from malignant melanoma. Am J Clin Pathol. 2004;122(4):499–505.
66. National Cancer Institute. SEER stat fact sheets: melanoma of the skin [Internet] [cited 2014 Feb 12]. Available from: http://seer.cancer.gov/statfacts/html/melan.html.

Melanoma In Situ Versus Paget's Disease

13

Jon A. Reed, Christopher R. Shea, and Victor G. Prieto

Introduction

Most patients with noninvasive malignant melanoma (melanoma in situ; MIS) present with a clinically atypical pigmented lesion. In many cases, MIS is suspected, and the biopsy is confirmatory. The histological differential diagnosis of MIS however, is more challenging when the clinical presentation is unusual. Occasionally, patients with MIS have an erythematous, eczematous scaly patch without obvious pigmentation. In this scenario, an inflammatory dermatosis or epithelial neoplasm may be considered more likely than MIS in the clinical differential diagnosis. Similarly, a diagnosis of MIS may be considered less likely when evaluating pigmented lesions from anatomic sites where an inflammatory dermatosis with pigmentary alteration or an epithelial malignancy such as intraepidermal adenocarcinoma (Paget's disease/ extramammary Paget's disease) is encountered more frequently.

This chapter will focus on the histological differential diagnosis of MIS vs. Paget's disease, but will include discussion of other lesions (pigmented and nonpigmented) histologically characterized by intraepidermal "pagetoid" scatter of atypical cells.

J.A. Reed, M.S., M.D. (✉)
Baylor College of Medicine,
1 Baylor Plaza, Houston, TX 77030, USA

CellNetix Pathology & Laboratories,
1124 Columbia St., Suite 200, Seattle,
WA 98117, USA
e-mail: jreed@bcm.edu; jreed@cellnetix.com

C.R. Shea, M.D.
University of Chicago Medicine,
5841 S. Maryland Ave., MC 5067, L502,
Chicago, IL 60637, USA

V.G. Prieto, M.D., Ph.D.
MD Anderson Cancer Center, University of Houston,
1515 Holcombe Blvd., Unit 85, Houston,
TX 77030, USA

Malignant Melanoma In Situ (Intraepidermal Melanoma)

Clinical Features

MIS usually presents as an asymmetrical, variably pigmented macule or patch with irregular borders. Lesions often are long-standing, but change in appearance over time. Although MIS occurs at any site, areas of skin with a history of chronic sun exposure are more frequently involved. MIS arising on chronically sun-exposed skin were originally termed Hutchinson's melanotic freckle or precancerous melanosis, and later, lentigo maligna to acknowledge their association with invasive melanoma [1–6]. The amelanotic variant of MIS presents as an erythematous scaly patch resembling an inflammatory dermatosis or epithelial neoplasm [7–12]. More recently, molecular cytogenetic studies have shown that mela-

C.R. Shea et al. (eds.), *Pathology of Challenging Melanocytic Neoplasms: Diagnosis and Management*,
DOI 10.1007/978-1-4939-1444-9_13, © Springer Science+Business Media New York 2015

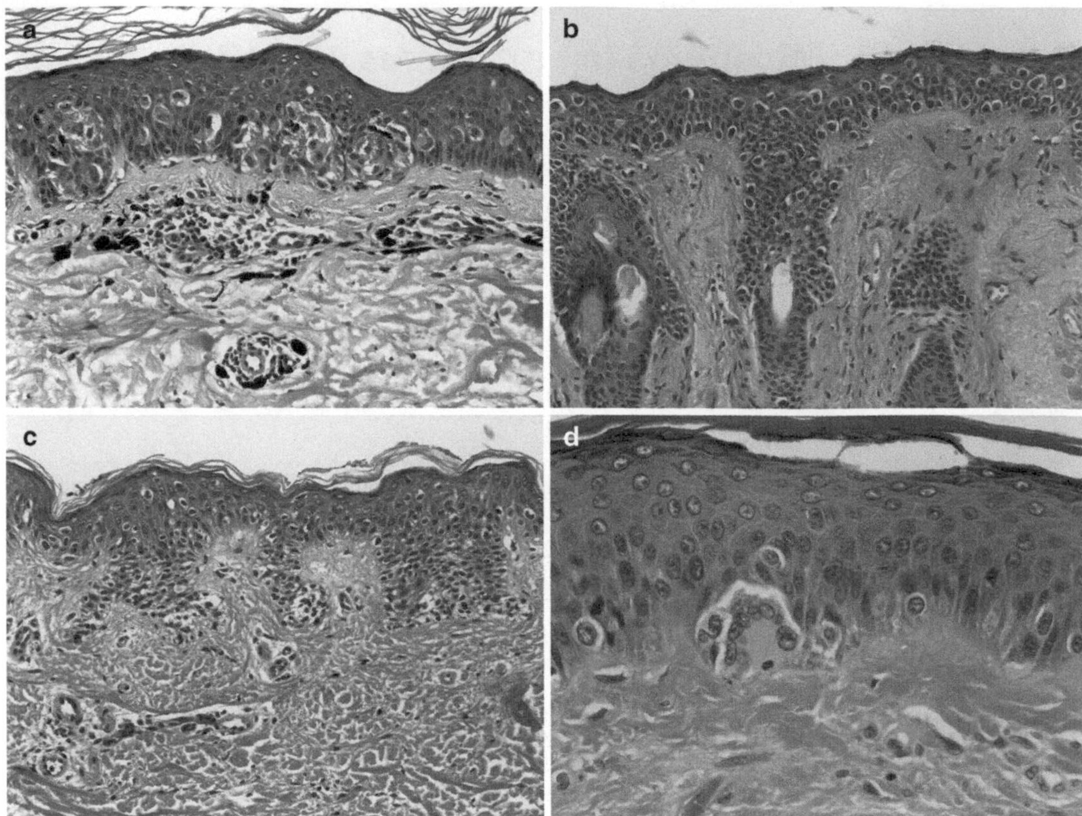

Fig. 13.1 The variable histological appearances of MIS. (**a**) Intraepidermal pagetoid scatter of cytologically atypical melanocytes containing abundant melanin (×10). (**b**) Intraepidermal pagetoid scatter of cytologically atypical, but less pigmented melanocytes (×10). (**c**) Intraepidermal pagetoid scatter of small, less atypical, and less pigmented melanocytes (×10). (**d**) Multinucleated starburst giant cell in a case of lentigo maligna (×40)

nomas arising in the setting of chronic exposure to ultraviolet light harbor nonrandom chromosomal aberrations different from those associated with melanomas involving skin with intermittent or low exposure [13–15].

Microscopic Features

MIS is characterized by a poorly circumscribed proliferation of cytologically atypical melanocytes in the epidermis (Fig. 13.1). The melanocytes often are disposed predominantly as single cells, although nests may be present as well. Rete ridges are elongated and distorted, but can be attenuated in lesions from chronically sun-exposed skin. Single melanocytes often form a confluent proliferation along the basal layer and involve adnexal structures. Atypical melanocytes are present in superficial epidermal layers, at least focally, in most lesions. This feature is less prominent in MIS arising from chronically sun-exposed skin. The melanocytes vary greatly in size, amount of cytoplasmic melanin, and by degree of nuclear atypia introducing the potential for sampling bias in small biopsies [16]. Multinucleated "starburst" giant cells may be present, especially in lentigo maligna [17]. MIS (and invasive melanoma) also can arise within a pre-existing atypical nevus [18].

MIS characterized by smaller, less atypical melanocytes may be partially obscured by surrounding pigmented basal keratinocytes on chronically sun-exposed skin. MIS also may be partially obscured by an associated interface/lichenoid inflammatory infiltrate, by an adjacent pigmented seborrheic keratosis, solar lentigo, or pigmented actinic keratosis [19]. The amelanotic

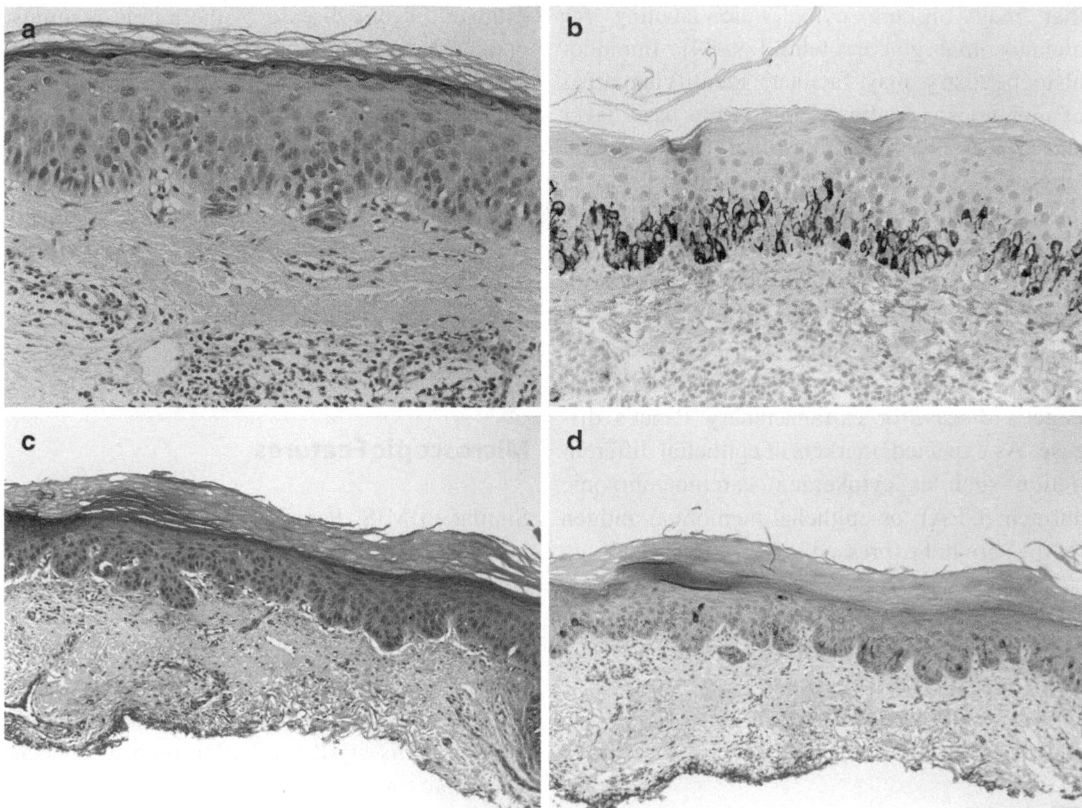

Fig. 13.2 Immunohistochemistry of melanoma in situ. (**a**) Amelanotic MIS on chronically sun-damages skin. Melanocytes are not easily recognized in the routine hematoxylin and eosin-stained section (×20). (**b**) Immunohistochemical labeling for gp100 (using HMB45) on the same amelanotic lentigo maligna (×20). (**c**) Actinic keratosis at the edge of MIS (×10). (**d**) Labeling for gp100 highlights atypical melanocytes, including cells in superficial layers of the actinic keratosis (×10)

variant of MIS also can be difficult to identify in routine hematoxylin- and eosin-stained sections (Fig. 13.2). Given the considerable variability of histological features, evaluation of MIS by frozen section without use of additional special studies, especially for the purposes of surgical margin assessment, is not recommended [20].

Immunohistochemical Features

Diagnosis of MIS is straightforward and special studies such as immunohistochemistry are not needed in most cases. Immunohistochemistry proves to be an invaluable diagnostic tool; however, for amelanotic MIS and for MIS in which melanocytes are partially obscured by an associated lichenoid inflammatory infiltrate or by an adjacent pigmented epithelial lesion [19, 21] (Fig. 13.2).

Markers of melanocyte differentiation such as melanosomal glycoproteins (e.g. gp100, gp75, or Melan A/MART-1) are commonly employed to better enumerate intraepidermal atypical melanocytes [21–25]. Some of these markers also have been advocated for improving accuracy of margin assessment in Mohs micrographic surgery [26, 27], although the specificity of labeling using Melan A/MART-1 has been questioned [28]. Immunohistochemistry also has been used to document expression of nuclear proteins microphthalmia transcription factor (MiTF) and SOX-10 for MIS containing abundant melanin that may obscure cytoplasmic labeling for melanosomal glycoproteins [29–34]. Immunohistochemistry may facilitate identifying areas of melanocyte confluence along the basal layer and "pagetoid" scatter regardless of the marker employed. S100 protein may be useful [35, 36], but is a less reliable marker for MIS because intraepidermal dendritic Langerhans cells also display labeling and some melanocytes on chronically sun-exposed skin are negative [22].

The absence of expression of melanocyte markers also is helpful to rule out MIS in cases of Paget's disease or extramammary Paget's disease. As expected, markers of epithelial differentiation such as cytokeratin, carcinoembryonic antigen (CEA), or epithelial membrane antigen (EMA) are not expressed in MIS [36–38].

Differential Diagnosis: Paget's Disease/Extramammary Paget's Disease (Intraepidermal Adenocarcinoma)

Clinical Features

Intraepidermal adenocarcinomas of the breast/nipple (Paget's disease) and other anatomic sites (extramammary Paget's disease), typically are characterized by an erythematous, eczematous patch, often with associated sero-sanguinous exudate. Paget's disease of the nipple is almost invariably associated with an underlying ductal carcinoma of the breast [39]. Extramammary Paget's disease often is associated with an underlying carcinoma of apocrine or eccrine sweat gland/duct origin [40]. Lesions arising on genital/perianal skin are most common; however, any site may be involved [41–45]. Genital/perineal lesions rarely may be associated with underlying carcinoma of Bartholin glands, rectal, urothelial, or even prostatic origin [46–49].

Microscopic Features

Similar to MIS, Paget's disease and extramammary Paget's disease are characterized by intraepidermal proliferation of cytologically atypical epithelial cells disposed singly and as clusters (Fig. 13.3). Larger clusters of cells may form luminal structures, but this feature is not prominent. The atypical cells are scattered throughout the epidermis at all levels, but tend to concentrate more toward the basal layer. Most cells have abundant slightly basophilic cytoplasm. Cytoplasmic melanin may be present in the atypical cells. Mitotic figures usually are present. Histochemical stains for epithelial mucin (Colloidal Iron, Alcian Blue pH 2.5, and Mucicarmine) are more strongly reactive in cases of extramammary Paget's disease.

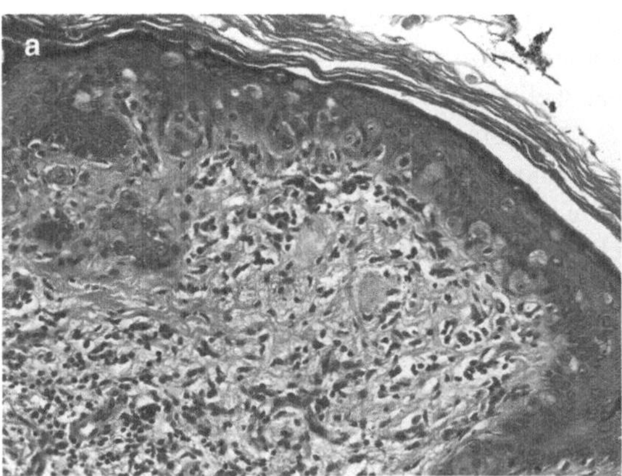

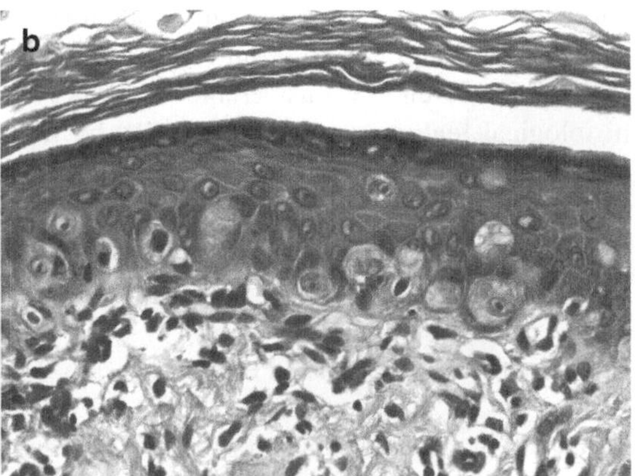

Fig. 13.3 Extramammary Paget's disease. (**a**) Cytologically atypical epithelioid cells are scattered throughout the epidermis (×20). (**b**) Note the basophilic vacuolated cytoplasm and nuclear atypia of the carcinoma cells (×40)

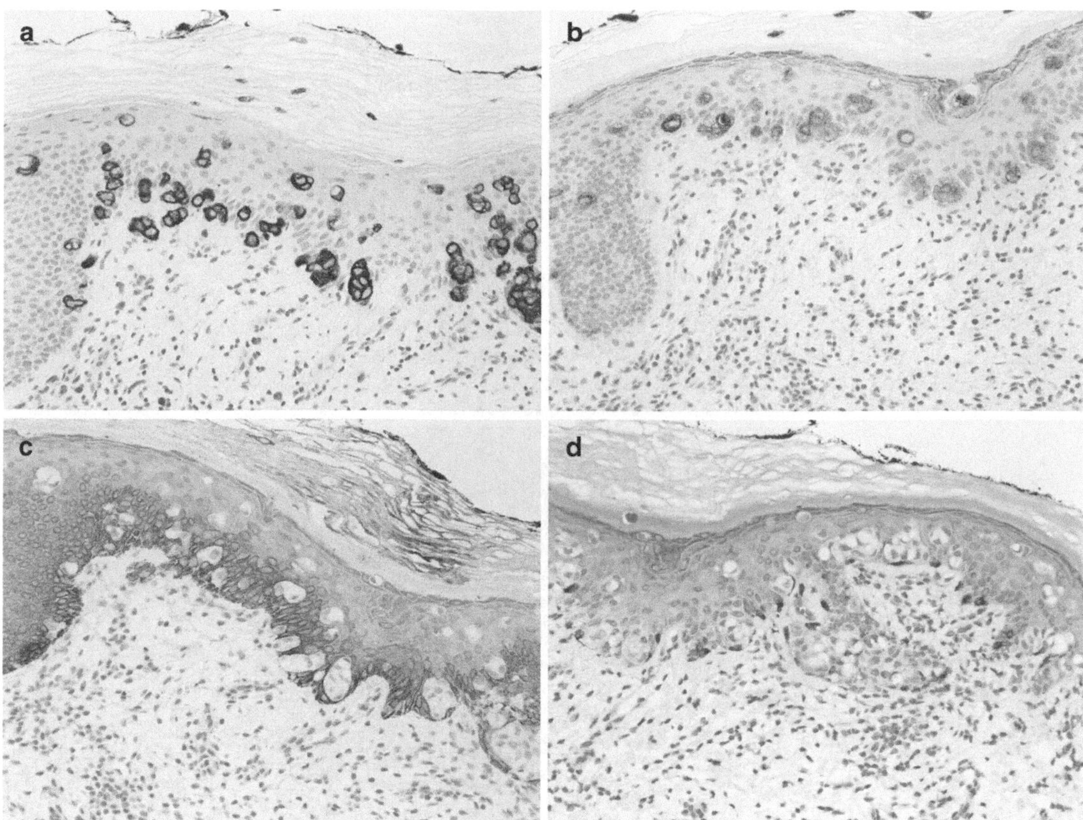

Fig. 13.4 Immunohistochemistry of Paget's disease. (**a**) Strong cytoplasmic labeling for CK7 (×20). (**b**) Strong labeling for CEA (×20). (**c**) Epidermis labeled for CK 5/6. Note the lack of labeling by the carcinoma cells. (**d**) Melan A/MART-1. Note the strong labeling of closely apposed dendritic melanocytes. The carcinoma cells are not labeled (×20)

Immunohistochemical Features

Epithelial markers, such as CEA, and cytokeratin 7 (CK7) are helpful to distinguish Paget's disease from MIS [23, 36–38, 50, 51] (Fig. 13.4). Labeling for melanocyte markers such as gp100 or Melan A/MART-1 must be interpreted with caution in pigmented lesions as labeled normal melanocytes may be closely apposed to clusters of carcinoma cells [52] (Fig. 13.4). Other markers also have been shown to reliably distinguish Paget's disease/extramammary Paget's disease from MIS [53, 54].

Differential Diagnosis: Pagetoid Bowen's Disease (Pagetoid Squamous Cell Carcinoma In Situ)

Clinical Features

Another important differential diagnosis for MIS includes pagetoid Bowen's disease (pagetoid squamous cell carcinoma in situ). Pagetoid Bowen's disease presents as an erythematous scaly patch, most often on chronically sun-exposed skin [55]. Other areas may be involved especially in the setting of

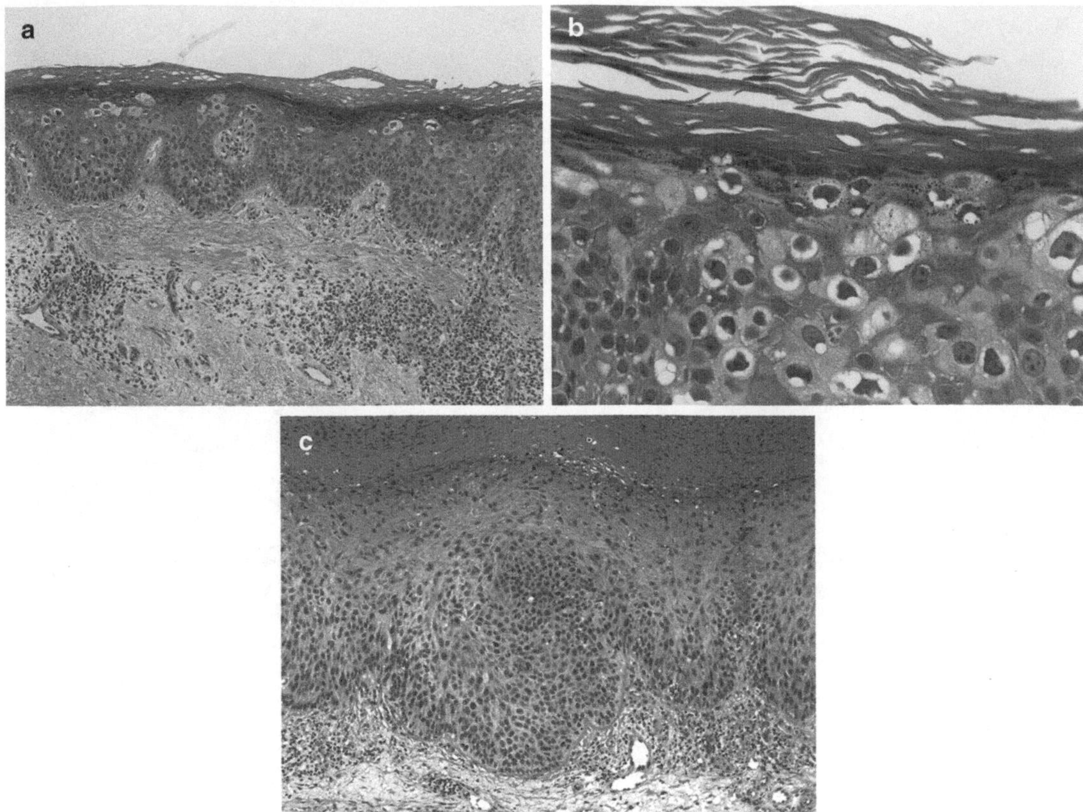

Fig. 13.5 Bowen's disease. (**a**) Cytologically atypical cells are scattered within the epidermis (×10). (**b**) Atypical cells in the granular layer contain keratohyaline granules (×40). (**c**) An adjacent focus of epidermis displaying cytologically atypical keratinocytes throughout its full thickness more typical of Bowen's disease (×10)

predisposing factors of prior immunosuppressive therapy for organ transplant or a history of exposure to certain environmental toxins such as arsenic [56, 57]. Occasionally, the scaly patch may be hyperpigmented raising the suspicion of MIS/lentigo maligna [58–64]. Most lesions have an ill-defined border and expand slowly over a period of many years.

Microscopic Features

Pagetoid Bowen's disease is characterized by large, often pale-staining atypical keratinocytes scattered within the epidermis at all levels (Fig. 13.5). The atypical keratinocytes are disposed singly and in small clusters resembling MIS or Paget's disease. Some of the atypical cells may contain notable cytoplasmic melanin. Mitotic figures and apoptotic cells are scattered in supra-basal layers as well. Clusters of atypical cells do not form luminal structures as in Paget's disease. Careful examination of the entire section often will reveal areas with cytologically atypical cells throughout the full thickness of the epidermis facilitating the diagnosis of squamous cell carcinoma in situ. Areas of full-thickness atypia may not be present in very small biopsies. In such cases, careful examination of the granular cell layer should be performed. The presence of atypical cells containing keratohyaline granules confirms a diagnosis of Bowen's disease. Unlike melanin, keratohyaline granules are not transferred between adjacent cells and their presence in a cytologically atypical cell serves as a valuable marker of keratinocyte differentiation.

Histochemical stains for epithelial mucin are negative, but this feature would not rule out MIS or Paget's disease. Stains for melanin may be positive or negative depending on the amount of melanin transfer from adjacent normal melanocytes, and as such, are not of value.

Immunohistochemical Features

Immunohistochemical labeling for cytokeratin (CK) 5/6 and other markers distinguish pagetoid Bowen's disease from Paget's disease and from MIS [53, 54, 65–67]. Recently, Bowen's disease has been shown to rarely express epithelial markers typical of Paget's disease such as CK7 and low molecular weight cytokeratin [68] underscoring the need for multiple immunohistochemical markers in some cases [69].

Differential Diagnosis: Irritated Seborrheic Keratosis with "Clonal Features"

Clinical Features

One histological sub-type of seborrheic keratosis (SK) is the so-called "clonal" variant. This histological variant is believed to result from chronic irritation/trauma and has recognizable changes on dermoscopy [70]. Irritated SKs often have a clinical differential diagnosis of squamous cell carcinoma, making their histological distinction from Bowen's disease most relevant.

Microscopic Features

The "clonal" variant of irritated SK is characterized by intraepidermal, circumscribed clusters of similar-appearing keratinocytes within a lesion architecturally compatible with ordinary SK (Fig. 13.6). Importantly, the keratinocytes within these clusters lack significant nuclear atypia or pleomorphism. Mitotic figures and dyskeratotic/apoptotic cells are rare. Pagetoid scatter of single atypical keratinocytes is not observed. The "clonal" cells lack keratohyaline granules and most usually contain very little cytoplasmic melanin. Histochemical stains for epithelial mucin are negative.

Immunohistochemical Features

Given the lack of significant cytologic atypia, immunohistochemistry usually is not needed to distinguish clonal SK from MIS or from most cases of Paget's disease. Documenting absence of immunohistochemical labeling for CK7 or for

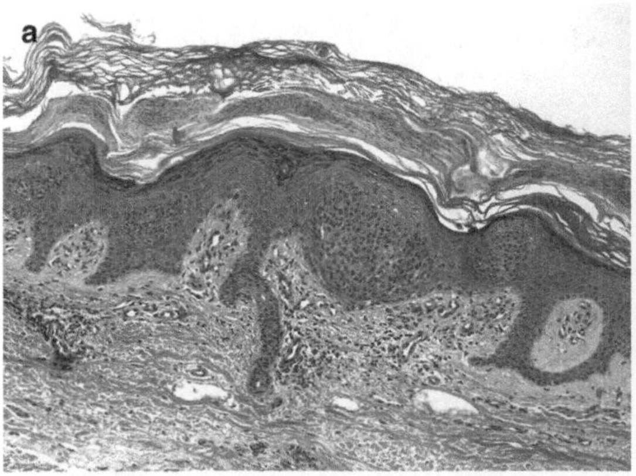

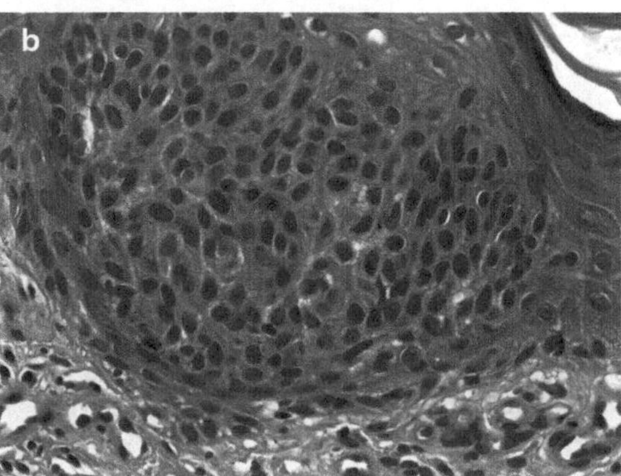

Fig. 13.6 Clonal seborrheic keratosis. (**a**) Well-circumscribed clusters of keratinocytes form "pseudonests" within the epidermis (×10). (**b**) Keratinocytes within the nest do not exhibit significant nuclear atypia. Dyskeratotic cells and mitotic figures are absent (×40)

CEA may be helpful to rule out Paget's disease/extramammary Paget's disease in exceptional cases. Similarly, immunohistochemistry can demonstrate lack of expression of melanocyte markers helping to rule out MIS.

Distinguishing clonal SK from pagetoid Bowen's disease may be more difficult. Recently it was shown that the expression of BCL-2 and absence of expression of CK10 distinguishes clonal SK from Bowen's disease [71].

Differential Diagnosis: Melanoacanthoma and Pigmented Seborrheic Keratosis

Clinical Features

Melanoacanthomas and pigmented SK have a similar clinical appearance to irritated/clonal SK, but are more pigmented [72–79]. The clinical differential diagnosis often includes an atypical nevus and melanoma in larger lesions. Larger ulcerated lesions are especially worrisome for melanoma.

Microscopic Features

Melanoacanthomas and pigmented SK display varying degrees of acanthosis, papillomatosis, and hyperkeratosis with associated horn pseudocyst formation (Fig. 13.7). Both lesions have an increased number of intraepidermal melanocytes. In melanoacanthomas, the melanocytes are enlarged, contain abundant cytoplasmic melanin, and have prominent dendritic processes that surround numerous adjacent keratinocytes. The keratinocytes themselves contain a sparse amount of cytoplasmic melanin suggesting an underlying defect in melanin transfer from the melanocytes [80, 81].

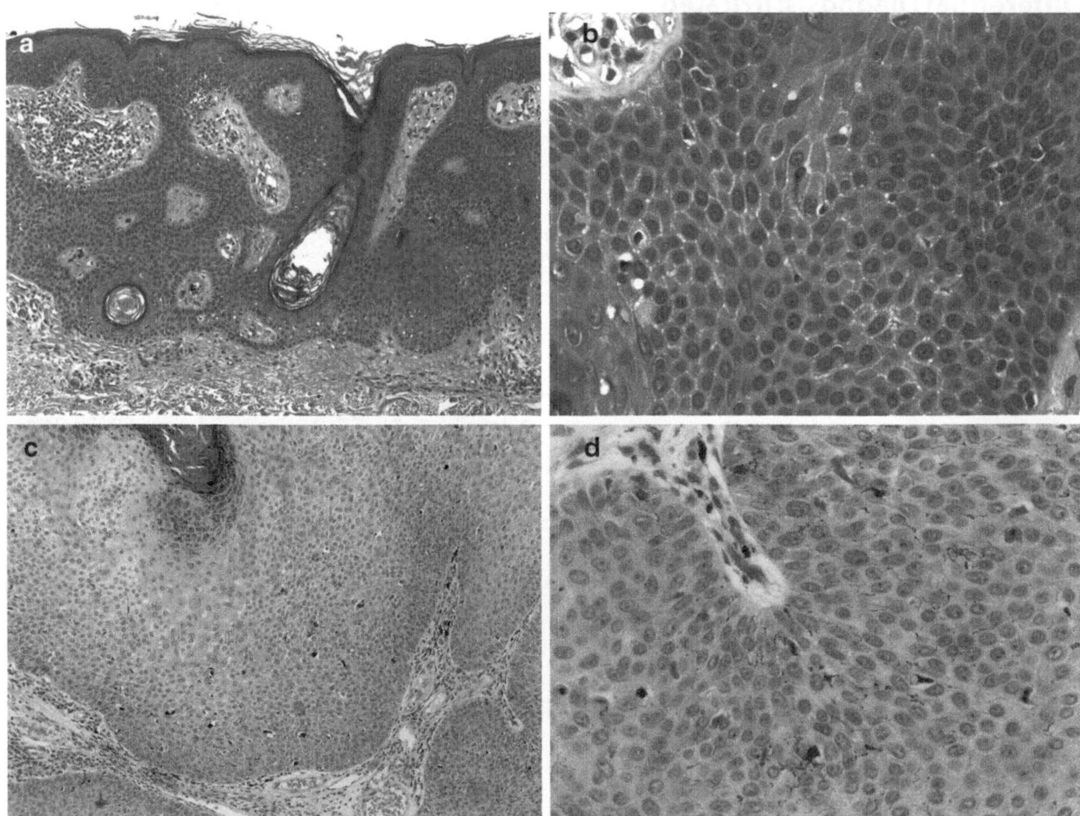

Fig. 13.7 Melanoacanthoma and pigmented seborrheic keratosis. (**a**) Pigmented SK displaying typical acanthosis, papillomatosis, and horn pseudocysts (×20). (**b**) A small dendritic melanocyte in the same pigmented SK. Note cytoplasmic melanin in adjacent keratinocytes (×40). (**c**) Large melanoacanthoma (×4). (**d**) Melanoacanthoma. Note the large, pigmented melanocytes with prominent dendrites and the adjacent keratinocytes without melanin (×40)

The melanocytes are scattered at all levels of the epidermis, but do not form nests. The prominent dendritic appearance of the melanocytes distinguishes them from most MIS. Pigmented SKs have similar architectural features, but keratinocytes contain more prominent cytoplasmic melanin and the melanocytes are smaller less, pigmented, and have less prominent dendritic processes.

Immunohistochemical Features

As expected, the pigmented dendritic melanocytes in melanoacanthomas and in pigmented SK express markers associated with melanosomal glycoproteins (gp100, Melan A/MART-1). The melanocytes lack expression of epithelial markers typical of Paget's disease and Bowen's disease.

Conclusions

The histological distinctions between MIS, Paget's disease, Bowen's disease, and certain subtypes of SK can be very challenging especially in the absence of clinical information. Conversely, clinical information can be misleading in cases of amelanotic MIS, pigmented Bowen's disease, and in lesions present at an unusual anatomic site. Careful consideration of the histological features and the selected use of histochemical and immunohistochemical studies should lead to accurate diagnosis in almost all cases.

References

1. Clark WHJ, Mihm MCJ. Lentigo maligna and lentigo-maligna melanoma. Am J Pathol. 1969;55:39–67.
2. Clark WHJ. Malignant melanoma in situ. Hum Pathol. 1990;21:1197–8.
3. Costello MJ, Fisher SB, Defeo CP. Melanotic freckle, lentigo maligna. Arch Dermatol. 1959;80:753–71.
4. Klauder JV, Beerman H. Melanotic freckle (Hutchinson), melanose circonscrite precancereuse (Dubreuilh). AMA Arch Derm. 1955;71:2–10.
5. McGovern VJ, Shaw HM, Milton GW, Farago GA. Is malignant melanoma arising in a Hutchinson's melanotic freckle a separate disease entity? Histopathology. 1980;4:235–42.
6. Mishima Y. Melanosis circumscripta praecancerosa (Dubreuilh), a non-nevoid premelanoma distinct from junction nevus. J Invest Dermatol. 1960;34:361–75.
7. Rahbari H, Nabai H, Mehregan AH, Mehregan DA, Mehregan DR, Lipinski J. Amelanotic lentigo maligna melanoma: a diagnostic conundrum—presentation of four new cases. Cancer. 1996;77: 2052–7.
8. Su WP, Bradley RR. Amelanotic lentigo maligna. Arch Dermatol. 1980;116:82–3.
9. Borkovic SP, Schwartz RA. Amelanotic lentigo maligna melanoma manifesting as a dermatitislike plaque. Arch Dermatol. 1983;119:423–5.
10. Kelly RI, Cook MG, Mortimer PS. Aggressive amelanotic lentigo maligna. Br J Dermatol. 1994;131: 562–5.
11. Pichler E, Fritsch P. Macular amelanotic melanoma in situ. Dermatologica. 1988;177:313–6.
12. Prieto VG, McNutt NS, Prioleau PG, Shea CR. Scaly erythematous lesion in a patient with extensive solar damage. Malignant melanoma in situ, amelanotic type. Arch Dermatol. 1996;132:1239, 1242.
13. Bastian BC, Olshen AB, LeBoit PE, Pinkel D. Classifying melanocytic tumors based on DNA copy number changes. Am J Pathol. 2003;163:1765–70.
14. Gerami P, Mafee M, Lurtsbarapa T, Guitart J, Haghighat Z, Newman M. Sensitivity of fluorescence in situ hybridization for melanoma diagnosis using RREB1, MYB, Cep6, and 11q13 probes in melanoma subtypes. Arch Dermatol. 2010;146:273–8.
15. Grammatico P, Modesti A, Steindl K, et al. Lentigo maligna. Cytogenetic, ultrastructural, and phenotypic characterization of a primary cell culture. Cancer Genet Cytogenet. 1992;60:141–6.
16. Stevens G, Cockerell CJ. Avoiding sampling error in the biopsy of pigmented lesions. Arch Dermatol. 1996;132:1380–2.
17. Katz SK, Guitart J. Starburst giant cells in benign nevomelanocytic lesions. J Am Acad Dermatol. 1998; 38:283.
18. Gruber SB, Barnhill RL, Stenn KS, Roush GC. Nevomelanocytic proliferations in association with cutaneous malignant melanoma: a multivariate analysis. J Am Acad Dermatol. 1989;21:773–80.
19. Helm K, Findeis-Hosey J. Immunohistochemistry of pigmented actinic keratoses, actinic keratoses, melanomas in situ and solar lentigines with Melan-A. J Cutan Pathol. 2008;35:931–4.
20. Prieto VG, Argenyi ZB, Barnhill RL, et al. Are en face frozen sections accurate for diagnosing margin status in melanocytic lesions? Am J Clin Pathol. 2003; 120:203–8.
21. Lane H, O'Loughlin S, Powell F, Magee H, Dervan PA. A quantitative immunohistochemical evaluation of lentigo maligna and pigmented solar keratosis. Am J Clin Pathol. 1993;100:681–5.
22. Bhawan J. Mel-5: a novel antibody for differential diagnosis of epidermal pigmented lesions of the skin in paraffin-embedded sections. Melanoma Res. 1997;7:43–8.
23. Kohler S, Rouse RV, Smoller BR. The differential diagnosis of pagetoid cells in the epidermis. Mod Pathol. 1998;11:79–92.

24. Reed JA, Shea CR. Lentigo maligna: melanoma in situ on chronically sun-damaged skin. Arch Pathol Lab Med. 2011;135:838–41.
25. Shah KD, Tabibzadeh SS, Gerber MA. Immunohistochemical distinction of Paget's disease from Bowen's disease and superficial spreading melanoma with the use of monoclonal cytokeratin antibodies. Am J Clin Pathol. 1987;88:689–95.
26. Kelley LC, Starkus L. Immunohistochemical staining of lentigo maligna during Mohs micrographic surgery using MART-1. J Am Acad Dermatol. 2002;46:78–84.
27. Menaker GM, Chiang JK, Tabila B, Moy RL. Rapid HMB-45 staining in Mohs micrographic surgery for melanoma in situ and invasive melanoma. J Am Acad Dermatol. 2001;44:833–6.
28. Demartini CS, Dalton MS, Ferringer T, Elston DM. Melan-A/MART-1 positive "pseudonests" in lichenoid inflammatory lesions: an uncommon phenomenon. Am J Dermatopathol. 2005;27:370–1.
29. Buonaccorsi JN, Prieto VG, Torres-Cabala C, Suster S, Plaza JA. Diagnostic utility and comparative immunohistochemical analysis of MITF-1 and SOX10 to distinguish melanoma in situ and actinic keratosis: a clinicopathological and immunohistochemical study of 70 cases. Am J Dermatopathol. 2014;36:124–30.
30. King R, Weilbaecher KN, McGill G, Cooley E, Mihm M, Fisher DE. Microphthalmia transcription factor. A sensitive and specific melanocyte marker for melanoma diagnosis. Am J Pathol. 1999;155:731–8.
31. King R, Page RN, Googe PB, Mihm MCJ. Lentiginous melanoma: a histologic pattern of melanoma to be distinguished from lentiginous nevus. Mod Pathol. 2005;18:1397–401.
32. Mohamed A, Gonzalez RS, Lawson D, Wang J, Cohen C. SOX10 expression in malignant melanoma, carcinoma, and normal tissues. Appl Immunohistochem Mol Morphol. 2013;21:506–10.
33. Ramos-Herberth FI, Karamchandani J, Kim J, Dadras SS. SOX10 immunostaining distinguishes desmoplastic melanoma from excision scar. J Cutan Pathol. 2010;37:944–52.
34. Shin J, Vincent JG, Cuda JD, et al. Sox10 is expressed in primary melanocytic neoplasms of various histologies but not in fibrohistiocytic proliferations and histiocytoses. J Am Acad Dermatol. 2012;67:717–26.
35. Glasgow BJ, Wen DR, Al-Jitawi S, Cochran AJ. Antibody to S-100 protein aids the separation of pagetoid melanoma from mammary and extramammary Paget's disease. J Cutan Pathol. 1987;14:223–6.
36. Rosen L, Amazon K, Frank B. Bowen's disease, Paget's disease, and malignant melanoma in situ. South Med J. 1986;79:410–3.
37. Guldhammer B, Norgaard T. The differential diagnosis of intraepidermal malignant lesions using immunohistochemistry. Am J Dermatopathol. 1986;8:295–301.
38. Reed W, Oppedal BR, Eeg LT. Immunohistology is valuable in distinguishing between Paget's disease, Bowen's disease and superficial spreading malignant melanoma. Histopathology. 1990;16:583–8.
39. Seetharam S, Fentiman IS. Paget's disease of the nipple. Womens Health (Lond Engl). 2009;5:397–402.
40. Vergati M, Filingeri V, Palmieri G, Roselli M. Perianal Paget's disease: a case report and literature review. Anticancer Res. 2012;32:4461–5.
41. Chilukuri S, Page R, Reed JA, Friedman J, Orengo I. Ectopic extramammary Paget's disease arising on the cheek. Dermatol Surg. 2002;28:430–3.
42. Cohen MA, Hanly A, Poulos E, Goldstein GD. Extramammary Paget's disease presenting on the face. Dermatol Surg. 2004;30:1361–3.
43. de Blois GG, Patterson JW, Hunter SB. Extramammary Paget's disease. Arising in knee region in association with sweat gland carcinoma. Arch Pathol Lab Med. 1984;108:713–6.
44. Hilliard NJ, Huang C, Andea A. Pigmented extramammary Paget's disease of the axilla mimicking melanoma: case report and review of the literature. J Cutan Pathol. 2009;36:995–1000.
45. Sawada Y, Bito T, Kabashima R, et al. Ectopic extramammary Paget's disease: case report and literature review. Acta Derm Venereol. 2010;90:502–5.
46. Hastrup N, Andersen ES. Adenocarcinoma of Bartholin's gland associated with extramammary Paget's disease of the vulva. Acta Obstet Gynecol Scand. 1988;67:375–7.
47. Inose T, Asao T, Nakamura J, Ide M, Fukuchi M, Kuwano H. Double anal canal cancers associated with a long history of perianal Paget's disease: report of a case. Surg Today. 2012;42:697–702.
48. Sleater JP, Ford MJ, Beers BB. Extramammary Paget's disease associated with prostate adenocarcinoma. Hum Pathol. 1994;25:615–7.
49. Wilkinson EJ, Brown HM. Vulvar Paget disease of urothelial origin: a report of three cases and a proposed classification of vulvar Paget disease. Hum Pathol. 2002;33:549–54.
50. Lanzafame S, Broggi B. Extramammary Paget's disease. Immunocytochemical study and histogenetic considerations. Pathologica. 1989;81:661–9.
51. Pizzichetta MA, Canzonieri V, Massarut S, et al. Pigmented mammary Paget's disease mimicking melanoma. Melanoma Res. 2004;14:S13–5.
52. Petersson F, Ivan D, Kazakov DV, Michal M, Prieto VG. Pigmented Paget disease—a diagnostic pitfall mimicking melanoma. Am J Dermatopathol. 2009;31:223–6.
53. Bayer-Garner IB, Reed JA. Immunolabeling pattern of syndecan-1 expression may distinguish pagetoid Bowen's disease, extramammary Paget's disease, and pagetoid malignant melanoma in situ. J Cutan Pathol. 2004;31:169–73.
54. Sellheyer K, Krahl D. Ber-EP4 enhances the differential diagnostic accuracy of cytokeratin 7 in pagetoid cutaneous neoplasms. J Cutan Pathol. 2008;35:366–72.
55. Bhawan J. Squamous cell carcinoma in situ in skin: what does it mean? J Cutan Pathol. 2007;34:953–5.

56. Bordea C, Wojnarowska F, Millard PR, Doll H, Welsh K, Morris PJ. Skin cancers in renal-transplant recipients occur more frequently than previously recognized in a temperate climate. Transplantation. 2004;77:574–9.
57. Yu HS, Liao WT, Chai CY. Arsenic carcinogenesis in the skin. J Biomed Sci. 2006;13:657–66.
58. Cicale L, Dalle S, Thomas L. Pigmented Bowen's disease. Ann Dermatol Venereol. 2008;135:334–6.
59. De Vries K, Lelie B, Habets WJ, De Bruijckere L, Prens EP. Pigmented Bowen's disease: a report of two cases. Dermatol Surg. 2011;37:1061–4.
60. Gahalaut P, Rastogi MK, Mishra N, Chauhan S. Multiple pigmented Bowen's disease: a diagnostic and therapeutic dilemma. Case Rep Oncol Med. 2012;2012:342030.
61. Krishnan R, Lewis A, Orengo IF, Rosen T. Pigmented Bowen's disease (squamous cell carcinoma in situ): a mimic of malignant melanoma. Dermatol Surg. 2001;27:673–4.
62. Lee JW, Hur J, Yeo KY, Yu HJ, Kim JS. A case of pigmented Bowen's disease. Ann Dermatol. 2009;21: 197–9.
63. Marschall SF, Ronan SG, Massa MC. Pigmented Bowen's disease arising from pigmented seborrheic keratoses. J Am Acad Dermatol. 1990;23:440–4.
64. Papageorgiou PP, Koumarianou AA, Chu AC. Pigmented Bowen's disease. Br J Dermatol. 1998; 138:515–8.
65. Chang J, Prieto VG, Sangueza M, Plaza JA. Diagnostic utility of p63 expression in the differential diagnosis of pagetoid squamous cell carcinoma in situ and extramammary Paget disease: a histopathologic study of 70 cases. Am J Dermatopathol. 2014;36:49–53.
66. Raju RR, Goldblum JR, Hart WR. Pagetoid squamous cell carcinoma in situ (pagetoid Bowen's disease) of the external genitalia. Int J Gynecol Pathol. 2003; 22:127–35.
67. Sakiz D, Turkmenoglu TT, Kabukcuoglu F. The expression of p63 and p53 in keratoacanthoma and intraepidermal and invasive neoplasms of the skin. Pathol Res Pract. 2009;205:589–94.
68. Clarke LE, Conway AB, Warner NM, Barnwell PN, Sceppa J, Helm KF. Expression of CK7, Cam 5.2 and Ber-Ep4 in cutaneous squamous cell carcinoma. J Cutan Pathol. 2013;40:646–50.
69. Wang EC, Kwah YC, Tan WP, Lee JS, Tan SH. Extramammary Paget disease: immunohistochemistry is critical to distinguish potential mimickers. Dermatol Online J. 2012;18:4.
70. Longo C, Zalaudek I, Moscarella E, et al. Clonal seborrheic keratosis: dermoscopic and confocal microscopy characterization. J Eur Acad Dermatol Venereol. 2013. Epub ahead of print. doi: 10.1111/jdv.12261
71. Boer-Auer A, Jones M, Lyasnichaya OV. Cytokeratin 10-negative nested pattern enables sure distinction of clonal seborrheic keratosis from pagetoid Bowen's disease. J Cutan Pathol. 2012;39:225–33.
72. Cashmore RW, Perry HO. Differentiating seborrheic keratosis from skin neoplasm. Geriatrics. 1985;40 (69–71): 74–5.
73. Cheng AG, Deubner H, Whipple ME. Melanoacanthoma of the external auditory canal: a case report and review of the literature. Am J Otolaryngol. 2007;28:433–5.
74. Jain S, Barman KD, Garg VK, Sharma S, Dewan S, Mahajan N. Multifocal cutaneous melanoacanthoma with ulceration: a case report with review of literature. Indian J Dermatol Venereol Leprol. 2011;77: 699–702.
75. Lambert WC, Lambert MW, Mesa ML, et al. Melanoacanthoma and related disorders. Simulants of acral-lentiginous (P-P-S-M) melanoma. Int J Dermatol. 1987;26:508–10.
76. Matsuoka LY, Barsky S, Glasser S. Melanoacanthoma of the lip. Arch Dermatol. 1982;118:290.
77. Rossiello L, Zalaudek I, Ferrara G, Docimo G, Giorgio CM, Argenziano G. Melanoacanthoma simulating pigmented spitz nevus: an unusual dermoscopy pitfall. Dermatol Surg. 2006;32:735–7.
78. Shankar V, Nandi J, Ghosh K, Ghosh S. Giant melanoacanthoma mimicking malignant melanoma. Indian J Dermatol. 2011;56:79–81.
79. Spott DA, Heaton CL, Wood MG. Melanoacanthoma of the eyelid. Arch Dermatol. 1972;105:898–9.
80. Prince C, Mehregan AH, Hashimoto K, Plotnick H. Large melanoacanthomas: a report of five cases. J Cutan Pathol. 1984;11:309–17.
81. Schlappner OL, Rowden G, Philips TM, Rahim Z. Melanoacanthoma. Ultrastructural and immunological studies. J Cutan Pathol. 1978;5:127–41.

Desmoplastic Nevus Versus Desmoplastic Melanoma

14

Victor G. Prieto, Penvadee Pattanaprichakul, Christopher R. Shea, and Jon A. Reed

Almost all melanocytic lesions may have some degree of fibrosis, but the term "desmoplastic" is left for those in which there is a predominance of a stroma composed of dense, thick collagen fibers. Some authors suggest the term "sclerotic" rather than "desmoplastic" when applied to benign lesions (i.e., sclerotic nevus). However, we think that if the same type of stroma is seen in both benign and malignant lesions, thus it is not necessary to use different words to describe it.

Within benign melanocytic lesions, there is a spectrum of lesions going from classic blue nevus to desmoplastic Spitz and desmoplastic nevus. In this chapter we will use the term "desmoplastic" nevus to describe lesions in which, in addition to the markedly fibrous stroma, there is a population of spindle melanocytes with only focal melanin pigment and with only scattered, large cells with prominent nucleoli (such benign lesions with prominent melanin pigment should be included within the group of blue nevi and lesions with numerous, large melanocytes with prominent nucleoli should be included within the group of desmoplastic Spitz nevi). An intermediate lesion has received the term "hypopigmented blue nevus" [1, 2], also commonly seen on the extremities and buttocks.

The main differential diagnosis of desmoplastic nevus is with desmoplastic melanoma. The distinction may be especially difficult in small superficial biopsies or lacking clinical history. Diagnostic features favoring desmoplastic melanoma include larger size, location in a sun-exposed area, infiltrative pattern of growth, asymmetric silhouette, and numerous cells with large, irregular, hyperchromatic nuclei with prominent nucleoli. Thus the morphology of the tumor cells closely resembles that of fibroblasts seen in a scar. Observation of the overlying epidermis may reveal increased, enlarged melanocytes consistent with melanoma in situ. Desmoplastic melanomas may show scattered dermal mitotic figures. It is important to apply strictly the histologic criteria of desmoplastic melanoma, since lesions with more than 90 % of

V.G. Prieto, M.D., Ph.D. (✉)
MD Anderson Cancer Center, University of Houston, 1515 Holcombe Blvd., Unit 85, Houston, TX 77030, USA
e-mail: vprieto@mdanderson.org

P. Pattanaprichakul
Faculty of Medicine Siriraj Hospital, Mahidol University, 2 Prannok Rd., Bangkoknoi, Bangkok 10700, Thailand

C.R. Shea
University of Chicago Medicine, 5841 S. Maryland Ave., MC 5067, L502, Chicago, IL 60637, USA

J.A. Reed
CellNEtix Pathology & Laboratories, 1124 Columbia St., Suite 200, Seattle, WA 98117, USA

C.R. Shea et al. (eds.), *Pathology of Challenging Melanocytic Neoplasms: Diagnosis and Management*, DOI 10.1007/978-1-4939-1444-9_14, © Springer Science+Business Media New York 2015

its invasive component being relatively hypocellular and showing dense fibrous stroma (i.e., desmoplastic melanoma), only rarely metastasize to lymph nodes and therefore are usually not considered for examination of sentinel lymph nodes [3, 4]. Poor prognostic indicators are high mitotic rate, tumor thickness, and inadequate excision [5, 6].

Desmoplastic nevi are usually wedge-shaped and circumscribed. However, when desmoplastic nevi are combined (standard junctional or compound nevus and desmoplastic nevus) such cases may appear asymmetrical. Commonly desmoplastic nevi display a junctional component, either nested or as single cells. The epidermis may be hyperplastic and may have focal pigmentation thus mimicking a dermatofibroma. Similar to desmoplastic melanoma, desmoplastic nevi have large, hyperchromatic spindle cells with focal nucleoli; such cells may be fairly numerous. A minority of lesions may display also epithelioid cells.

Similar to desmoplastic melanoma, desmoplastic nevi show small aggregates of lymphocytes in the dermis, next to the tumor cells, as well as perineural involvement. However, in contrast, dermal mitotic figures are exceptional in desmoplastic nevi.

Other, non-melanocytic lesions that may resemble desmoplastic nevus/melanoma, include dermatofibroma, scar, malignant peripheral nerve sheath tumor, and dermatofibrosarcoma protuberans. In such cases immunohistochemistry is especially helpful in the differential diagnosis (see next paragraph).

Dermatofibromas show epidermal hyperpigmentation with elongation of rete ridges, and even adnexal induction. The latter is not seen in desmoplastic nevus or melanoma. In the dermis there are interstitial spindle and epithelioid cells, also mixed with occasional multinucleated and foamy cells. Although mitotic figures are frequent they are of benign shapes. Intervening stroma has thick, kelloidal collagen, mostly at the periphery of the lesion.

Although many of the melanocytic markers are either negative or only weakly expressed by some of the cells in desmoplastic melanoma, most of the tumor cells in desmoplastic melanomas express S100 protein. Therefore, anti-S100 may help delineate the extent of the lesion and thereby determine the depth of invasion (Dermatofibromas are negative for S100 (see Chap. 4 for possible impaired expression of S100 protein due to technical reasons).

Desmoplastic melanomas usually display high numbers of Ki67-positive cells and may show rare cells labeled with HMB-45 [7], often with a "maturation" pattern [8] (Fig. 14.1). In contrast, desmoplastic nevi show low numbers of Ki-67 positive cells (in a range between 1 and 18/mm^2) [7]. Another marker that may be helpful to distinguish desmoplastic nevus from desmoplastic melanoma is MART1. As mentioned in Chap. 4, most melanocytic lesions express this marker, with the notable exception of spindle-cell melanoma. Therefore, a spindle-cell melanocytic lesion that does not express MART1 is more likely to be a melanoma than a nevus (Fig. 14.2). However, a possible pitfall is the reduced pattern of expression of MART1 in neurotized nevi [9]. Even so, neurotized nevi lack the degree of cytologic atypia and stromal desmoplasia seen in desmoplastic melanoma. Similar to dermatofibromas, desmoplastic nevi may have numerous dendritic cells expressing Factor XIIIa.

To distinguish between desmoplastic melanoma and malignant peripheral nerve sheath tumor, S-100 protein is uniformly positive in melanoma and it is usually patchy or negative in malignant peripheral nerve sheath tumor. MITF is focally positive in both lesions. All other melanocytic markers are uniformly negative in both lesions.

Also, it has been proposed that immunohistochemical labeling for p16 may be helpful in such distinction, as the majority of desmoplastic melanomas show loss of labeling with p16. In our opinion, there is significant overlap between nevi

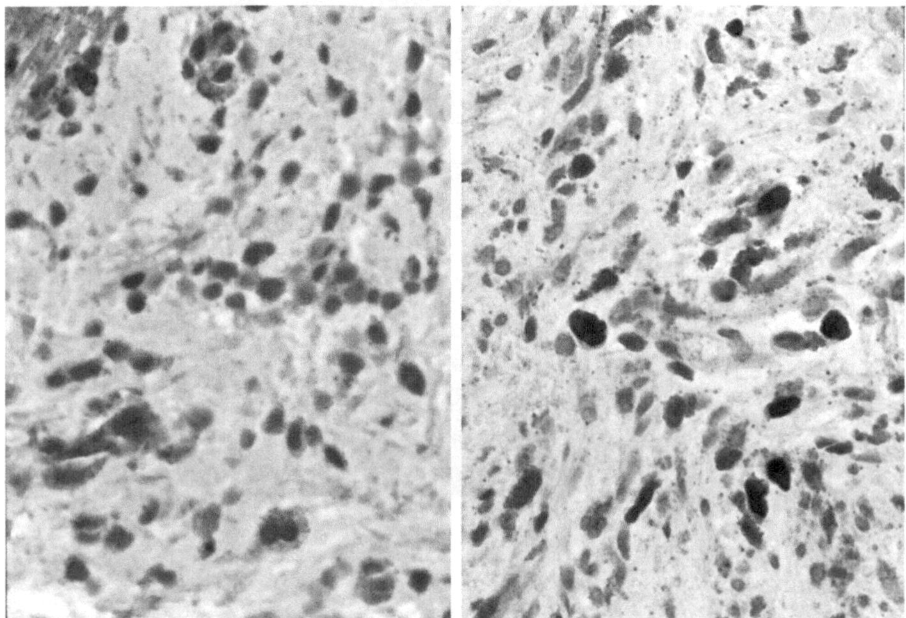

Fig. 14.1 Comparison of desmoplastic nevus (left) and desmoplastic melanoma (right). Desmoplastic nevus, as some Spitz nevi do, may show many cells expressing HMB45 antigen in the dermis; however, anti-Ki67 shows very rare dermal cells. In contrast, desmoplastic melanoma is usually negative with HMB45 and shows numerous cells expressing Ki67, usually more than 20/mm^2 (H) (HMB-45 and anti-Ki67, aminoethylcarbazol and diaminobencidine, respectively, with light hematoxylin as counterstain)

and melanoma regarding p16 expression, also seen in Spitz lesions [10]; therefore we do not consider p16 to be a very useful marker in this differential diagnosis.

Immunohistochemistry is also helpful in the diagnosis of desmoplastic melanoma and scar, since the tumor cells will express S100 protein. Even though scar tissue has scattered S100-positive cells [11, 12] (Fig. 14.3), when compared with scars, desmoplastic melanomas will have many more cells positive for this marker. Other markers expressed in desmoplastic melanoma and not in scars are p75 [13] and SOX10 [14] (Fig. 14.4). The latter appears to be a very promising marker since in our experience the vast majority of melanomas express this marker, regardless of the histologic subtype.

A recent study using fluorescence in situ hybridization (FISH) targeting RREB1, MYB, Cep6, and CCND1 showed that 47 % of desmoplastic melanoma contained detectable aberrations in the probe sites by FISH, while none of sclerosing melanocytic nevi (including sclerosing blue nevi) showed any [15]. Thus a positive FISH result strongly supports the diagnosis of desmoplastic melanoma and makes a diagnosis of a sclerosing melanocytic nevus unlikely.

In summary, immunohistochemistry plays a very important role in the differential diagnosis of desmoplastic melanocytic lesions. In general, a diagnosis of desmoplastic nevus is favored in younger individuals, outside the head and neck area, without mitotic figures and very low Ki-67 expression.

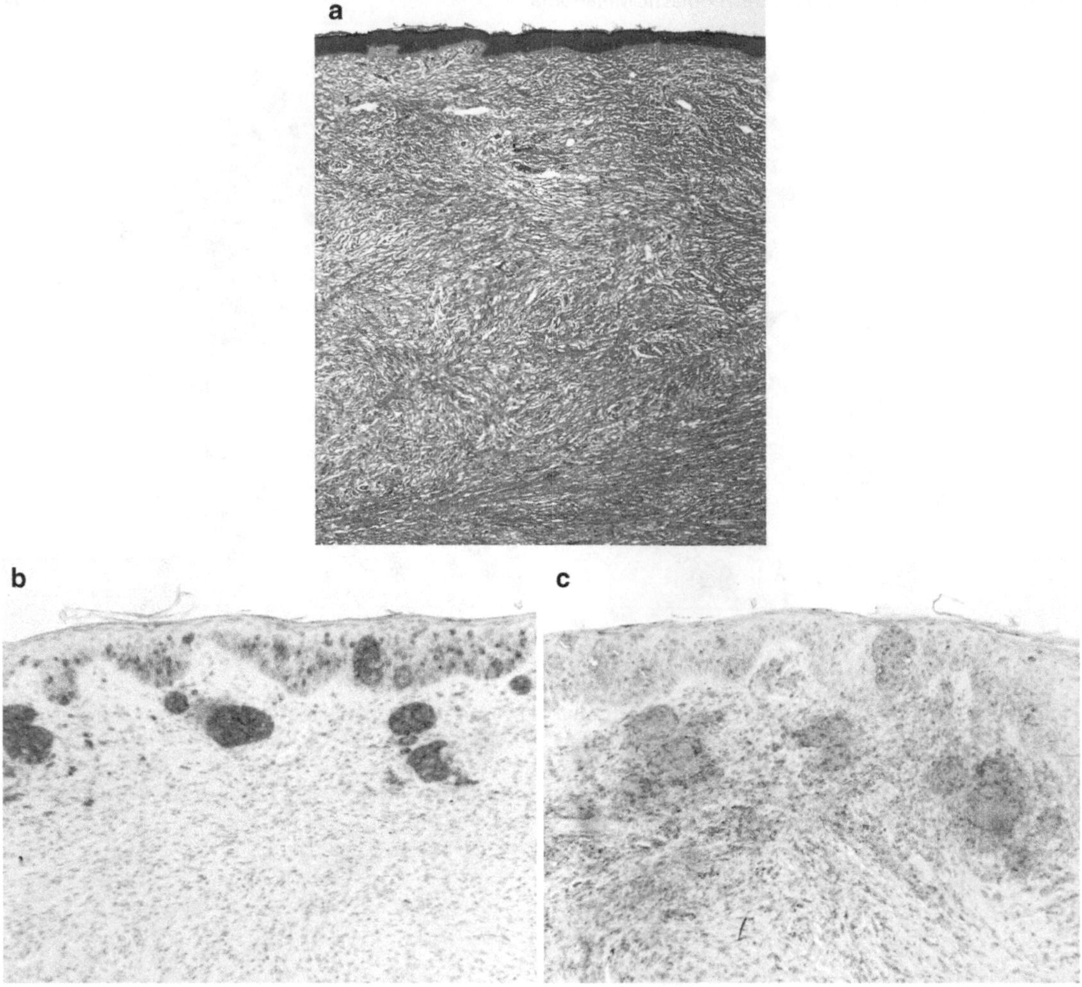

Fig. 14.2 Desmoplastic melanoma Illustration of the use of anti-MART1 in the differential diagnosis of desmoplastic lesions. Flat epidermis with hyperchromatic cells in the dermis (**a**). Only intraepidermal cells and very rare, superficial dermal cells express MART1 (**b**). In contrast, both the intraepidermal and dermal components are strongly positive for S100 protein (**c**) (**a**: hematoxylin and eosin; **b**: anti-MART1; **c**: anti-S-100 protein; both **b** and **c**, aminoethylcarbazol, with light hematoxylin and eosin)

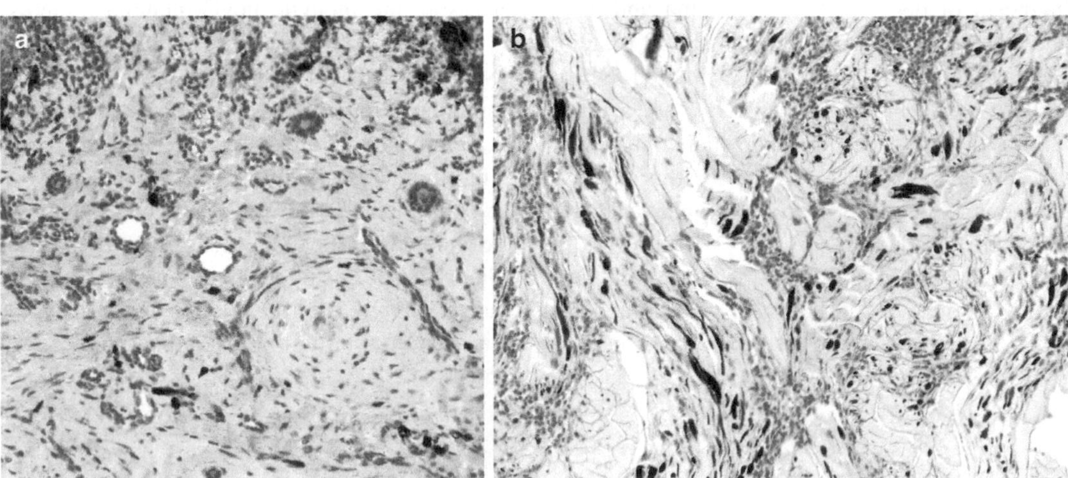

Fig. 14.3 In contrast with dermal scars (**a**), desmoplastic melanoma (**b**) shows numerous S100-positive cells (dendritic cells) (anti-S100; diaminobencidine and light hematoxylin as counterstain)

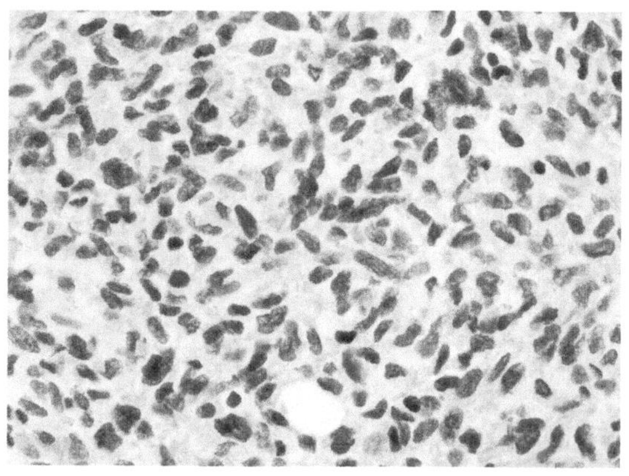

Fig. 14.4 Strong expression of SOX10 by many melanoma cells in this lesion (anti-SOX10; diaminobencidine and light hematoxylin as counterstain)

References

1. Carr S, See J, Wilkinson B, Kossard S. Hypopigmented common blue nevus. J Cutan Pathol. 1997;24(8):494–8.
2. Zembowicz A, Granter SR, McKee PH, Mihm MC. Amelanotic cellular blue nevus: a hypopigmented variant of the cellular blue nevus: clinicopathologic analysis of 20 cases. Am J Surg Pathol. 2002;26(11):1493–500.
3. Pawlik TM, Ross MI, Prieto VG, et al. Assessment of the role of sentinel lymph node biopsy for primary cutaneous desmoplastic melanoma. Cancer. 2006; 106(4):900–6.
4. Gyorki DE, Busam K, Panageas K, Brady MS, Coit DG. Sentinel lymph node biopsy for patients with cutaneous desmoplastic melanoma. Ann Surg Oncol. 2003;10(4):403–7.
5. McCarthy SW, Scolyer RA, Palmer AA. Desmoplastic melanoma: a diagnostic trap for the unwary. Pathology. 2004;36(5):445–51.
6. de Almeida LS, Requena L, Rutten A, et al. Desmoplastic malignant melanoma: a clinicopathologic analysis of 113 cases. Am J Dermatopathol. 2008;30(3):207–15.
7. Harris GR, Shea CR, Horenstein MG, Reed JA, Burchette Jr JL, Prieto VG. Desmoplastic (sclerotic) nevus: an underrecognized entity that resembles dermatofibroma and desmoplastic melanoma. Am J Surg Pathol. 1999;23(7):786–94.
8. Prieto VG, Shea CR. Immunohistochemistry of melanocytic proliferations. Arch Pathol Lab Med. 2011;135(7):853–9.
9. Henderson SA, Kapil J, Prieto VG. Immunohistochemical expression of neurotized nevi. J Cutan Pathol. 2014;41(2):215.
10. Mason A, Wititsuwannakul J, Klump VR, Lott J, Lazova R. Expression of p16 alone does not differentiate between Spitz nevi and Spitzoid melanoma. J Cutan Pathol. 2012;39(12):1062–74.
11. Trejo O, Reed JA, Prieto VG. Atypical cells in human cutaneous re-excision scars for melanoma express p75NGFR, C56/N-CAM and GAP-43: evidence of early Schwann cell differentiation. J Cutan Pathol. 2002;29(7):397–406.
12. Chorny JA, Barr RJ. S100-positive spindle cells in scars: a diagnostic pitfall in the re-excision of desmoplastic melanoma. Am J Dermatopathol. 2002;24(4): 309–12.
13. Kanik AB, Yaar M, Bhawan J. p75 nerve growth factor receptor staining helps identify desmoplastic and neurotropic melanoma. J Cutan Pathol. 1996; 23(3):205–10.
14. Ramos-Herberth FI, Karamchandani J, Kim J, Dadras SS. SOX10 immunostaining distinguishes desmoplastic melanoma from excision scar. J Cutan Pathol. 2010;37(9):944–52.
15. Gerami P, Beilfuss B, Haghighat Z, Fang Y, Jhanwar S, Busam KJ. Fluorescence in situ hybridization as an ancillary method for the distinction of desmoplastic melanomas from sclerosing melanocytic nevi. J Cutan Pathol. 2011;38(4):329–34.

Cutaneous Metastatic Melanoma Versus Primary Cutaneous Melanoma

15

Jamie L. Steinmetz, Victor G. Prieto, Jon A. Reed, and Christopher R. Shea

It is of critical importance to differentiate between primary and metastatic melanoma because of the large implications for clinical management and prognosis. Many primary melanomas are curable by wide local excision, whereas metastatic tumors generally cannot be cured surgically, often require additional therapy, and usually have a much worse prognosis. Patients with invasive melanoma confined to the skin have a 5-year survival rate exceeding 90 % compared to 60 % in those with regional lymph node metastases and 5 % in those with distant metastases [1]. However, it can sometimes be difficult for the pathologist to distinguish with confidence between primary and metastatic melanoma of the skin; while many features are suggestive and helpful, no criteria for this determination are absolutely reliable.

One feature favoring primary rather than metastatic melanomas is the presence of an associated nevus. Ten to thirty-five percent of primary malignant melanomas are associated with an adjacent melanocytic nevus, frequently a dysplastic nevus, whereas this is an extremely rare finding in metastatic melanoma [2]. This association is explained by the fact that while most melanomas arise de novo, some do arise from preexisting nevi [3] with an annual transformation rate of any single nevus into melanoma of 0.0005 % or less for both women and men under 40 years of age [4] [Fig. 15.1].

Another criterion favoring the interpretation of a primary rather than metastatic melanoma is the presence of regressive features, including an inflammatory infiltrate composed predominately of T-lymphocytes and plasma cells, melanophages, lamellar fibroplasia, and vascular proliferation [Fig. 15.2]. Complete regression of primary cutaneous melanoma is uncommon, occurring in 2.4–8.7 % of cases, while partial regression has been reported in 10–35 % of cases [5]. Evidence of spontaneous regression of metastatic melanoma is present in only 0.23 % of cases [6]. Regression is an immune-mediated phenomenon in which the patient's T-cells recognize antigens on certain clones of the tumor cells while other clones go unrecognized. It is thought that these surviving clones are more prone to metastasize to distant sites where they will continue to evade the immune response, explaining the low incidence of spontaneous regression of metastatic lesions [5, 6]. This theory is supported by the fact that in-transit metastases are clonal in origin [7].

J.L. Steinmetz • C.R. Shea, M.D. (✉)
University of Chicago Medicine,
5841 S. Maryland Ave., MC 5067, L502,
Chicago, IL 60637, USA
e-mail: cshea@medicine.bsd.uchicago.edu

V.G. Prieto
MD Anderson Cancer Center, University of Houston,
1515 Holcombe Blvd., Unit 85, Houston,
TX 77030, USA

J.A. Reed
CellNEtix Pathology & Laboratories,
1124 Columbia St., Suite 200, Seattle,
WA 98117, USA

C.R. Shea et al. (eds.), *Pathology of Challenging Melanocytic Neoplasms: Diagnosis and Management*,
DOI 10.1007/978-1-4939-1444-9_15, © Springer Science+Business Media New York 2015

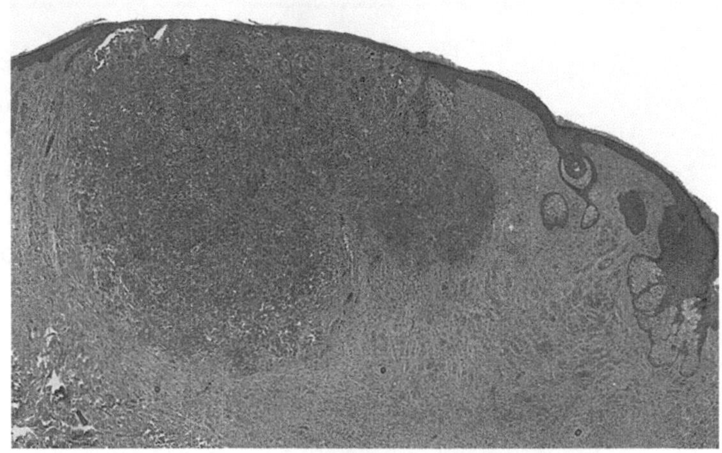

Fig. 15.1 Nodular malignant melanoma with an adjacent associated nevus

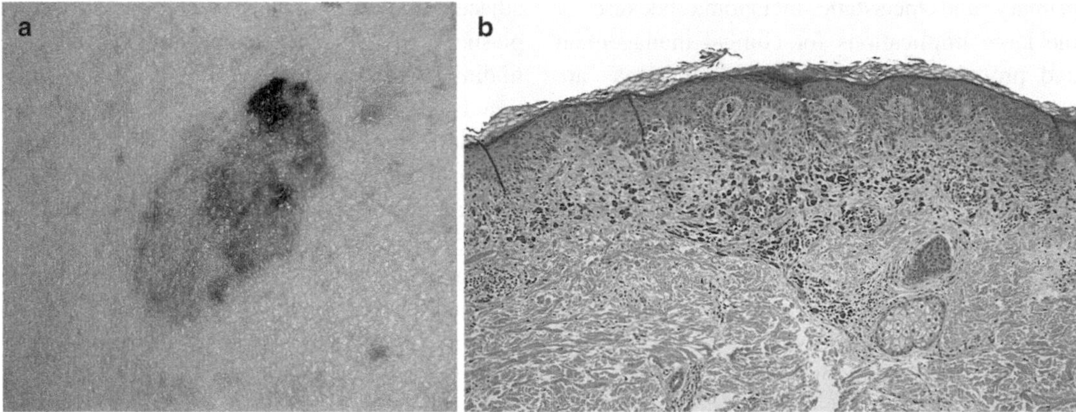

Fig. 15.2 (**a**) Primary melanoma with partial regression, seen grossly as an area of depigmentation within the melanoma; (**b**) Microscopic features of partial regression are seen here including the presence of a lymphocytic infiltrate, melanophages, and fibrosis

Probably the most important histopathologic feature favoring that a cutaneous melanoma is a primary and not a metastatic lesion is the presence of an intraepidermal (in situ) component, especially one extending beyond the lateral edge of the dermal component. However, even in some primary melanomas it can be difficult or even impossible to identify a definitive in situ lesion; this situation may arise due to sampling error, ulceration, regression, or effects of previous biopsy. If no in situ component can be identified, it is best to raise the possibility that the lesion could represent a metastasis.

To add a further complication, rare cases of epidermotropic metastatic malignant melanoma (EMMM) closely mimic primary melanoma. The histopathologic criteria originally proposed in 1978 for distinguishing EMMM from primary melanoma included the presence of an epidermal collarette; a dermal component extending beyond the intraepidermal component; and invasion of the lymphovascular space [8]. However, subsequently many cases of EMMM have been reported in which these criteria were not met and it has become clear that no set of histopathologic criteria can consistently discriminate between EMMM and primary melanoma. EMMM can even in some cases be completely confined to the epidermis, simulating an in situ melanoma [Fig. 15.3]. In such cases, histopathologic clues

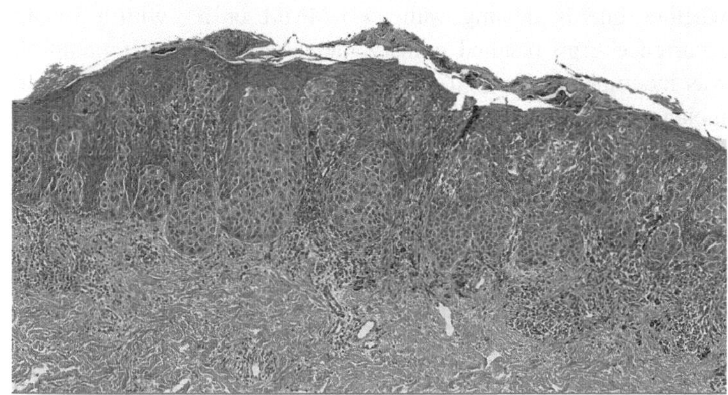

Fig. 15.3 Epidermotropic metastatic melanoma with prominent pagetoid spread mimicking a primary cutaneous melanoma

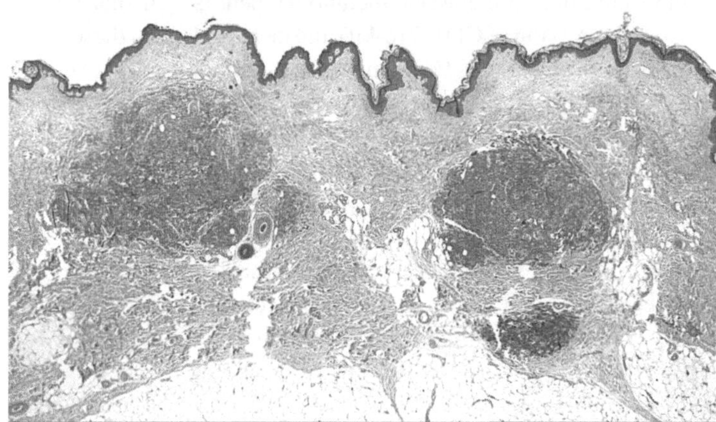

Fig. 15.4 Multiple nodules of cutaneous metastatic melanoma are seen here in the dermis

to the diagnosis of EMMM include relatively small size, symmetry, extensive pagetoid spread, and involvement of the adnexal epithelium. When a dermal component is also present, angiotropism is a strong indicator of metastatic disease [9].

Cutaneous melanoma metastasis classically presents as a well-circumscribed dermal or subcutaneous nodule of atypical, mitotically active melanocytes [Fig. 15.4]. Additional histopathologic characteristics in favor of cutaneous melanoma metastasis include a lack of involvement of the epidermis and absence of an inflammatory response. Metastatic lesions are more likely than primary tumors to be monomorphic [10], reflecting the frequent clonality of metastatic melanoma tumors [7]. The presence of angiotropism (melanoma tumor cells surrounding the external surface of vessels) and lymphatic invasion also supports a diagnosis of metastatic melanoma [9] [Fig. 15.5].

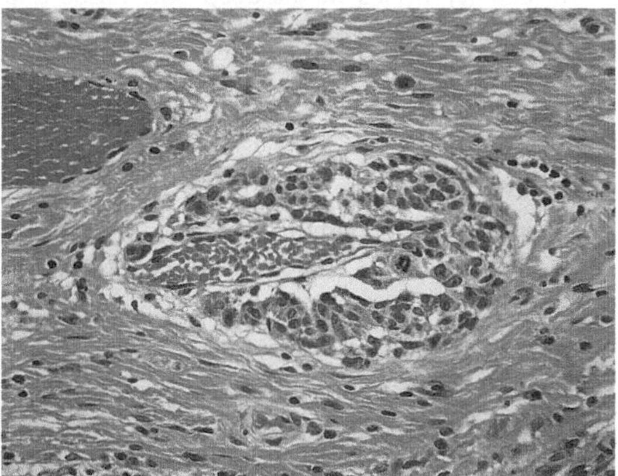

Fig. 15.5 Angiotropic spread of melanoma cells around a dermal blood vessel

Another diagnostic dilemma comes into play when the lesion in question is within or adjacent to the scar of a previously excised primary melanoma. In this instance it can be difficult to determine whether one is dealing with an EMMM or a recurrence from residual primary melanoma that was incompletely excised. Interestingly, recurrent melanoma arising within an excision scar has the same prognosis as melanoma with nodal metastasis, suggesting that many such cases may actually be metastatic lesions [9]. Histopathologically, a clue to recognizing cutaneous metastatic melanoma is the pattern of infiltration of the scar by small groups, strands, and individual melanoma cells.

There is no immunohistochemical stain that has been shown to differentiate absolutely between primary and metastatic melanoma (however one group found that in metastatic melanoma there is a loss of expression of CD117 (c-kit) and increased expression of p53 (54 % in metastatic tumors versus 9 % in primary tumors) and Ki67 (21 % in metastatic tumors versus 6 % in primary melanomas). One exception is that metastatic tumors from an ocular primary tend to retain CD117 expression [11].

To complicate matters further, when presented with lesions located entirely in the dermis or subcutis, in addition to metastatic melanoma one must also consider the possibilities of clear cell sarcoma (melanoma of soft parts) and the very rare primary dermal melanoma. Clear cell sarcoma usually arises in the deep soft tissue and extends up into the dermis; therefore, although it may be difficult to assess on biopsy specimens, the tissue plane involved by the tumor should be considered when possible. As melanoma and clear cell sarcoma have significant morphologic and immunohistochemical overlap, molecular studies may be necessary in order to distinguish between them. The characteristic t(12;22)(q13;q12) translocation resulting in EWSR1-ATF1 fusion is present in up to 90 % of clear cell sarcomas and has never been found in melanoma [12, 13]. Therefore, the presence of this translocation firmly establishes a diagnosis of clear cell sarcoma.

Primary dermal melanoma (PDM) is another important consideration as these tumors are reported to behave in a more indolent fashion with a 5-year survival rate approaching 100 %. Histopathologically PDM is characterized by a well-circumscribed nodule of malignant melanocytes located in the deep dermis and/or subcutis. There are no histopathologic or immunohistochemical features that can be used to definitively distinguish PDM from metastatic melanoma, both of which usually do not show ulceration, regression, or an in situ component. However, PDMs typically have a lower proliferative index by MIB-1 stain than metastatic melanoma. PDMs are often initially misdiagnosed as cutaneous metastatic melanoma, the prognosis of which is dismal with a median survival of 7–15 months. As these two tumors have a completely different prognosis it is important to consider the diagnosis of PDM in patients with a solitary cutaneous malignant melanoma with no known primary [14].

Clinical correlation is crucial as a history of a primary melanoma elsewhere may be the most important factor favoring that a lesion is metastatic as opposed to primary. While it is possible for a patient to have two synchronous primary cutaneous melanomas, this is a rare event and happens most often in the setting of multiple atypical/dysplastic nevi. One must also recognize that it is not uncommon to diagnose metastatic melanoma in the absence of a known primary lesion, with up to 10 % of patients initially presenting with metastases [1, 2]. In these instances the primary tumor may be a completely regressed cutaneous melanoma or may be in a non-cutaneous site such as the eye, meninges, or mucosa of the nasopharynx, intestine, or vagina.

In conclusion, while primary and metastatic melanoma can in some instances be histopathologically identical, many cases exhibit features that can help in distinguishing between the two. These include the presence or absence of an intraepidermal component, inflammatory response, adjacent nevus, features of regression and involvement of the appendages. It is important to distinguish between the two whenever possible because of the differences in management and prognosis.

References

1. Levine S, Shapiro R. Surgical treatment of malignant melanoma: practical guidelines. Dermatol Clin. 2012; 30:487–501.
2. Zurac S, Andrei R, Pestakos G, Nichita L, Bastian A, Micu G, Gramada E, Popp C, Staniceanu F, Petruscu S, Negroiu G, Giurcaneanu D, Chitu V. Cutaneous metastases of malignant melanoma—how difficult can it be? Rom J Intern Med. 2008;46(4):375–8.
3. Bevona C, Goggins W, Quinn T, Fullerton J, Tsao H. Cutaneous melanomas associated with nevi. Arch Dermatol. 2003;139:1620–4.
4. Tsao H, Bevona C, Goggins W, Quinn T. The transformation rate of moles (melanocytic nevi) into cutaneous melanoma. Arch Dermatol. 2003;139:282–8.
5. Blessing K, McLaren KM. Histological regression in primary cutaneous melanoma: recognition, prevalence and significance. Histopathology. 1992;20:315–22.
6. Bramhall RJ, Mahady K, Peach AHS. Spontaneous regression of metastatic melanoma—clinical evidence of the abscopal effect. EJSO. 2014;40:34–41.
7. Nakayama T, Taback B, Turner R, Morton DL, Hoon D. Molecular clonality of in-transit melanoma metastasis. Am J Pathol. 2001;158:1371–8.
8. Abernethy JL, Soyer P, Kerl H, Jorizzo JL, White WL. Epidermotropic metastatic melanoma simulating melanoma in situ: a report of 10 examples from two patients. Am J Surg Path. 1994;18(11):1140–9.
9. Gerami P, Shea C, Stone MS. Angiotropism in epidermotropic metastatic melanoma: another clue to diagnosis. Am J Dermatopathol. 2006;28(5):429–33.
10. Plaza JA, Torres-Cabala C, Evans H, Diwan HA, Suster S, Prieto VG. Cutaneous metastases of malignant melanoma: a clinicopathologic study of 192 cases with emphasis on the morphologic spectrum. Am J Dermatopathol. 2010;32:129–36.
11. Guerriere-Kovach PM, Hunt EL, Patterson JW, Glembocki DJ, English JC, Wick MR. Primary melanoma of the skin and cutaneous melanomatous metastases. Am J Clin Pathol. 2004;122:70–7.
12. Dim DC, Cooley LD, Miranda RN. Clear cell sarcoma of tendons and aponeuroses: a review. Arch Path Lab Med. 2007;131:152–6.
13. Sandberg AA, Bridge JA. Updates on the cytogenetics and molecular genetics of bone and soft tissue tumors: clear cell sarcoma (malignant melanoma of soft parts). Cancer Genet Cytogenet. 2001;130:1–7.
14. Cassarino DS, Cabral ES, Kartha RV, Swetter SM. Primary dermal melanoma. Arch Dermatol. 2008; 144(1):49–56.

16 Acral Nevus Versus Acral Melanoma

Penvadee Pattanaprichakul, Christopher R. Shea, Jon A. Reed, and Victor G. Prieto

Melanocytic lesions of the palms and soles may cause diagnostic difficulties [1]. This appears to be related in this special anatomic site to the presence of skin markings (dermatoglyphics) with the pattern of ridges and furrows. When the sections are cut perpendicular, rather than parallel to the dermatoglyphics, the histologic features suggesting nevus (symmetry and circumscription with columns of melanin) are more evident [2–4]. Therefore, pathologists should keep in mind when interpreting melanocytic lesions in acral sites that the plane of section could affect the morphology. Similarly, the clinical and dermoscopic findings will be helpful in the differential diagnosis.

Most acquired acral nevi are clinically recognized as single, symmetrical, well-defined macules or papules, less than or equal to 7 mm in diameter on palms and soles (acral congenital nevi may be larger) [5]. They are uniformly pigmented, brown to black, occasionally with irregular margins. Plantar is more common than palmar location, and acral nevi may occur on both pressure-bearing and pressure-spared surfaces. Similar lesions may also be found on the dorsal surfaces of hands, feet, and subungual region. For subungual nevi or subungual lentigines, there may be longitudinal melanonychia (melanonychia striata) *without* extension of the pigmentation into the proximal or lateral nail folds (absence of Hutchinson sign). Typically, benign acral nevus occurs in young individuals in contrast to acral melanoma, which tends to develop in the elderly. Moreover, dermoscopy becomes a useful tool in this diagnosis. Pigmentation on the ridges of the surface skin markings is detected in early melanoma, whereas pigmentation along the furrows of the skin markings is seen in acral nevus. These special patterns are termed "parallel ridge pattern" in acral melanoma and "parallel furrow pattern" in acral nevi where pigment distributed in relation to the deep furrows of the dermatoglyphics. Also, pigmentation in the sulci is more characteristic of a benign process [6]. These features have been reported to have high sensitivity (86 %) and high specificity (99 %) in diagnosing early acral melanoma [7]. Thus combination of age of onset, dermoscopy, and histologic features is crucial for the accurate diagnosis. Clinical characteristics and dermoscopic finding of acral

P. Pattanaprichakul
Faculty of Medicine Siriraj Hospital, Mahidol University, 2 Prannok Rd., Bangkoknoi, Bangkok 10700, Thailand

C.R. Shea
University of Chicago Medicine, 5841 S. Maryland Ave., MC 5067, L502, Chicago, IL 60637, USA

J.A. Reed
CellNEtix Pathology & Laboratories, 1124 Columbia St., Suite 200, Seattle, WA 98117, USA

V.G. Prieto, M.D., Ph.D. (✉)
MD Anderson Cancer Center, University of Houston, 1515 Holcombe Blvd., Unit 85, Houston, TX 77030, USA
e-mail: vprieto@mdanderson.org

C.R. Shea et al. (eds.), *Pathology of Challenging Melanocytic Neoplasms: Diagnosis and Management*, DOI 10.1007/978-1-4939-1444-9_16, © Springer Science+Business Media New York 2015

Table 16.1 Clinical and dermoscopic findings in acral nevus versus acral lentiginous melanoma

Clinical and dermoscopic findings	Acral nevus	Acral lentiginous melanoma
Onset	Childhood and adolescence	Middle-aged adult and elderly
Symmetry (A)	Symmetry	Asymmetry
Border (B)	Sharp, irregular	Irregular
Color (C)	Homogeneous or irregular pigmented	Inhomogeneous
Diameter (D)	≤7 mm	>7 mm
Evolution (E)	Stable, long-standing lesion	Abruptly enlarged, ulcerated
Dermoscopic findings [5, 7]	Parallel furrow pattern (pigment is in the sulci)	Parallel ridge pattern (pigment is in the ridges)
	Lattice-like pattern (parallel lines along the sulci as well as lines bridging the parallel lines)	
	Fibrillary pattern (lines of pigment across sulci and ridges)	

nevus and acral lentiginous melanoma are shown in Table 16.1.

Histologically, acral nevus is characterized by a circumscribed and usually symmetrical, lentiginous, and nested pattern. Melanocytes are arranged mostly in well-demarcated nests mainly located at the dermoepidermal junction. The nests are variable in size and often vertically oriented. However, solitary arranged melanocytes can be found in the lower epidermis and occasionally even in the upper epidermis. It was reported that random single cells arrangement could be prominent in acral nevi and was termed Melanocytic Acral Nevus with Intraepidermal Ascent of Cells ("MANIAC mole") [8]. This is an example of pagetoid melanocytosis, also known as transepidermal migration of melanocytes which is a process seen in melanoma and some nevi at special sites [9, 10] (between 38 % and 61 % of acral nevi) [11, 12]. However, when there is pagetoid infiltration of the epidermis by single atypical cells, or small groups of atypical cells with pale cytoplasm, particularly at the periphery of the lesion, such melanocytic proliferations should be carefully evaluated to rule out melanoma [11–13]. It should be taken into consideration, as mentioned above, that such features can be seen in acral nevi cut parallel to the skin marking (dermatoglyphics) [2]. The nevus cells may show conspicuous pale-staining cytoplasm and hyperchromatic to vesicular nuclei, sometimes with mild cytological atypia. Nucleoli may be prominent. The rete ridges may be elongated and narrow. In addition, melanocytes along the dermoepidermal junction frequently display dendritic morphology. Involvement of eccrine ducts (acrosyringium) by melanocytic nests occurs, but is usually limited to upper portions of ducts. Pigmentary incontinence is generally present and there may be mild dermal fibrosis with a sparse lymphocytic infiltrate. A dense lymphocytic infiltrate in the dermis should raise the possibility of melanoma [13]. The dermal component will show maturation, bland cytology, and lack mitotic activity (Fig. 16.1f–i).

The vast majority of subungual nevi occur in children with a well-demarcated, uniformly pigmented, single, longitudinal band. Histologically they are junctional, characterized by several, well-formed nests, with only focal, solitary melanocytes and without atypia. Occasionally, there may be asymmetry, confluence, and with angulation and distortion of the junctional nests; such features should not be overinterpreted as diagnostic of melanoma [14]. As mentioned earlier, pagetoid epidermal migration is commonly seen in acral nevi but the pattern of pagetoid spread is usually orderly and confined to the central portion of the nevi.

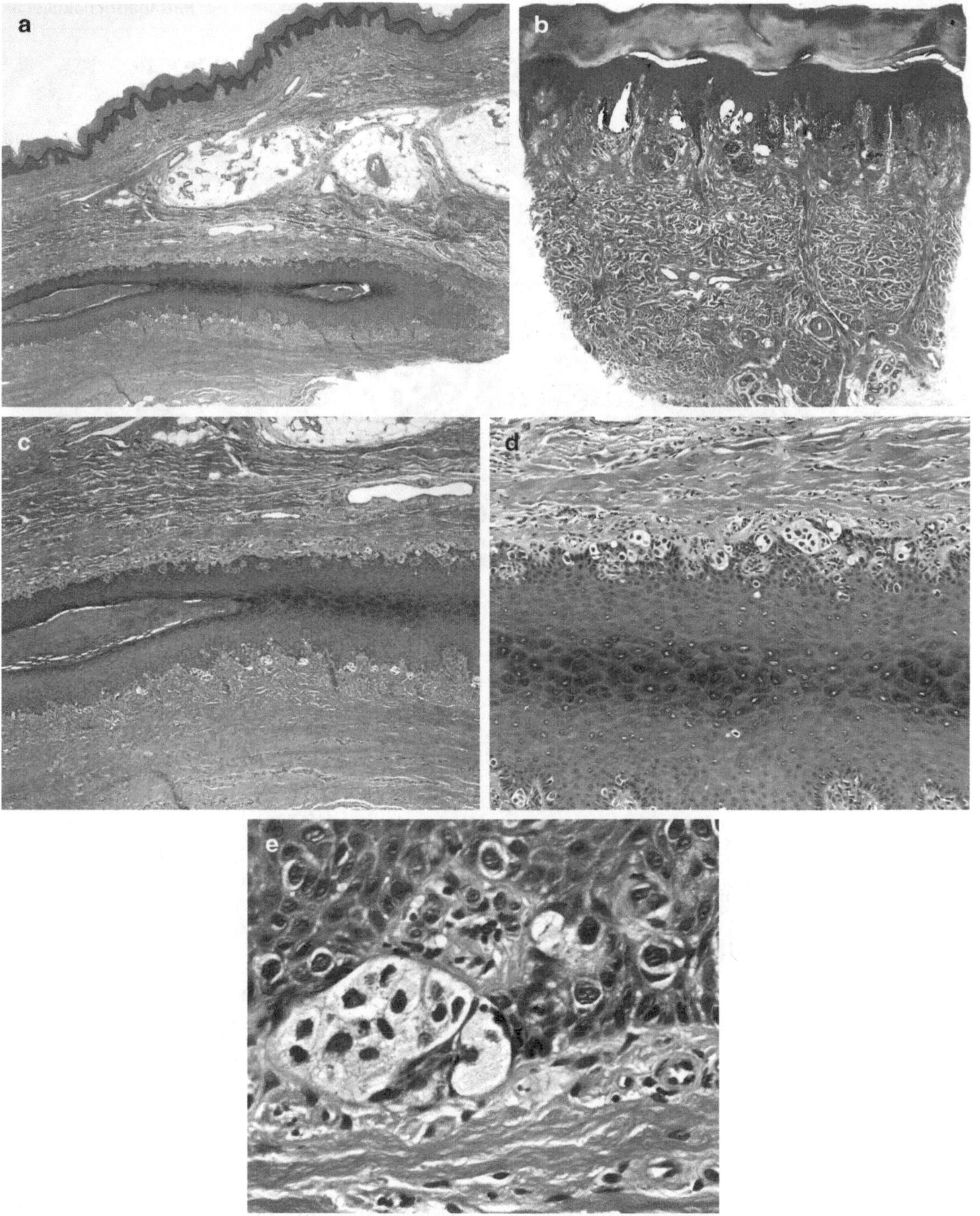

Fig. 16.1 (**a**) Melanoma of nail matrix (acral lentiginous melanoma): Atypical melanocytic proliferation along dermoepidermal junction with irregular acanthosis of nail matrix and proximal nail fold as compared with compound melanocytic proliferation on acral skin in compound acral nevus. Higher magnification demonstrates large irregular melanocytic nests and atypical epithelioid melanocytes with pale cytoplasm and single cell growth along dermoepidermal junction, some pagetoid upward migration of single cells is observed. This pattern of growth can be focal or skipped area within the lesion (**b**). Melanocytic nests showing severe cytological atypia with pale cytoplasm and enlarged hyperchromatic and vesicular nuclei. There is no invasive component with sparse superficial dermal lymphocytic infiltrate. The diagnosis is melanoma in situ, acral lentiginous subtype (**c**–**e**). In acral melanocytic nevi, compound type; the melanocytes arrange along dermoepidermal junction in nests and single cells with minimal pagetoid upward migration in the center of nevus without cytological atypia. Dermal nests are composed of small round melanocytes showing maturation pattern. There is no lymphocytic infiltrate and no dermal mitoses (**f**–**g**). Maturation pattern of HMB-45 which is positive in scattered cells in the epidermis and negative Ki-67 in dermal components support banal acral nevi (**h**–**i**)

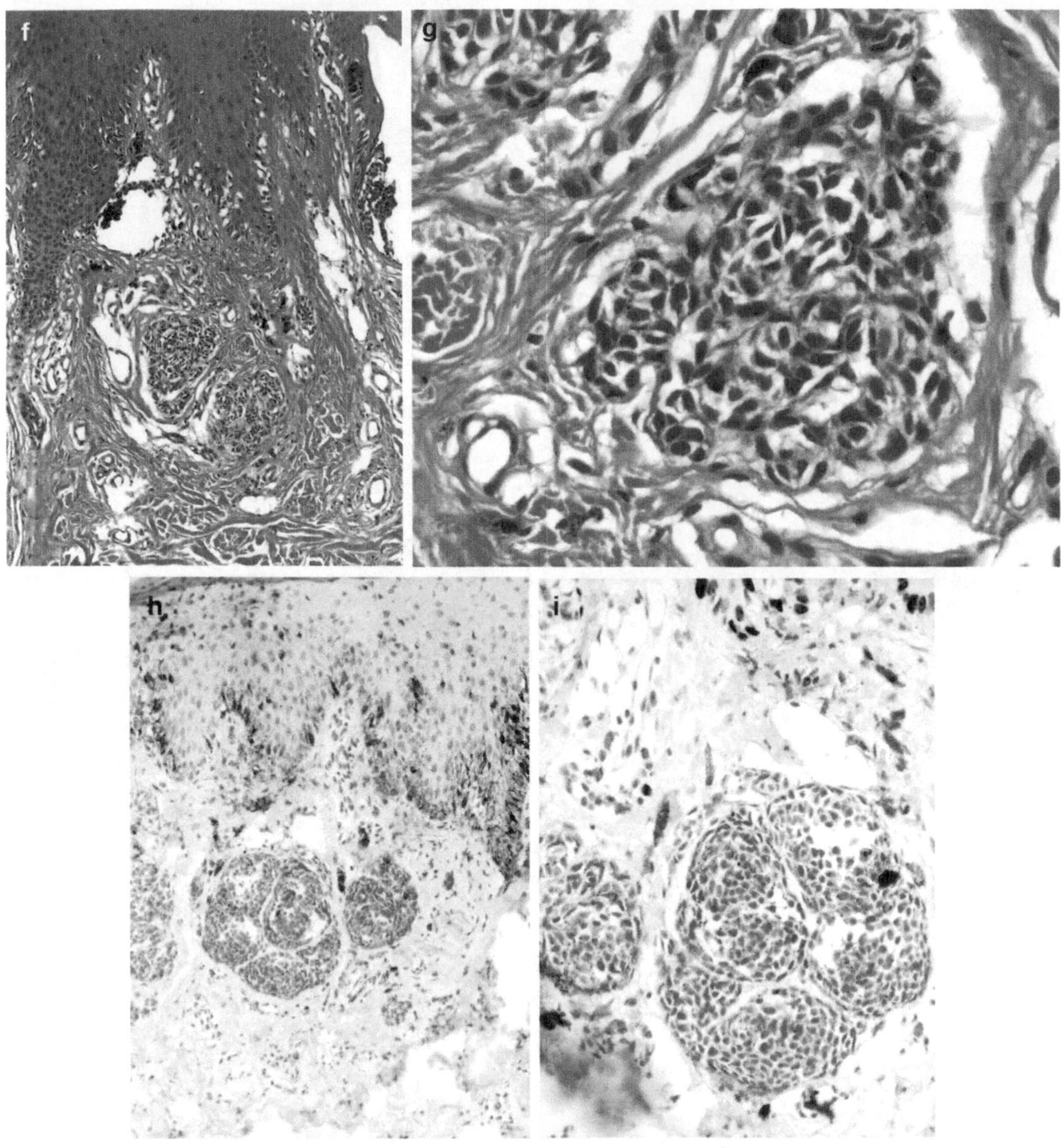

Fig. 16.1 (continued)

Differential Diagnosis

Clinically, standard acral nevi should be relatively easy to diagnose. However, the differential diagnosis includes a spectrum of other melanocytic lesions such as acral lentigo, acral dysplastic nevi, acral Spitz nevi, and acral congenital melanocytic nevi. The most important differential diagnosis is acral lentiginous melanoma (ALM), especially in the early stage or ALM in situ. Other non-melanocytic pigmented lesions in the differential diagnosis include seborrheic keratosis, pigmented basal cell carcinoma, squamous cell carcinoma, palmoplantar warts, and traumatic inoculation (graphite). Also included are flat, pigmented lesions of tinea nigra (superficial fungal infection by *Hortaea werneckii*) and intracorneal hemorrhage post trauma.

Acral dysplastic nevi are distinguished from acral standard nevi by the presence of shoulder, dusty pigmentation, and bridging nests, in addition to lamellar and eosinophilic fibrosis. A host inflammatory response is generally absent in acral standard nevi. They differ from acral lentiginous melanoma by the absence of irregular epidermal acanthosis, only mild cytological atypia, rare mitotic figures, and by the presence of maturation of the dermal component (when present). The presence of a dense lymphocytic infiltrate is highly suspicious for melanoma and should prompt careful examination of additional sections. Nevi on the distal lower extremity (ankle), with female predominance, may have moderate to severe architecture but only mild to moderate cytological atypia [15]. As such, they share features with acral nevi, dysplastic nevi, and melanoma in situ. However, these lesions show benign clinical course without recurrence after complete excision. This subgroup of ankle-located nevi might represent early dysplastic nevi [16] or may be part of "special" nevi.

Spitz nevi of acral skin can demonstrate extensive pagetoid spread of large epithelioid atypical melanocytes in symmetrical fashion. These lesions are usually small, circumscribed, in children and adolescents, composed of junctional nests of epithelioid and spindle-shaped melanocytes with scattered Kamino bodies. Dermal melanocytic nests can be present with pattern of maturation and exceptional, superficial mitotic figures. Since the most common site of acral lentiginous melanoma is the sole, acral Spitz nevus occurring on the sole should be studied with special care [17].

Acral congenital melanocytic nevi are comparatively less common than in other locations. They may be small, medium, or giant (>20 cm) with tendency to develop malignant transformation in larger lesions [18, 19]. Histologic features include benign-appearing melanocytes involving around skin appendages. There is maturation in the deeper areas and melanocytes disperse among collagen bundles rather than showing a "pushing" border with the adjacent dermis.

Acral lentiginous melanoma (ALM) is a distinct variant that occurs on the palms, soles, and subungual sites. ALM was proposed as the fourth subtype by Reed in 1976 [20]. ALM accounts for approximately 8–10 % of all melanomas in Caucasians. It is, however, the predominant subtype affecting Afro-Caribbeans and Asians. The tumor is particularly common on the digits (especially beneath the nails) and on weight-bearing sites; plantar tumors are most common, with the heel being the most frequently affected region. ALM usually presents as irregular, gradually enlarging, and variable pigmented macules (Fig. 16.2a). With progression to vertical growth phase, there is relatively frequent ulceration. In Caucasians, ALM presents most often in the seventh decade, has an equal incidence in both sexes, and it is generally associated with a poor prognosis since tumors are generally thick by the time of diagnosis. Mucosal melanomas are often classified within the acral lentiginous subtype, given a partial morphologic and molecular overlap. Clinically, acral nevus is usually small sized (less than or equal to 7 mm) with a light to dark brown striated macular component. As mentioned above, on dermoscopic examination, the pigmentation of acral nevi is accentuated in dermatoglyphic furrows and occasionally around eccrine ostia, thereby creating reproducible patterns. In contrast, in ALM the pigment is distributed along the dermatoglyphic ridges.

Subungual ALM, which most commonly affects the great toe and the thumb, is a rare tumor, accounting for only 2 % of all cutaneous melanoma. There is a female preponderance and ALM presents most often in the elderly. Longitudinal melanonychia is relatively common, a single pigmented nail streak that enlarges in size and varies in color. The lesion may extend onto the proximal or lateral nail fold (Hutchinson sign) (Fig. 16.2b). Other clinical changes are nail dystrophy (thickening and splitting) in early lesions and ulceration and hemorrhage in late stage lesions [21, 22]. Several studies have found that 46–60 % of the patients with subungual ALM report a history of antecedent trauma [23].

Histologically, distinction of acral nevi form ALM in early stage can be troublesome because both may have overlapping features such as asymmetry, poor circumscription, and focal

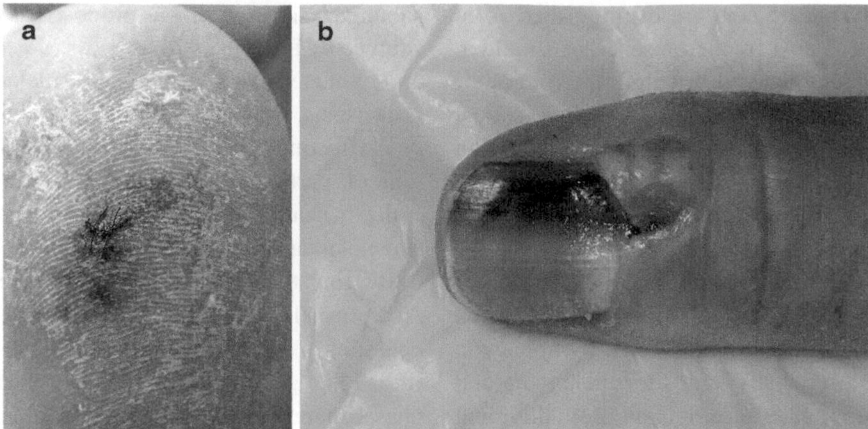

Fig. 16.2 (**a**) Acral lentiginous melanoma on the heel: poorly circumscribed, irregularly pigmented, hyperkeratotic brownish plaques, a commonly affected site; (**b**) subungual melanoma: longitudinal melanonychia (melanonychia striata) on the right thumb nail. The broad, irregularly pigment band on the nail plate with minimal extension of brown pigmentation into the adjacent lateral nail fold. (Hutchinson sign)

pagetoid upward migration. Suprabasal melanocytes in acral nevi are relatively more columnar, circumscribed, and less prominent than in melanomas. Signoretti et al. [2] reported that symmetry, circumscription, the columnar ascending melanocytes and organization of the junction component are all influenced by the histologic plane of section when nevi sectioned perpendicular to dermatoglyphics are more likely to have benign attributes. Furthermore, in acral sites, upward migration of single melanocytes into the spinous and granular layers of the epidermis is considered a common phenomenon. On the other hand, severe melanocytic atypia and a dense lymphocytic infiltrate have been found to be reliable features indicative of melanoma [13]. The most useful clue indicating the benign nature of the lesion is the maturation of melanocytes as they reach the dermis (transition between larger cells at the junction toward small nevoid cells at the base of the lesion) (Fig. 16.1f–g).

The invasive component of ALM may consist of epithelioid cells, spindle cells, small nevus-like cells or highly pleomorphic cell type [24]. In a significant number of these cases, the dermal component shows an unusual morphology including the presence of giant, nevoid, and clear cells (Fig. 16.3a–c). Neural differentiation and perineural infiltration may also occur [25]. Phan et al. [26] reported the presence of small nevus cells in dermal component in association with a worse prognosis and they also found that a minority of ALM (4 % of cases) had desmoplastic stromal response. Moreover, it is not uncommon for tumor cells to have infiltrated the deep dermis or subcutaneous tissue by the time of diagnosis [27]. Furthermore, the presence of a deep-seated nodules of pale-staining epithelioid to spindle-shaped cells (clear cells) with positive melanocytic markers (S100, HMB-45, and MART-1) and lack of epidermal or junctional melanocytic component on the acral location of young individuals, should raise the suspicion for clear cell sarcoma (Fig. 16.4a–e). Tumor-infiltrating lymphocytes (TILs) were often present in the series of subungual melanomas reported from the Sydney Melanoma Unit [28]. Therefore, the presence of TILs favors melanoma over acral nevi. Features that distinguish subungual melanoma in situ form subungual melanocytic macules include pagetoid spread, multinucleated melanocytes, lichenoid inflammatory reaction, and the presence of confluent stretches of solitary unit of melanocytes in melanoma in situ (Figs. 16.1a–e and 16.5a–c) [14]. In addition to the most common acral lentiginous pattern, subungual or acral melanomas may rarely represent superficial spreading and nodular

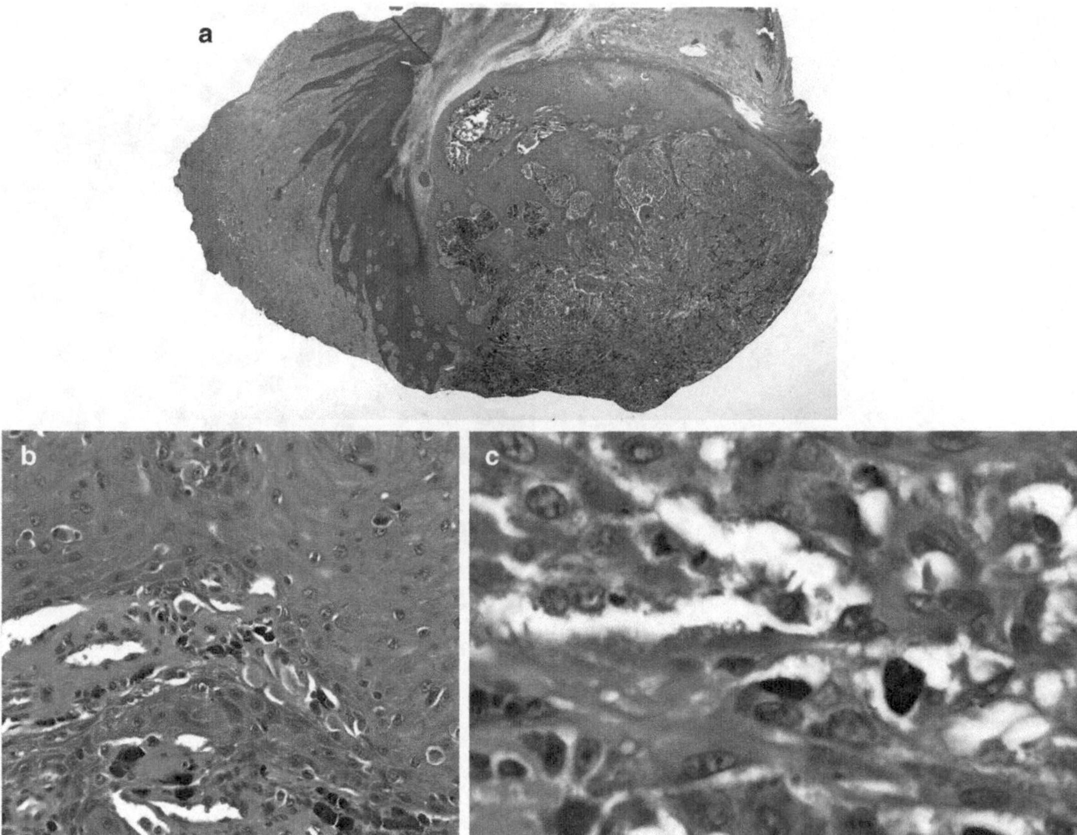

Fig. 16.3 (**a**) Invasive acral lentiginous melanoma with vertical growth phase, tangentially cut specimen, reveals the intraepidermal large atypical melanocytic nests and marked pagetoid migration of single atypical cells with hyperchromatic nuclei and prominent nucleoli in markedly hyperplastic epidermis. Scattered melanophages in the papillary dermis are observed (**b–c**)

histological variants. Nevoid and desmoplastic melanoma are unusual on volar skin but represent disproportionate sources of diagnostic errors. ALM typically have a lentiginous in situ component as opposed to the obvious pagetoid upward spreading as in other non-acral melanomas, and melanoma arising at the site of an acral nevus is uncommon. Mild lentiginous growth can be expected in acral nevi, its presence at the margin of the specimen should raise the concern of either a potential precursor for ALM or the inability to assess the adjacent area to exclude melanoma, especially in the nail matrix biopsies. Despite acral nevi are more common than ALM [29], in doubt of peripheral margin involvement, re-excision to perform the complete histologic evaluation and removal should be recommended in such cases. Comparison between histopathologic findings between acral nevus and acral lentiginous melanoma are shown in Table 16.2.

Immunohistochemistry

In acral lentiginous melanoma, immunohistochemistry can be helpful in problematic cases but is usually not necessary due to their characteristic histologic findings. As in other types of melanoma, HMB-45, and anti-MART-1 (Melan A) are of great diagnostic value in ALM. HMB-45 has been reported to have 80 % sensitivity in ALM. Lack of maturation pattern and focal/patchy positivity of HMB-45 in dermal components supports the diagnosis of ALM over acral nevus.

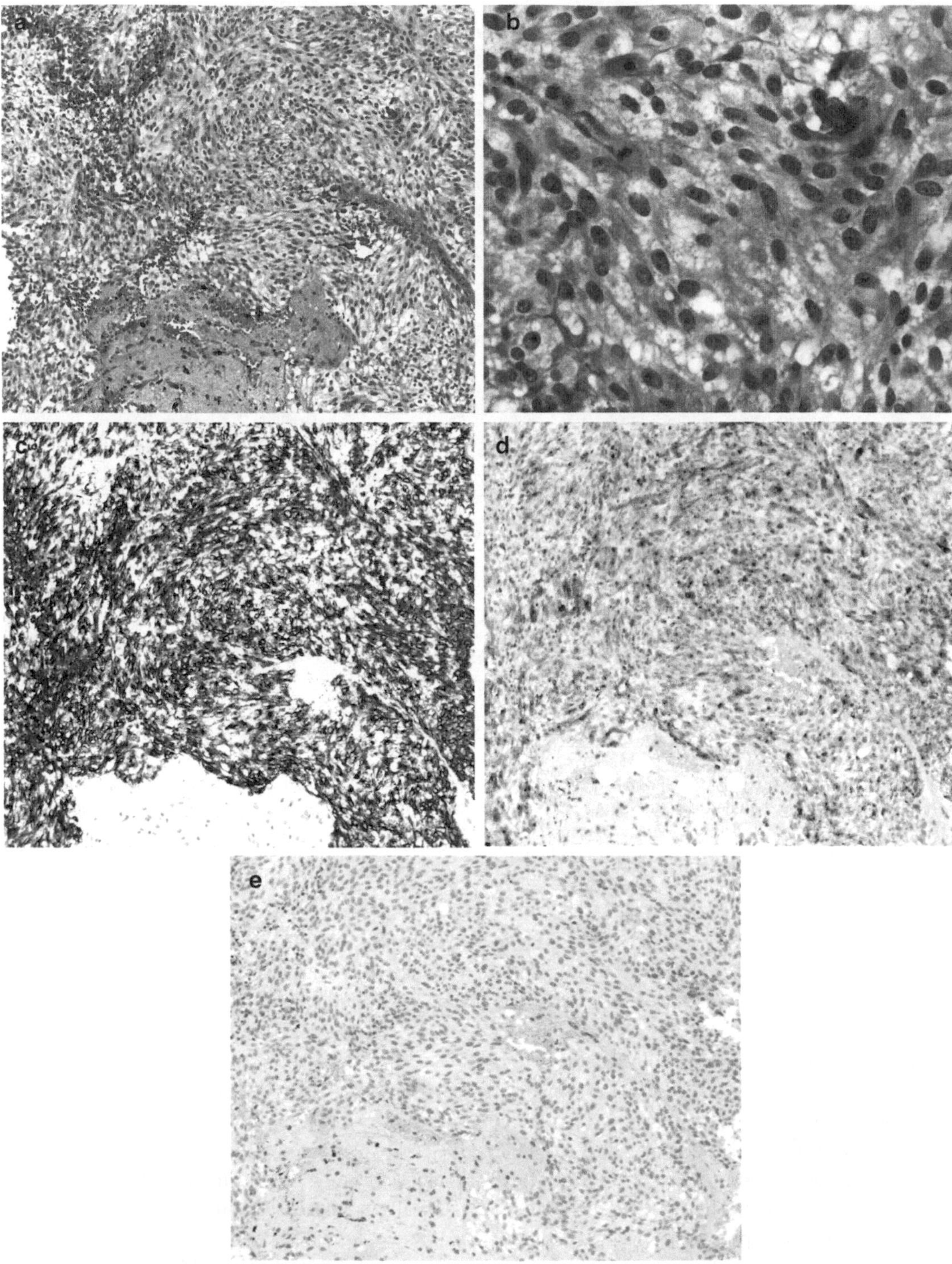

Fig. 16.4 (**a**) The presence of nests of spindle or epithelioid clear cells in the dermis with focal melanin pigment and no epidermal connection on the acral location raise the differential diagnosis of clear cell sarcoma. The cellular components are composed of clear cells with cytological atypia, variably prominent nucleoli, and increased mitotic figures (**b**). These cells stain with melanocytic markers such as HMB-45 (**c**) and MART-1 (**d**), but are negative for tyrosinase (**e**) in this case. The diagnosis of clear cell sarcoma (melanoma of soft part) is confirmed by the detection of t(12;22)(q13;q12) resulting in a fusion transcript of EWSR1/ATF1 gene

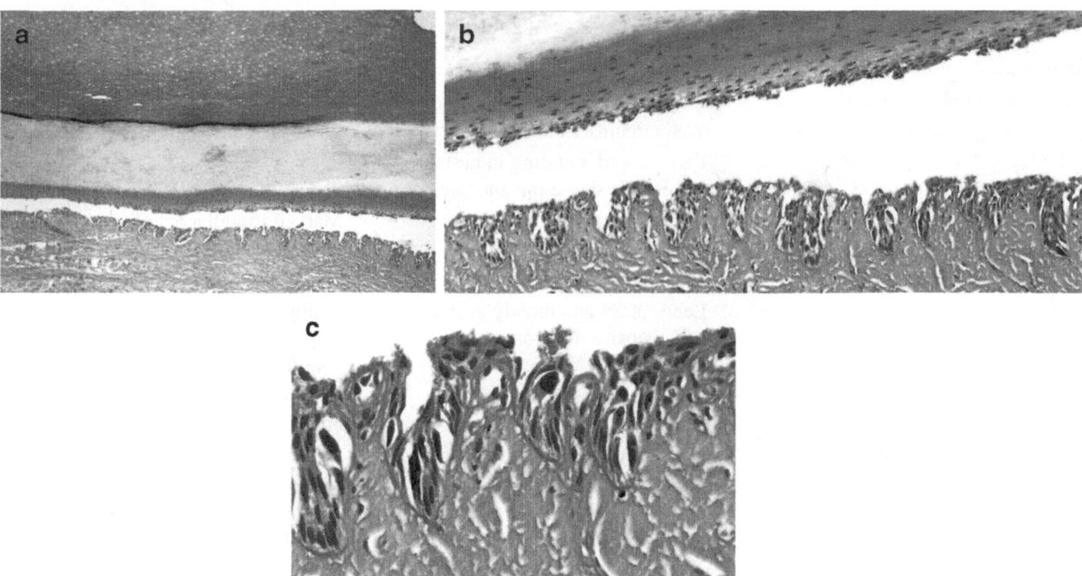

Fig. 16.5 (**a**) Melanoma in situ, acral lentiginous type of subungual region. Thick stratum corneum represents the area of nail plate. The separation of nail plate is shown with contiguous proliferation of single cells with marked atypia along dermoepidermal junction (**b**–**c**)

Ki-67, a proliferative marker, can be helpful to determine the mitotic activity of the dermal component. The use of Ki-67/MART-1 double immunostaining can be useful to distinguish between proliferating melanocytes and intermixed lymphocytes.

Occasionally, ALM can express epithelial markers (EMA and low-molecular weight keratins with CAM5.2). However, in this circumstance, those malignant melanocytes also express one or more melanocytic markers. Therefore, in poorly differentiated neoplasms of this location, pathologists should probably use a panel of antibodies to determine the likely pattern of differentiation [30].

Molecular Findings

There have been no specific reports evaluating the presence of chromosomal changes in acral nevi, but one study that included 54 benign nevi from different parts of the body, only 7 (13 %) showed chromosomal aberrations, and most of those (6 of 7; 86 %) were Spitz nevi with isolated gains involving the entire short arm of chromosome 11 [31].

In contrast to acral nevi and nevi of other locations, comparative genomic hybridization (CGH) of melanoma on acral, non-hair bearing skin showed distinct difference to melanoma on non-acral skin [32]. The most common amplified region is chromosome 11q13 (CCND1 gene amplification), which occurs in 50 % of cases, and therefore, remains the molecular hallmarks of ALM along with somatic mutations in c-KIT [32–34].

BRAF mutations were less frequent in ALM than in other subtypes of cutaneous melanoma at other locations, especially in skin without chronic sun damage, and in non-ALM subtypes, with frequency ranging from 10 % to 20 % for ALM to more than 50 % the other cutaneous locations without chronic sun damage and non-ALM subtypes [35–38].

Table 16.2 Histopathologic features in acral nevus versus acral lentiginous melanoma

Histologic features	Acral nevus	Acral lentiginous melanoma
Size (maximum diameter)	≤7 mm	>7 mm
Circumscription and symmetry	Well circumscribed, symmetrical	Poorly circumscribed, asymmetrical
	Lateral border ending in nests rather than single melanocytes	
Epidermal change	Normal or regular acanthosis	Marked irregular acanthosis
Melanin in stratum corneum	Linear arrangement in column above the furrows	Dispersed, heavily pigmented along the entire lesion
Melanocytic proliferation	Lentiginous and mostly nested and cohesive, not confluent	Lentiginous pattern with confluent single melanocytes predominate over focally non-cohesive nests
Junctional melanocytic distribution	Mostly under the furrows	Mostly under the crests or ridges and around acrosyringium
Cytological features and atypia	Small, round, epithelioid, focally mild to moderate cellular atypia	In late lesion; widespread cellular atypia with elongated, large cells with hyperchromatic nuclei, surrounding halo, and dusty melanin
Intraepidermal melanocyte with visible dendrites	No dendrites or few short, thin, with regular length, located at basal layer with no web formation throughout the entire nevus	Dendrites ascend into upper epidermis and they are thick, long, variable in length, and tend to form a web around the basal cells
Pagetoid spread	Scattered, more orderly, centrally located, maybe nested	Prominent in a late lesion
Appendageal involvement	Rarely	Common
Dermal component	Maturation as descent, small round melanocytes	Lack of maturation, nest formation in a late development, epithelioid or spindle cells morphology, presence of a desmoplastic stroma
Dermal mitoses	Absent	Presence of deep dermal mitoses
Lymphocytic infiltrate	Unusual	Usually present
Ulceration	Unusual	Usually present

Prognosis and Prognostic Factors of Acral Lentiginous Melanoma

As compared with cutaneous melanoma of other subtypes and locations, ALM has the worse prognosis, mainly as a consequence of delayed diagnosis leading to more advance tumors in thickness and stage at diagnosis [38–42]. Breslow thickness and ulceration are the main prognostic factors, but seem less reliable for prediction outcome than in other types of cutaneous melanoma. In the study by Gershenwald et al., while increasing Breslow thickness was an important factor in those patients with acral melanoma who underwent sentinel lymph node (SLN) biopsy, and confirmed the prognostic significance of SLN biopsy in acral melanoma patients [43]. The more recent study reported that the most important predictor of prognosis in acral lentiginous melanoma is the status of the SLN biopsy. All patients with ALM with a Breslow thickness of 1.0 mm or greater are recommended to be staged with a SLN biopsy. Primary tumor factors such as Breslow thickness and ulceration are less important predictors of prognosis [44]. Recurrent disease occurs mostly in the involved primary extremity, these sites should be monitored carefully during the follow-up period by clinical examination. Overall survival rate among all racial groups does not show statistically significant when controlled for Breslow thickness and tumor stage at diagnosis [45, 46]. Early diagnosis of melanoma with lower tumor thickness correlates with a better overall survival [45, 47].

Management

Careful evaluation should be taken with benign-looking lesions that are incompletely excised or when lentiginous component trailing the biopsy margin. ALM often has skip areas lacking an obvious melanocytic proliferation, which could limit the chance to make a diagnosis of melanoma in such a small biopsy. Therefore, if the clinician suspects melanoma but biopsy findings are negative or equivocal, additional biopsies should be considered. For most patients with ALM, complete excision with wide margin is recommended, including amputation [21, 48, 49]. Higher stages at diagnosis correlate with systemic metastases [50]. ALM seems to have important molecular genetic significance which could lead to the use of specific target therapies. Other treatments that have been used for treatment of ALM are chemotherapy, immunotherapy, radiation therapy, and Mohs micrographic surgery (MMS). These recommendations are discussed elsewhere [48, 50]. Overall, acral melanoma represents a particular subgroup of cutaneous melanoma, which could require specific management in the future, form prevention up to treatment.

References

1. Jaramillo-Ayerbe F, Vallejo-Contreras J. Frequency and clinical and dermatoscopic features of volar and ungual pigmented melanocytic lesions: a study in schoolchildren of Manizales, Colombia. Pediatr Dermatol. 2004;21(3):218–22.
2. Signoretti S, Annessi G, Puddu P, Faraggiana T. Melanocytic nevi of palms and soles: a histological study according to the plane of section. Am J Surg Pathol. 1999;23(3):283–7.
3. Song JY, Kim MY, Kim HO, Park YM. Melanocytic naevus of the palm resembling callus. Br J Dermatol. 2004;151(1):230–1.
4. Ferrara G, Argenziano G, Soyer HP. Melanocytic nevi of palms and soles. Am J Surg Pathol. 2003;27(3): 411–2.
5. Saida T. Malignant melanoma on the sole: How to detect the early lesions efficiently. Pigment Cell Res. 2000;13:135–9.
6. Saida T, Oguchi S, Miyazaki A. Dermoscopy for acral pigmented skin lesions. Clin Dermatol. 2002;20(3): 279–85.
7. Saida T, Koga H, Uhara H. Key points in dermoscopic differentiation between early acral melanoma and acral nevus. J Dermatol. 2011;38(1):25–34.
8. LeBoit PE. A diagnosis for maniacs. Am J Dermatopathol. 2000;22(6):556–8.
9. Petronic-Rosic V, Shea CR, Krausz T. Pagetoid melanocytosis: when is it significant? Pathology. 2004; 36(5):435–44.
10. Kerl K, Kempf W, Kamarashev J, et al. Constitutional intraepidermal ascent of melanocytes: a potential pitfall in the diagnosis of melanocytic lesions. Arch Dermatol. 2012;148(2):235–8.
11. Boyd AS, Rapini RP. Acral melanocytic neoplasms: a histologic analysis of 158 lesions. J Am Acad Dermatol. 1994;31(5 Pt 1):740–5.
12. Haupt HM, Stern JB. Pagetoid melanocytosis. Histologic features in benign and malignant lesions. Am J Surg Pathol. 1995;19(7):792–7.
13. Fallowfield ME, Collina G, Cook MG. Melanocytic lesions of the palm and sole. Histopathology. 1994; 24(5):463–7.
14. Amin B, Nehal KS, Jungbluth AA, et al. Histologic distinction between subungual lentigo and melanoma. Am J Surg Pathol. 2008;32(6):835–43.
15. Khalifeh I, Taraif S, Reed JA, Lazar AF, Diwan AH, Prieto VG. A subgroup of melanocytic nevi on the distal lower extremity (ankle) shares features of acral nevi, dysplastic nevi, and melanoma in situ: a potential misdiagnosis of melanoma in situ. Am J Surg Pathol. 2007;31(7):1130–6.
16. Torres-Cabala CA, Plaza JA, Diwan AH, Prieto VG. Severe architectural disorder is a potential pitfall in the diagnosis of small melanocytic lesions. J Cutan Pathol. 2010;37(8):860–5.
17. Jang YH, Lee JY, Kim MR, Kim SC, Kim YC. Acral pigmented spitz nevus that clinically mimicked acral lentiginous malignant melanoma. Ann Dermatol. 2011;23(2):246–9.
18. Tannous ZS, Mihm Jr MC, Sober AJ, Duncan LM. Congenital melanocytic nevi: clinical and histopathologic features, risk of melanoma, and clinical management. J Am Acad Dermatol. 2005;52(2):197–203.
19. Saida T, Yoshida N. Guidelines for histopathologic diagnosis of plantar malignant melanoma. Two-dimensional coordination of maximum diameters of lesions and degrees of intraepidermal proliferation of melanocytes. Dermatologica. 1990;181(2):112–6.
20. Reed R. Acral lentiginous melanoma. In: Harmann W, Reed RJ, editors. New concepts in surgical pathology of the skin. New York: Wiley; 1976. p. 89–90.
21. Harmelin ES, Holcombe RN, Goggin JP, Carbonell J, Wellens T. Acral lentiginous melanoma. J Foot Ankle Surg. 1998;37(6):540–5.
22. Kato T, Kumasaka N, Suetake T, Tabata N, Tagami H. Clinicopathological study of acral melanoma in situ in

44 Japanese patients. Dermatology. 1996;193(3): 192–7.

23. Green A, McCredie M, MacKie R, et al. A case-control study of melanomas of the soles and palms (Australia and Scotland). Cancer Causes Control. 1999;10(1): 21–5.
24. Barnhill RL, Mihm Jr MC. The histopathology of cutaneous malignant melanoma. Semin Diagn Pathol. 1993;10(1):47–75.
25. Hayashi K, Okubo S, Watanabe T, Yamazaki Y, Horiuchi N, Saida T. Malignant melanoma on the sole showing prominent neural differentiation and perineural infiltration. Int J Dermatol. 2002;41(4):247–9.
26. Phan A, Touzet S, Dalle S, Ronger-Savle S, Balme B, Thomas L. Acral lentiginous melanoma: histopathological prognostic features of 121 cases. Br J Dermatol. 2007;157(2):311–8.
27. Feibleman CE, Stoll H, Maize JC. Melanomas of the palm, sole, and nailbed: a clinicopathologic study. Cancer. 1980;46(11):2492–504.
28. Tan KB, Moncrieff M, Thompson JF, et al. Subungual melanoma: a study of 124 cases highlighting features of early lesions, potential pitfalls in diagnosis, and guidelines for histologic reporting. Am J Surg Pathol. 2007;31(12):1902–12.
29. Tosti A, Baran R, Piraccini BM, Cameli N, Fanti PA. Nail matrix nevi: a clinical and histopathologic study of twenty-two patients. J Am Acad Dermatol. 1996;34(5 Pt 1):765–71.
30. Kim YC, Lee MG, Choe SW, Lee MC, Chung HG, Cho SH. Acral lentiginous melanoma: an immunohistochemical study of 20 cases. Int J Dermatol. 2003;42(2):123–9.
31. Bastian BC, Olshen AB, LeBoit PE, Pinkel D. Classifying melanocytic tumors based on DNA copy number changes. Am J Pathol. 2003;163(5): 1765–70.
32. Bastian BC, Kashani-Sabet M, Hamm H, et al. Gene amplifications characterize acral melanoma and permit the detection of occult tumor cells in the surrounding skin. Cancer Res. 2000;60(7):1968–73.
33. Takata M, Goto Y, Ichii N, et al. Constitutive activation of the mitogen-activated protein kinase signaling pathway in acral melanomas. J Invest Dermatol. 2005;125(2):318–22.
34. Curtin JA, Busam K, Pinkel D, Bastian BC. Somatic activation of KIT in distinct subtypes of melanoma. J Clin Oncol. 2006;24(26):4340–6.
35. Curtin JAFJ, Kageshita T, Pated HN, Busam KJ, Kutzner H, Cho KH, Aiba S, Brocker EB, LeBoit PE, Pinkel D, Bastian BC. Distinct sets of genetic alteration in melanoma. N Engl J Med. 2005;353(20): 2135–47.
36. Saldanha G, Potter L, Daforno P, Pringle JH. Cutaneous melanoma subtypes show different BRAF and NRAS mutation frequencies. Clin Cancer Res. 2006;12(15):4499–505.
37. Maldonado JL, Fridlyand J, Patel H, et al. Determinants of BRAF mutations in primary melanomas. J Natl Cancer Inst. 2003;95(24):1878–80.
38. Durbec F, Martin L, Derancourt C, Grange F. Melanoma of the hand and foot: epidemiological, prognostic and genetic features. A systematic review. Br J Dermatol. 2012;166(4):727–39.
39. Soudry E, Gutman H, Feinmesser M, Gutman R, Schachter J. "Gloves-and-socks" melanoma: does histology make a difference? Dermatol Surg. 2008; 34(10):1372–8.
40. Hsueh EC, Lucci A, Qi K, Morton DL. Survival of patients with melanoma of the lower extremity decreases with distance from the trunk. Cancer. 1999;85(2):383–8.
41. Nagore E, Oliver V, Botella-Estrada R, Moreno-Picot S, Insa A, Fortea JM. Prognostic factors in localized invasive cutaneous melanoma: high value of mitotic rate, vascular invasion and microscopic satellitosis. Melanoma Res. 2005;15(3):169–77.
42. Barnes BC, Seigler HF, Saxby TS, Kocher MS, Harrelson JM. Melanoma of the Foot. J Bone Joint Surg Am. 1994;76A(6):892–8.
43. Gershenwald JE, Mansfield PF, Lee JE, Ross MI. Role for lymphatic mapping and sentinel lymph node biopsy in patients with thick (>or =4 mm) primary melanoma. Ann Surg Oncol. 2000;7(2):160–5.
44. Egger MEMK, Callender GG, Quillo AR, Martin II RC, Stromberg AJ, Scoggins CR. Unique prognostic factors in acral lentiginous melanoma. Am J Surg. 2012;204:874–80.
45. Bradford PT, Goldstein AM, McMaster ML, Tucker MA. Acral lentiginous melanoma: incidence and survival patterns in the United States, 1986–2005. Arch Dermatol. 2009;145(4):427–34.
46. Phan A, Touzet S, Dalle S, Ronger-Savle S, Balme B, Thomas L. Acral lentiginous melanoma: a clinicoprognostic study of 126 cases. Br J Dermatol. 2006;155(3):561–9.
47. Kogushi-Nishi H, Kawasaki J, Kageshita T, Ishihara T, Ihn H. The prevalence of melanocytic nevi on the soles in the Japanese population. J Am Acad Dermatol. 2009;60(5):767–71.
48. Tseng JF, Tanabe KK, Gadd MA, et al. Surgical management of primary cutaneous melanomas of the hands and feet. Ann Surg. 1997;225(5):544–50. discussion 550–543.
49. Stalkup JR, Orengo IF, Katta R. Controversies in acral lentiginous melanoma. Dermatol Surg. 2002;28(11): 1051–9. discussion 1059.
50. Gray RJ, Pockaj BA, Vega ML, et al. Diagnosis and treatment of malignant melanoma of the foot. Foot Ankle Int. 2006;27(9):696–705.

Capsular (Nodal) Nevus Versus Metastatic Melanoma

17

Victor G. Prieto, Christopher R. Shea, and Jon A. Reed

Sentinel lymph node (SLN) biopsy is a relatively minimally invasive technique. When applied to melanoma patients considered at risk of regional metastatic disease, it permits accurate staging and thereby provides critical prognostic information. Moreover, a positive SLN biopsy result provides the basis for performing a therapeutic completion lymphadenectomy and allows stratification for possible clinical trials.

Since lymphatic drainage cannot always be accurately predicted on anatomic grounds alone, the technique of SLN biopsy currently requires combined detection markers, usually two, which are injected into the skin site of the primary melanoma. A radioactive tracer, assessed by Geiger counter, localizes the relevant node basin(s) to which lymphatic drainage occurs, and a blue dye permits the surgeon to visualize the SLN(s).

V.G. Prieto, M.D., Ph.D. (✉)
MD Anderson Cancer Center, University of Houston, 1515 Holcombe Blvd., Unit 85, Houston, TX 77030, USA
e-mail: vprieto@mdanderson.org

C.R. Shea
University of Chicago Medicine, 5841 S. Maryland Ave., MC 5067, L502, Chicago, IL 60637, USA

J.A. Reed
CellNEtix Pathology & Laboratories, 1124 Columbia St., Suite 200, Seattle, WA 98117, USA

The main indications for examination of SLN are for melanomas of Breslow thickness $\geq$1.00 mm, or having an ulcerated surface, or with dermal mitotic figures [1]. In addition, the presence of vascular invasion, satellites, or extensive regression is considered as relative indication for SLN biopsy in some centers.

Regarding processing of SLN biopsies, use of frozen sections is strongly discouraged; such specimens often have suboptimal morphologic detail, lead to loss of precious tissue as the frozen section remnants are prepared for permanent slides, and are prone to miss the crucial subcapsular region, precisely the location in which early metastatic deposits are most likely to occur [2]. The entire specimen should be grossed and submitted in order to detect even minimal disease (i.e., isolated tumor cells). At our institution we recommend breadloafing of the SLN to allow examination of a large area of the subcapsular region in a single block [3]. Then we study one H&E slide; if this is positive we report it as such. If negative, we order a new H&E deeper section slide (~200 μm deeper in the block) and two unstained slides for immunohistochemistry [3, 4] (see below).

Approximately 20 % of patients with cutaneous melanoma show deposits of melanoma cells in the SLN. Metastatic melanoma cells may be epithelioid or spindled, pigmented or amelanotic. However, most commonly metastatic melanoma cells resemble the cells in the primary lesion. Thus, when examining SLN, it may be very

C.R. Shea et al. (eds.), *Pathology of Challenging Melanocytic Neoplasms: Diagnosis and Management*, DOI 10.1007/978-1-4939-1444-9_17, © Springer Science+Business Media New York 2015

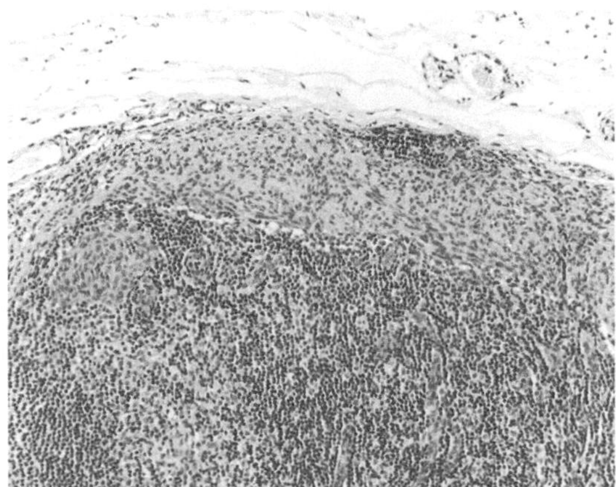

Fig. 17.1 Metastatic melanoma involving the subcapsular sinus

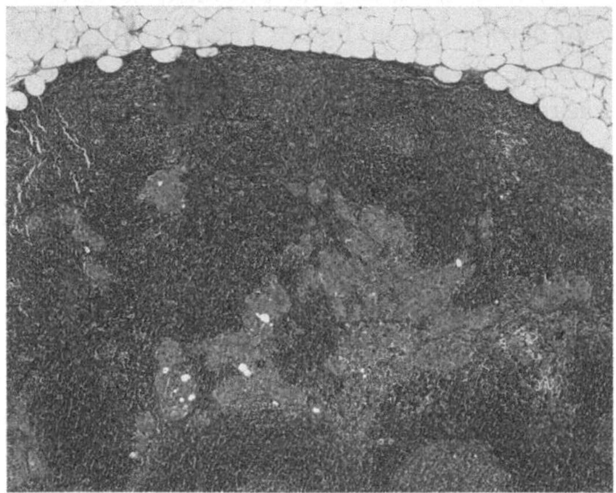

Fig. 17.2 Metastatic melanoma involving the lymph node parenchyma

important to study the original melanoma, to compare the morphologic features, particularly to distinguish metastatic cells from macrophages or nevus cells. By morphology only, it may be difficult to distinguish pigmented melanoma cells from melanophages; however, pigment granules are usually coarser and larger in macrophages than in melanoma cells.

In general, melanoma cells in the SLN usually are located in the subcapsular sinus (Fig. 17.1), as single cells, small nests, or large, expansile clusters. Less frequently the metastasis is located within the parenchyma (Fig. 17.2). Very rarely do melanoma cells involve the fibrous capsule, and in such cases it is likely secondary to involvement of intracapsular lymphatic vessels (see below). There may be (fewer than 5 % of cases) extracapsular extension into the perinodal fibroadipose tissues. A recent study has indicated that nodal nevi are more commonly seen in SLN from melanomas occurring in the lower extremities [5].

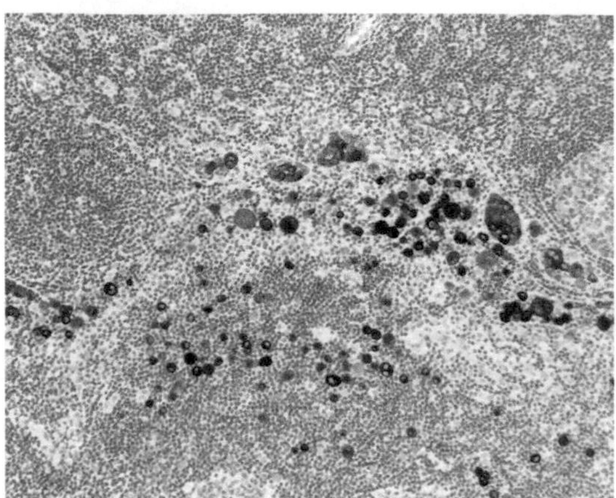

Fig. 17.3 Melanoma metastatic to a lymph node highlighted by an immunohistochemical cocktail against melanocytic markers (anti-MART1, HMB45, and anti-tyrosinase; diaminobencidine; hematoxylin as counterstain)

Immunohistochemistry may be very helpful when examining SLN. As with melanomas at other anatomic sites, use of a panel of antibodies directed at various melanoma-associated antigens (usually a combination of anti-MART1, HMB45, and anti-tyrosinase) (Fig. 17.3) helps detecting melanoma cells. As mentioned in Chap. 4, S-100 protein is a very sensitive but relatively nonspecific marker for melanocytic tumors including melanoma (since there are S100+ dendritic cells in lymph nodes). The antigen gp100 (detected with HMB-45 antibody) is very specific but is less sensitive (~75 %) than S-100; on the other hand, gp100 is usually not expressed in most benign melanocytic lesions including nodal nevi (see below). Tyrosinase has value similar to gp100. MART-1/ Melan-A expression is both very specific and very sensitive for melanocyte-lineage cells (although it can occur also in macrophages, especially when DAB chromogen is utilized). Microphthalmia transcription factor (MiTF) and SOX10 are relatively recent melanocyte markers with good sensitivity and specificity, and the quite useful property of nuclear

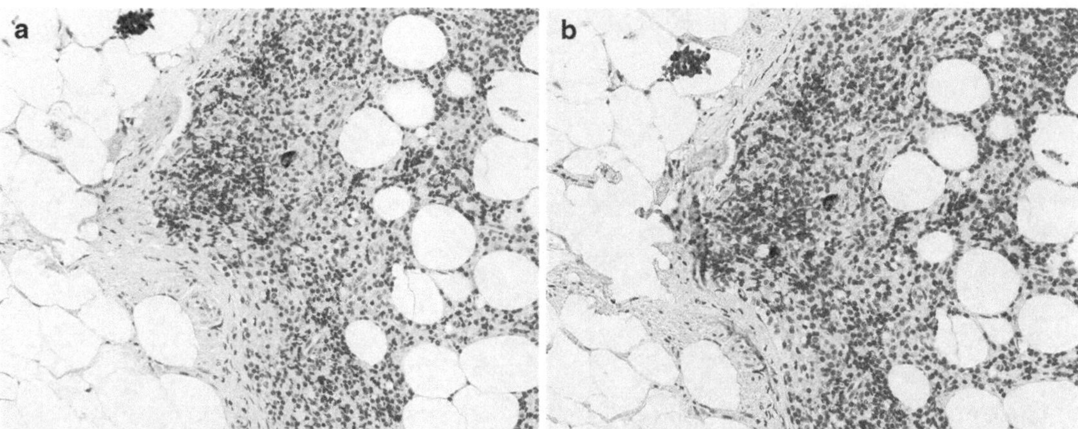

Fig. 17.4 Sentinel lymph with a single cell in the subcapsular area labeled with the anti-melanocytic cocktail (**a**). By morphologic features alone it is difficult to determine if this cell is a melanoma cell or a macrophage. After removing the coverslip, this cell is negative for SOX10 (nuclear marker) (**b**), thus supporting the interpretation of being a macrophage and not a melanoma cell. The cytoplasmic labeling seen in b is the leftover of the anti0melanocytic cocktail after de-coversliping the slide and relabel it with anti-SOX10

localization, permitting assessment of nuclear size and of coexpression with cytoplasmic markers such as gp100.

Pitfalls in the application of IHC to melanoma SLN biopsy include the occurrence of spindle-cell forms of melanoma, which characteristically are strongly S100+ but usually lack consistent expression of the more sensitive markers such as gp100 and MART-1. For such cases we recommend anti-SOX10 [6]. Other hazards include the presence of intranodal pigment (include melanin and exogenous substances) that may be mistaken for veritable IHC chromogen, and the occurrence of necrosis, which may cause misleading IHC results.

To help distinguish between macrophages and melanoma cells, since MART1 can be expressed by macrophages [7], we use HMB45 by itself or anti-SOX10 (HMB45 or anti-SOX10 usually do not label macrophages). Our approach is to first examine the anti-melanocytic cocktail (anti-MART1, HMB45, and anti-tyrosinase). If there are cells in which morphology does not clearly distinguish between melanoma and macrophages we then do an HMB45 or anti-SOX10 (both usually negative in melanoma) (Fig 17.4).

A potentially vexing phenomenon is the nodal nevus. Benign melanocytes are detectable in up to 20 % of lymphadenectomies performed for melanoma. To complicate things further, they are more common in cases where the primary melanoma was associated with a nevus [8]. The location of melanocytes in the node is a critical consideration; most nevi are situated within the capsule (Fig. 17.5) (although rare cases of intraparenchymal nodal nevi do occur); in contrast, melanoma characteristically affects the subcapsular sinus and node parenchyma, and true capsular involvement by melanoma usually occurs as extension from an obvious parenchymal metastasis.

IHC provides very helpful data; in particular, the expression of gp100 (HMB-45) is generally supportive of melanoma rather than nevus. Similarly, analysis of Ki67 expression is important in this differential diagnosis since it will be almost completely negative in the nodal nevus while it is expected to be at least focally positive in the metastatic melanoma cells [9] (Fig. 17.5). A very unusual situation is that of observing melanocytes with cytologic atypia within the capsule. Due to the anatomic location, such cells are much more likely to be nevus cells. However, it is possible that they correspond to metastatic melanoma involving the lymphatic vessels within the capsule (Fig. 17.6). In such cases, anti-D2–40 may be very helpful since it would highlight the endothelial cells of those vessels and thus would

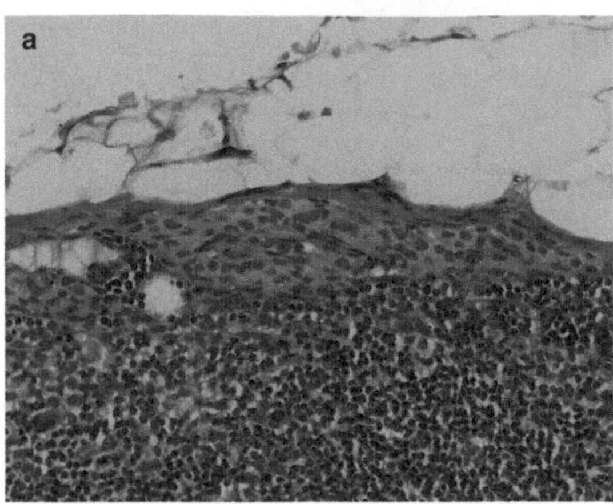

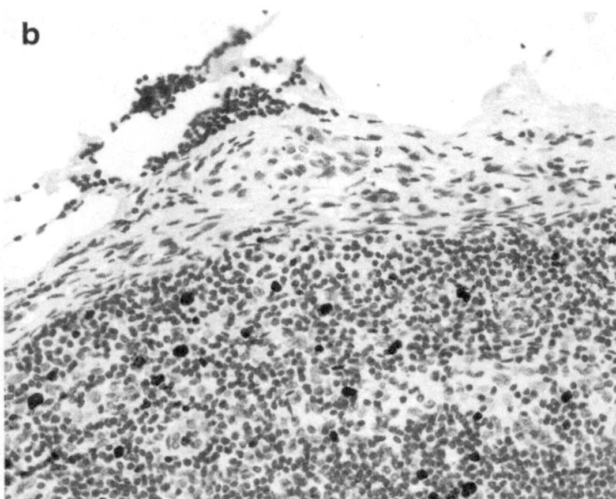

Fig. 17.5 (**a**) Benign-appearing melanocytes in the fibrous capsule of this sentinel lymph node. (**b**) The cells in this capsular nevus do not express Ki67 (note the adjacent lymphocytes with focal expression) (Anti-Ki67; diaminobencidine; hematoxylin as counterstain)

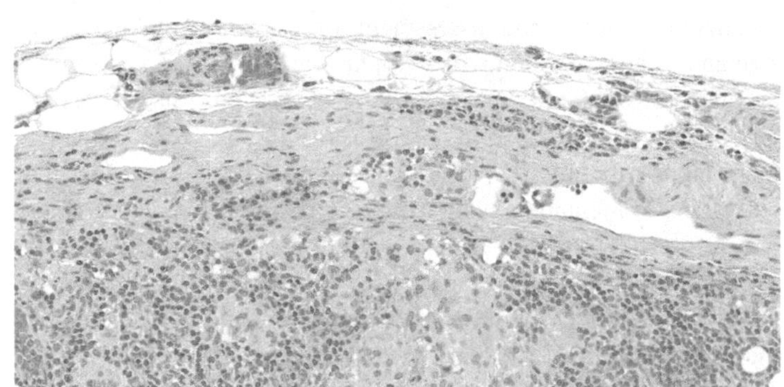

Fig. 17.6 Cluster of melanoma cells both within the capsule (intravascular, black arrow) and in the parenchyma (white arrow)

support the diagnosis of metastatic melanoma [10]. It has been suggested that nestin and SOX2 may also be helpful since they are reportedly positive in metastatic melanoma and negative nodal nevi [11]. Also possibly useful may be FISH [12]. At any rate, as mentioned before, probably the most useful method to distinguish between metastatic melanoma and nodal nevus would be comparison of cytomorphologic features with the primary cutaneous melanoma.

In summary, SLN biopsy is a valuable technique for the management of patients with melanoma. Careful histopathologic assessment, including use of a panel of IHC reagents, is the key to accurate diagnosis.

References

1. Balch CM, Gershenwald JE, Soong SJ, Thompson JF. Update on the melanoma staging system: the importance of sentinel node staging and primary tumor mitotic rate. J Surg Oncol. 2011;104(4):379–85.
2. Prieto VG. Use of frozen sections in the examination of sentinel lymph nodes in patients with melanoma. Semin Diagn Pathol. 2008;25(2):112–5.
3. Prieto VG, Clark SH. Processing of sentinel lymph nodes for detection of metastatic melanoma. Ann Diagn Pathol. 2002;6(4):257–64.
4. Prieto VG. Sentinel lymph nodes in cutaneous melanoma. Clin Lab Med. 2011;31(2):301–10.
5. Gambichler T, Scholl L, Stucker M, et al. Clinical characteristics and survival data of melanoma

patients with nevus cell aggregates within sentinel lymph nodes. Am J Clin Pathol. 2013;139(5): 566–73.
6. Ramos-Herberth FI, Karamchandani J, Kim J, Dadras SS. SOX10 immunostaining distinguishes desmoplastic melanoma from excision scar. J Cutan Pathol. 2010;37(9):944–52.
7. Trejo O, Reed JA, Prieto VG. Atypical cells in human cutaneous re-excision scars for melanoma express p75NGFR, C56/N-CAM and GAP-43: evidence of early Schwann cell differentiation. J Cutan Pathol. 2002;29(7):397–406.
8. Holt JB, Sangueza OP, Levine EA, et al. Nodal melanocytic nevi in sentinel lymph nodes. Correlation with melanoma-associated cutaneous nevi. Am J Clin Pathol. 2004;121(1):58–63.
9. Biddle DA, Evans HL, Kemp BL, et al. Intraparenchymal nevus cell aggregates in lymph nodes: a possible diagnostic pitfall with malignant melanoma and carcinoma. Am J Surg Pathol. 2003; 27(5):673–81.
10. Prieto VG. Sentinel lymph nodes in cutaneous melanoma: handling, examination, and clinical repercussion. Arch Pathol Lab Med. 2010;134(12):1764–9.
11. Chen PL, Chen WS, Li J, Lind AC, Lu D. Diagnostic utility of neural stem and progenitor cell markers nestin and SOX2 in distinguishing nodal melanocytic nevi from metastatic melanomas. Mod Pathol. 2013; 26(1):44–53.
12. Fang Y, Dusza S, Jhanwar S, Busam KJ. Fluorescence in situ hybridization (FISH) analysis of melanocytic nevi and melanomas: sensitivity, specificity, and lack of association with sentinel node status. Int J Surg Pathol. 2012;20(5):434–40.

Index

C.R. Shea et al. (eds.), *Pathology of Challenging Melanocytic Neoplasms: Diagnosis and Management*, DOI 10.1007/978-1-4939-1444-9, © Springer Science+Business Media New York 2015

CPSIA information can be obtained at www.ICGtesting.com
Printed in the USA
LVOW02*0523221114

415074LV00005BA/386/P

9 781493 914432